AF352368

Short Dialysis

# Topics in Renal Medicine

Vittorio E. Andreucci, *series editor*

V.E. Andreucci, ed., The Kidney In Pregnancy. ISBN 0-89939-741-8
A.R. Clarkson, ed., IgA Nephropathy. ISBN 0-89838-839-2

# Short Dialysis

*Editor:*

VINCENZO CAMBI, M.D.
*Professor of Nephrology*
*University of Parma*
*Parma, Italy*

MARTINUS NIJHOFF PUBLISHING
A Member of the Kluwer Academic Publishers Group
Boston/Dordrecht/Lancaster

RC
901
.7
.H45
S56
1987

**Distributors**

*for the United States and Canada*: Kluwer Academic Publishers, 101 Philip Drive, Assinippi Park, Norwell, MA 02061
*for the UK and Ireland*: Kluwer Academic Publishers, MTP Press Limited, Falcon House, Queen Square, Lancaster LA1 1RN, UK
*for all other countries*: Kluwer Academic Publishers Group, Distribution Centre, P.O. Box 322, 3300 AH Dordrecht, The Netherlands

**Library of Congress Cataloging-in-Publication Data**

Short dialysis.

   (Topics in renal medicine)
   Includes bibliographies and index.
   1. Hemodialysis.  I. Cambi, Vincenzo.  II. Series.
[DNLM:  1. Hemodialysis.  WJ 378 S559]
RC901.7.H45S56  1986      617′.461059      86-33192
ISBN 0-89838-858-9

**Copyright**

© 1987 by Martinus Nijhoff Publishing, Boston.

All rights reserved. No part of this publication may be reproduced, stored in a retrieval system, or transmitted in any form or by any means, mechanical, photocopying, recording, or otherwise, without the prior written permission of the publishers,
Martinus Nijhoff Publishing, 101 Philip Drive, Assinippi Park, Norwell, MA 02061

PRINTED IN THE UNITED STATES

# Contents

To Belding H. Scribner,
    Luigi Migone,
        and Graziella

# Foreword

Vittorio E. Andreucci

Initially created with the purpose of keeping alive patients in terminal chronic renal failure, dialysis has undergone improvements in methodology, and its final goal has become complete health rehabilitation and optimization of the quality of life of chronic dialysis patients. To achieve this, many investigators have attempted to increase dialysis efficiency and at the same time shorten dialysis time. Their main concern was, obviously, patient safety: the Latin proverb *'primum non nocere'* is still valid all over the world. Thus, when clinical observations of the first patients on regular dialysis therapy suggested an inverse relationship between duration of dialysis sessions and severity of peripheral neuropathy, long and frequent dialysis sessions were considered the only way to prevent the catastrophic consequences of nerve damage and underdialysis syndrome. It was then, in 1971, when dialysis duration was 8–12 hours per session, that Vincenzo Cambi started a 'short dialysis' trial, i.e., 4 hours 3 times weekly or 3 hours every second day. For the first time, dialysis was shortened from 24–36 hours weekly to 10.5–12 hours weekly [1, 2].

In 1971 I was still at the Parma University Hospital. We had both just returned from the United States, and Dr. Cambi was responsible for the dialysis unit. The 'low-flow dialysis' trial seemed to have demonstrated that uremic toxicity could be prevented despite a significant increase in serum concentration of small molecules, suggesting a key role of middle molecules in the toxicity of uremia [3]. If this was true, then it stood to reason that a shorter dialysis time, even with high blood flow and coil dialysers used to obtain low predialysis blood urea-nitrogen, would lead to inefficient removal of middle molecules and therefore cause severe peripheral neuropathy. Cambi thus decided to monitor nerve function by measuring motor nerve conduction velocity and motor nerve action potentials of ulnar and peroneal nerves in all patients every other month. *Primum non nocere* was always kept in mind: should any deterioration of nerve function occur, even without symptoms, patients would immediately be switched back to traditional dialysis.

But Cambi was right: the shortened dialysis time caused no deterioration — either in nerve function or in overall clinical status of the patients [1, 2, 4].

Cambi's discovery was initially accepted with reluctance and sometimes actually criticized. In the 1982 European Dialysis and Transplant Association report [5], short dialysis was even indicated as responsible for a significant increase in mortality of dialysis patients, especially from myocardial infarction. This was then demonstrated to be an erroneous conclusion based on an incorrect definition of short dialysis [2]. The reality is that short dialysis as initiated by Cambi in 1971 is a dialysis treatment of 4 hours 3 times weekly. As such, short dialysis has now become the traditional regular dialysis therapy used all over the world. As readers will find in this book, shortening dialysis duration is becoming even more necessary today so that treatment-related complications, such as carpal tunnel syndrome, can be avoided. New techniques — hemofiltration and hemodiafiltration, etc. — are also being developed in this direction. But the pioneer of short dialysis treatment was Cambi. His merit, however, has not been recognized even in detailed historical reviews of dialysis [6]. And this is a pity, indeed.

## References


1. Cambi, V., Dall'Aglio, P., Savazzi, G., Arisi, L., and Migone, L. (1972) Clinical assessment of haemodialysis patients with reduced small molecules removal. Proc. Europ Dial. Transp. Ass. 9: 67.
2. Cambi, V., Arisi, L., Bignardi, L., Bruschi, G., Rossi, E., Savazzi, G. and Migone, L. (1974) Short dialysis schedules: finally ready to become a routine? Proc. Europ. Dial. Transpl. Ass. XI: 112–120.
3. Christopher, T.G., Cambi, V., Haker, L.A., Hurst, P., Popovic, R.P., Babb, A.L. and Scribner, B.H. (1971) A study of haemodialysis with lowered dialysate flow rate. Proc. Am. Soc. Art. Int. Org. 17: 92.
4. Cambi, V., Savazzi, G., Arisi, L., Buzio, C., Dall'Aglio, P., Rossi, E. and Migone, L. (1973) Dialysis schedules and peripheral neuropathy. Proc. Europ. Dial. Transpl. Ass. X: 271.
5. Broyer, M, Brunner, F.P., Brynger, H., Donckerwolcke, R.A., Jacobs, C., Kramer, P., Selwood, N.H. and Wing, A.J. (1982) Combined report on regular dialysis and transplantation in Europe, XII, 1981. Proc. Europ. Dial. Transpl. Ass. XIX: 2.
6. Drukker, W., Parsons, F.M. and Maher, J.F. (1983) Replacement of renal function by dialysis. Martinus Nijhoff.

# Preface

In 1960, the efficiency of the artificial kidney could obviously not be conceptually separated from the fact that the human kidney works 24 hours a day. Thus, the concept of dialysis was necessarily correlated to normal kidney function, and dialysis duration was not even taken into consideration.

Since the first trials with short dialysis (chapter 1 and 2), several years elapsed before this treatment modality became common in Europe. In fact, by 1977 37% of patients were still treated with 14–15 hours in 3 runs per week [1].

Only by 1984 were over 50% of the entire hospital population in Europe receiving 12 hours per week dialysis in 3 runs [2]; however, it is also very interesting to observe that this modality has been adopted independently of the type of dialyzer utilized (parallel flow or capillary kidney), membrane quality (cuprophan or other membranes), and most of all body weight of the patients. Wing (chapter 3) describes the different methods of dialysis therapy in Europe.

The development of short dialysis has been closely followed in our institution for over 15 years by several students belonging to the school of nephrology created in Parma by Luigi Migone: Buzio (chapter 4) analyzes the problem of uremic toxicity, making a very extensive contribution to the debate on the middle molecules; in chapter 5, Savazzi discusses the peripheral nerve function which he followed closely in the first years of the trial, with very sophisticated tests, in order to detect the earliest signs of peripheral neuropathy; Arisi (chapter 6) examines the relationship between nitrogen metabolism and dialysis treatment. The problem of nutrition and acid-base equilibrium in dialysis patients and, on the other hand, urea modeling, clearly represent the most rational approach to the unresolved problem of uremic toxicity. Chapter 7 (Maschio and associates), chapter 8 (Mion and associates), and chapter 9 (Farrell) cover this important topic.

In the eighties, the term 'short dialysis' has become synonymous with 'efficient' and 'effective' dialysis. Highly permeable membranes play a key role in the majority of the most recent treatment modalities. Considering the importance of water quality in the future of the substitutive therapy, two chapters have been devoted to standard water treatment for dialysis solution

(Davison, chapter 11), and to the preparation of sterile pyrogen free water for hemofiltration and hemodiafiltration (Mion, chapter 12).

Finally, two important chapters have been devoted to the dialysis strategies most intensively studied at present: hemodiafiltration (chapter 13, Wizemann) and hemofiltration (chapter 14, Baldamus and associates). The present availability of sterile pyrogen free solutions and high flux membranes will probably exert a paramount influence on the dialysis modalities of the nineties, and will certainly accelerate the optimization of clinical application of other modalities of therapy.

This book is dedicated to two masters who have had a paramount influence in promoting culture and human solidarity and, last but not least, who have also played crucial roles in the development of my academic formation: Belding H. Scribner and Luigi Migone. Scribner's discovery acquires increasing universal significance as the years pass. He has restored hope and trust in life to a multitude of disabled human beings, much beyond the great achievement of chronic dialysis. I was privileged to spend the most important period of my professional life in his division. Luigi Migone has dedicated his acute intelligence to a generation of Italian nephrologists, including myself, and has given all of us intellectual freedom, genuine culture, and by his example, the possibility to mature both academically and spiritually.

A special acknowledgment to Nancy Birch Podini who tried, we hope successfully, to improve the quality of most of the Italian chapters.

## References


1. Wing, A.J., Brunner, F.P., Brynger, H., Chantler, C., Donckerwolcke, R.A., Gurland, H.J., Hathaway, R.A. and Jacobs, C. (1978) Combined report on regular dialysis and transplantation in Europe Proceedings of the VIII Congress of EDTA, 1977.
2. Qulès et al. (1986) Combined report on regular dialysis and transplantation in Europe. XXIII Congress of EDTA-ERA (in press).

# List of contributors

LUCA ARISI, Department of Internal Medicine and Nephrology, Parma, Italy.

BALDAMUS C.A., Dept. of Nephrology, University Hospital, Cologne, West Germany.

ROBERTA BARANI, Department of Internal Medicine and Nephrology, Parma, Italy.

FABIO BONO, Department of Internal Medicine and Nephrology, Parma, Italy.

FELIX P. BRUNNER, EDTA Registry, St. Thomas Hospital, London, Great Britain.

CARLO BUZIO, Department of Internal Medicine and Nephrology, Parma, Italy.

VINCENZO CAMBI, Chair of Nephrology, University of Parma, Italy.

BERNARD CANAUD, Division of Nephrology, Lapeyronie Hospital, Montpellier, France.

CASTIGLIONI A., Department of Internal Medicine and Nephrology, Parma, Italy.

SABRI CHALLAH, EDTA Registry, St. Thomas Hospital, London, Great Britain.

ALEXANDER M. DAVISON, St. James' Hospital, Leeds, Great Britain.

PETER C. FARRELL, University of New South Wales and Travenol Centre for Medical Research, Sydney, Australia.

ANTONINO FAVAZZA, Division of Nephrology, City Hospital, Udine, Italy.

MARIA ELENA FERRARI, Department of Internal Medicine and Nephrology, Parma, Italy.

KOCH K.M., Department of Nephrology, Medical School, Hannover, West Germany.

GIUSEPPE MASCHIO, Division of Nephrology, University Hospital, Verona, Italy.

ROBERTO MENTA, Chair of Nephrology, University of Parma, Italy.

PIERGIORGIO MESSA, Division of Nephrology, City Hospital, Udine, Italy.

CHARLES MION, Division of Nephrology, Lapeyronie Hospital, Montpellier, France.

GIUSEPPE MIONI, Division of Nephrology, City Hospital, Udine, Italy.

PANZETTA G., Division of Nephrology, University Hospital, Verona, Italy.

GIORGIO M. SAVAZZI, Department of Internal Medicine and Nephrology Parma, Italy.

STANLEY SHALDON, Division of Nephrology, Université de Nimes, Nimes, France.

ANTHONY J. WING, EDTA Registry, St. Thomas Hospital, London, Great Britain.

VOLKER WIZEMANN, Dept. of Internal Medicine, J. Liebig University, Giessen, West Germany.

Short Dialysis

# 1. Short dialysis 1971–1986: the first experience

Vincenzo Cambi

One of the main reasons preventing hemodialysis from escaping from empiricism is our inability to shed more light on the problem of uremic toxicity. Technological advances have decurred which have in common a trend to the production of dialyzers whose efficiency is relatively independent of the surface area. However, while for some patients it is possible to predict life expectancy of over two decades, we continue to observe that the problems regarding the central nervous system, erythropoiesis and hemostasis, carbohydrate and lipid metabolism, divalention metabolism, etc., have only been partially corrected.

In the sixties, the relationship between the duration of dialysis sessions and peripheral neuropathy, made on the basis of clinical observations of the first patients receiving intermittent dialysis therapy, influenced the choice and development of new dialysis strategies. However, at that time, the importance of residual kidney function, as well as the long-term consequences of solute retention, were largely misunderstood. Subsequently, clinical and experimental data have allowed for modifications of dialysis strategies. At present, the maintenance or improvement of erythropoiesis is obtained without resorting to blood transfusion; a normal blood pressure is achieved in almost all patients by drug therapy, and bilateral nephrectomy is practically abandoned. Dialysis cachexia has disappeared, thanks to an awareness of the need for correct nutrition; thus, the improvement in the general well-being of patients, as shown by improved rehabilitation and survival, must be considered the consequence of better prevention of complications rather than therapeutic improvement of uremia.

In summary, whereas dialysis treatment cannot bring about the metabolic rehabilitation of a patient, it can lead to important improvements in specific areas such as hypertension, anemia, hemostasis, and peripheral neuropathy.


**The history of short dialysis**

The first rational attempt at a considerable reduction of the dialysis session (to 3–4 hours per session) was made in Parma in 1971 [1]. The first trial was

*Vincenzo Cambi (editor) Professor of Nephrology*
© *1987 Martinus Nijhoff Publishing, Boston. ISBN 0-89838-858-9. Printed in The United States.*

actually aimed at gaining a deeper understanding of the potential toxicity of uraemic metabolites of large molecular weight, the so-called middle molecules hypothesized by Scribner.

Scribner based the middle molecules hypothesis [2] on the premise that the well-being of peritoneal dialysis patients might be related to the removal, through the peritoneal membrane, of large-sized toxic solutes with molecular weight between 300 and 1,500 (middle molecules). However, independently of Scribner's hypothesis, it was also noticed that 'underdialysis syndrome' was little correlated with the height of blood urea and creatinine (small molecules = substances with molecular weight <300) and occurred more frequently where PT300 cellophane was used for dialysis (i.e., all forms of coil dialysis) than with PT150 cellophane (cuprophane) using the Kiil dialyzer. On the basis of this observation Shaldon made the hypothesis that 'inadequate dialysis results from retention of larger molecular compounds which are cleared by prolonged dialysis with a thin-membrane dialyzer, but not by either short or prolonged dialysis with a thick-membrane dialyzer' [3].

The middle molecules hypothesis later developed to the square meter/hour hypothesis [4] was formulated to reproduce, by means of cuprophane membrane in a Kiil dialyzer, the hypothetical condition of a patient in peritoneal dialysis, i.e., easy removal of larger solutes at the expense of a reduced removal of small molecules. However, the comparison of hemodialysis with peritoneal dialysis did not take into account the relationship between uremic toxicity and protein metabolism. In fact, obligatory protein loss during peritoneal dialysis actually modifies the genesis of uremic toxicity and paradoxically improves treatment efficacy despite a reduced urea clearance.

The clinical trial to test the square meter/hour hypothesis was conducted during the course of a standard Kiil dialysis with a cuprophan dialyzer and operated on a single variable: the reduction of the dialysate flow from 500 to 100 ml/min. Blood flow was maintained by Scribner's artero-venous shunt, and dialysis duration remained 8–10 hours [5]. According to Scribner's hypothesis, this 'low flow dialysis' strategy was capable of maintaining the same removal of large-sized toxic metabolites without jeopardizing the safety of treatment. This method could not prevent urea and creatinine accumulation, and indeed, there was an increase of about 30% in patients who underwent the clinical trial. Yet a retrospective analysis of low flow dialysis showed that this dialysis strategy did not challenge the potential toxicity of middle molecules because their blood concentration remained unchanged. On the contrary, low flow dialysis only demonstrated that patients were able to tolerate higher concentrations of urea and creatinine in comparison to their baseline values (actually not too high) without apparent harm. In conclusion, this dialysis modality had essentially no influence on clinical condition. It should also be noted that careful analysis of the experiment indicated that patients receiving 30 hours of 1 m standard Kiil were overdialyzed.

Low flow dialysis, however, gave some unanticipated results: during the one-year trial in Seattle, improvement in platelet function and a reduction of

2

postdialysis fatigue were observed [6]. Identical results were obtained in Parma when the same dialysis modality was used [1].

The next step in understanding the role of middle molecules in uremic toxicity seemed to be to maintain a conceptual approach identical to that of low flow dialysis but to create a mirror-image trial, i.e., to let the theoretical middle molecules concentration increase as much as possible. In fact, according to the middle molecules hypothesis, the only way to increase the serum concentration of middle molecules and maintain the same predialysis urea and creatinine levels was to make a drastic reduction in duration of the dialysis session but keep the same dialyzer surface area.

Since theoretically, the shorter the treatment time, the lower the removal of middle molecules, we devised several methodological changes, aimed at reducing the standard duration of a dialysis session from 8–12 hours to 3–4 hours. The main technical modifications were [1, 7]:

1. The patients chosen for the trial switched from the Scribner external shunt to an arterio-venous fistula: a blood flow of at least 250 ml/min was thus obtained.

2. Sodium concentration of the dialysate was increased from 130 to 137 mEq/l and, a year later, to 140 mEq/l.

3. Predialysis BUN and creatinine concentration identical to those obtained during low flow dialysis (i.e., 30% higher than standard Kiil dialysis in the same patient) were maintained.

4. The cuprophane membrane of 1 m$^2$ (i.e., identical surface area as that used in the low flow dialysis trial) was also kept, but the more efficient coil dialyzer replaced the standard Kiil dialyzer, despite the thicker membrane.

This combination permitted a reduction of the dialysis session to 4 hours 3 times weekly or 3 hours every second day (10.5 hours weekly) [7].

Short dialysis was then carried out for 3 years with the entire population of our dialysis center. The results were presented in 1974 at the 11th European Congress of Dialysis and Transplantation [7], and a year later at the International Congress of Nephrology [8, 9].

At that time, peripheral nerve conduction velocity was the most important measurable parameter of patient well-being: in fact, during the first decade of dialysis, peripheral neuropathy was considered the most dreadful complication as well as the most evident sign of treatment inadequacy. In 1971, these considerations stimulated us to begin a long-term study of the peripheral nerve [10]. This research, conducted by Savazzi, is reported later in detail in chapter 5. The premise that short dialysis was clinically safe, and that middle molecules toxicity did not influence the patient condition, was supported chiefly by the continuous and detailed observation of the peripheral nerve status.

The first clinical impact of short versus long dialysis was impressive. Improved well-being, apparently due to the psychological advantage of a shorter session, was actually confirmed by significantly improved erythropoiesis and by a complete lack for the need of blood transfusions (figure 1–1).

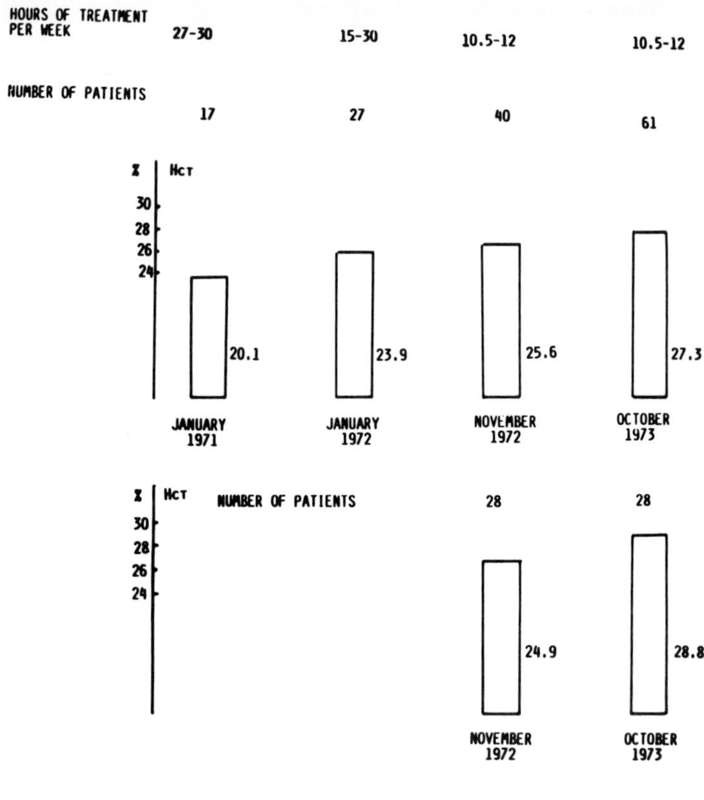


*Figure 1–1.* Relationship between hematocrit and weekly dialysis duration. The above part of the figure refers to the hematocrit of the growing population of the unit initially treated with standard Kill (January 1971) and progressively transferred to short dialysis (November 1972–October 1973). The lower part of the figure shows the hematocrit of 28 patients exclusively and uninterruptedly treated with short dialysis for a period of 4 months (1972) and 15 months (1973).

At the same time (see chapter 5), peripheral nerve status either improved or remained stable.

In spite of this, however, a pyrotechnic series of dialysis techniques was devised beginning with the mid-seventies. It was claimed that short dialysis was 'only' feasible if larger surface areas or more permeable membranes or sorbents were used [11, 12]. However, in no cases were clinical results from the use of larger dialyzer superior to the data we presented regarding a population of mostly anuric patients.

Reduced postdialysis fatigue was observed in the pioneering low flow dialysis trial. At that time, this result was attributed to a higher retention of 'vital metabolites' of small molecular weight [6]. Later on Shaldon confirmed

4

that low flow dialysis reduces postdialysis fatigue, but he attributed this clinical observation to an improved vascular stability [13].

If, on the one hand, the middle molecules theory has been one of the most fascinating and stimulating working hypothesis during the last two decades, on the other hand, several important considerations limit their importance in formulating future dialysis treatment.

Recently our center evaluated middle molecule removal in the course of long-term hemofiltration (Buzio and Barani, chapter 4). Five patients on chronic hemodialysis with cuprophane were transferred to hemofiltration with polyamide filters. The serum concentration and removal of solutes with m.w. ranging from 300–1,500 D were measured in both treatments. After 11–15 months of hemofiltration several middle molecules 'peaks' — which were absent or in low concentration during intermittent hemodialysis — appeared ex novo or, if already present, evidenced paradoxically increased concentration during convective treatment with high permeability membranes (figure 1–2; see also chapter 4). This original observation, together with evidence of a continuous increase in middle molecules concentration during long-term hemodalysis (after 10 years of dialysis treatment serum middle molecules concentrations are higher than after 5 years — table 1–1), raise several questions and doubts about middle molecules toxicity. Clearly serum urea concentration always correlates with urea generation and remains stable when nutritional intake and protein catabolic rate do not change. On the contrary, the progressive increased concentrations of solutes of larger

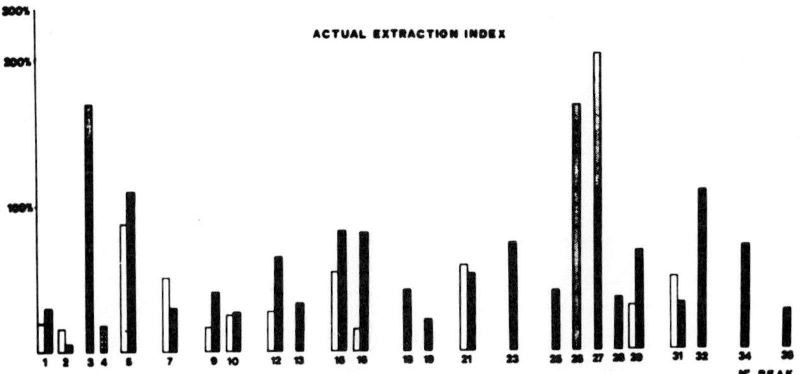


*Figure 1–2.* Peaks of middle molecules in dialysis (HD) and hemofiltration (HF) fluid. ▢ dialysis fluid; ▮ hemofiltration fluid; ▨ dialysis fluid only: absent in HF; ▤ hemofiltration only: new in HF. For a better understanding see figure 4–8, which evaluates the blood concentration of the same peaks. Total removal of MM is higher in HF than in HD. From direct comparison of blood and HD — HF fluid concentrations the following observation can be made: (1) peak 24–35 are 'new' in HF, do not cross the membrane, and are absent in HF fluid; (2) peak 3-26-27 'new' in HF absent in dialysis, do cross the membrane, and are present in HF fluid; (3) the intradialytic generation of removed solutes is testified by an extraction index exceeding 100%.

*Table 1–1.* Serum concentration of middle molecules in four different populations

| Population | N | Total Area of Chromatographic Peaks G 15 Gelfiltration | P Value |
|---|---|---|---|
| Normal Subjects | 10 | $0.3 \pm 0.2$ cm$^2$ | |
| | | | <0.001 |
| Uremic patients on conservative treatment | 6 | $1.56 \pm 0.32$ cm$^2$ | |
| | | | <0.01 |
| Uremic patients on hemodialysis for 5 years | 5 | $3.35 \pm 0.68$ cm$^2$ | |
| | | | <0.05 |
| Uremic patients on hemodialysis for 10 years | 10 | $4.675 \pm 1.02$ cm$^2$ | |

Serum concentrations of middle molecules (expressed as total area of chromatographic peak G15 gelfiltration) in four different populations, homogeneous with regard to age, body weight, blood pressure, hematocrit, serum creatinine. Only 2 patients on regular dialysis treatment (RDT) presented a residual renal function: one had a FGR of 0.18 ml/min. after 10 years of RDT, the other one a GFR of 0.17 after 5 years of RDT.

molecular weight after long-term treatment not only imply that middle molecules are not toxic in themselves but also suggest the possibility that dialysis or hemofiltration membranes may stimulate the generation of a new family of solutes. In the latter case, the introduction of biocompatibility as a new variable in the ongoing debate over uremic toxicity may invalidate any relationship between dialysis strategies and mathematical models. In the early seventies, Gotch and associates began a very important study aimed at modelling dialysis treatment as a pharmacokinetic phenomenon [14]. Given the relationship between protein intake and uremic toxicity, the urea model was chosen due to the fact that the urea generation rate could be used as an indicator of protein catabolism in dialysis patients. Using this pharmacokinetic approach, Gotch concluded in 1973 that in a patient with a residual renal function of 1 ml/min., a dialysis treatment of 4 hours 3 times a week using a Cordis-Dow Model 4 containing an active 1.3 m$^2$, membrane was equivalent to 8 hours 3 times a week with a D-1 Kiil dialyzer. Gotch's and our observations, although different in practice and approach, confirmed the total absence of clinical relevance of middle molecules in the genesis of uremic toxicity as well as the fact that a 1 m$^2$ dialyzer was sufficient to maintain patient well-being. Nevertheless, the common opinion among nephrologists was that a short dialysis session might be acceptable, but that longer sessions were preferable [15]. In any case, the debate on the duration of the dialysis session is still open [16, 17].

It is, however, becoming evident that the duration of a dialysis session can no longer be planned only in relation to the treatment efficiency. Recent research shows that blood contamination with particulates (i.e., silicon spallation) coming from the tubing set is directly proportional to dialysis

6

duration [18]. The associated clinical damage can be very serious [19]. Gutierrez and associates [20] investigated free aminoacid balance across the leg of fasting normal subjects before and after passage of blood through a cuprophane dialyzer without circulating the dialysis solution. The authors observed that the release of thyrosine, an aminoacid not metabolized in the muscle, increased by about 100%, suggesting the possibility that intradialytic protein catabolism can be stimulated by blood-membrane interaction when the membrane is made of cuprophane. This observation confirms that the duration of a dialysis session should not be unnecessarily prolonged if treatment-related complications are to be avoided.

In a recent debate regarding the adequate duration of the dialysis session, Guy Laurent and associates [15] observed that the incidence of carpal tunnel syndrome (CTS) in their population treated with standard Kiil dialysis, for at least 8 hours each run, was high. More recently Charra and colleagues [21] studied the same population and confirmed an exceptionally high incidence of CTS. The pathogenesis of CTS is certainly multifactorial and several variables are involved. However, the observation that CTS increases in parallel to long-term dialysis treatment seems to us particularly important [22]. In fact, it is very difficult to separate the role of dialysis aging per se from potential problems related to biocompatibility: in the latter case the increasing frequency of CTS in the older dialysis population should not be considered a late complication of uremia. On the contrary, the relationship we found between the duration of the dialysis session and CTS [22] after an identical period of dialysis treatment confirms that CTS is a 'dialysis disease' and stresses unequivocally the importance of biocompatibility problems. Once again traditional technology, i.e., nonsterile solutions, tubing sets, and cuprophane membranes, may be the direct or indirect cause of an unpredicted large category of diseases related to treatment itself.

Residual renal function, even at a very low level, and independently of daily urine volume, continues to be considered very important, and the implications regarding the role of middle molecules are always present. On the other hand, anuric patients show no deterioration in clinical indices with respect to patients who have conserved a certain amount of residual renal function. However, the condition of renal parenchyma independent of residual filtration might be of notable importance. The function of the peripheral nerve in the transplanted patient tends to become normalized more quickly than does residual renal function. Recently Teschan [23] evaluated the effects of reduced dialysis on several neurobehavioral functions and suggested that the presence of residual renal function per se may positively influence these parameters beyond the significance of vitamin B12 clearance rates. These findings imply that the presence of kidney tissue, even with almost negligible function, improves patient response independently of dialysis efficiency.

Moreover, the fact that middle molecules can be generated during a dialysis session raises the suspicion that dialysis membranes trigger and/or modify the metabolism of some retained solutes and actively contribute to their production. Thus it seems extremely limiting and misleading to attribute to the residual renal function of a dialysis patient only the role of middle molecules excreting. On the contrary, our observations exclude any relationship of middle molecules with uremic toxicity and emphasizes the potential danger of unnecessarily prolonged dialysis sessions.

**Hemodiafiltration**

In 1976, while we were critically evaluating the results of five years of short dialysis [7, 8, 9], a new treatment was described: the postdilution hemofiltration [24]. The difference between short dialysis and hemofiltration was extremely relevant. Short dialysis, using the diffusion mode, emphasized the importance of water and electrolyte balance, as well as the removal of small molecules; the role of retained solutes of high molecular weight was considered of minor importance. On the contrary, hemofiltration, originated by the wish to imitate the human glomerulus [25], considered the removal of middle molecular weight solutes to be of primary importance.

However, at that time both short dialysis and hemofiltration presented several lacunae that kept them from being adequate dialysis treatments. Hemofiltration was inefficient in removing small molecules; short dialysis was characterized by a high degree of cardiovascular instability. The recently discovered possibility of obtaining asymptomatic fluid removal from overhydrated patients by means of ultrafiltration followed by sequential diffusion described by Bergström [26] stimulated a renewed interest in the mechanisms regulating hemodynamic changes in dialysis treatment.

In the meantime the unappropriate loss of bicarbonate, potassium, and amino acids in the course of every dialysis session required the verification of the rational of a schedule of 3 times a week. In fact, this observation justifies reduction of either dialysis frequency or fluid in order to minimize the losses of several important metabolites.

We thus combined a reduction of dialysis duration and frequency within experimented limits (4 hours every third day, i.e., 7 hours per week), with a reduction of the dialysate flow to 200–250 ml/min. Thus only 36–40 litres of dialysate were used, but this reduction was compensated for an increased convection due to intravenous infusion of 2.5 litres of a bicarbonate, glucose, and amino acid solution throughout the 4-hour session. The dialyzer area was 1.5 m$^2$ blood flow 250 ml/min. Ultrafiltration rate during the entire session was 25–30 ml/min. We called this dialysis modality 'hemodiafiltration with reduced dialysis fluid' (HDF) [27].

The concept of HDF presented in 1977 at the Second Garda Meeting on New Dialysis Techniques and Haemoperfusion [27] did not come about as a means of increasing dialyzer efficiency. It was simply used to replace all the solutes and water necessary to correct 'dialysis unphysiology' with a sufficient amount of isotonic fluid. In other words, the main goal of hemodiafiltration

8

with reduced dialysis fluid was to obtain an overall positive balance of some important metabolic factors without impairing the removal of uremic toxins guaranteed by elevated convection.

Interestingly, at the same Garda Meeting, Leber, Wizemann, and coworkers [28] presented hemodiafiltration with a different philosophy, i.e., combining convection and diffusion to obtain the advantage of hemofiltration and hemodialysis and to increase efficiency. They suggested the new dialysis schedule of 3 × 3 hours weekly, as method of choice to shorten dialysis time. In both cases the dialysis duration was very short, respectively 9 hours (Leber's trial) and 7 hours (Cambi's trial) per week, despite the fact that our goal was mainly to reduce some treatment-related complications, whereas the Leber group's goal was to increase the overall efficiency of dialysis treatment. Clearly the improved clinical tolerance we obtained thanks to the use of bicarbonate allowed better utilization of the dialysis session without the interference of hypotensive episodes.

An interesting observation during hemodiafiltration with reduced dialysis fluid concerned the behavior of creatinine, phosphate, and potassium. The expected consequences of the dialysate flow reduction to 200–250 ml/min were, in fact, a parallel increase in the serum concentration of these solutes. On the contrary a significant rise of serum creatinine (around 23%) did occur but in the presence of a stable level of phosphate and potassium and, of course, optimal correction of acid base equilibrium [27]. However, it must also be emphasized that 4 patients were withdrawn from the trial after 4 weeks because of an increase in blood pressure.

In conclusion, this experience offered several clinical indications and allowed us to develop a new treatment modality: ultra-short dialysis.

Hemodiafiltration has had in the subsequent years a great success and is presently stimulating a large deal of research. In chapter 13 Wizemann describes his pioneering experience and examines the new advances in this area.


**Ultra-short dialysis**

In 1977 the advantages in terms of cardiovascular stability obtained by Scribner's group in Seattle with the introduction of bicarbonate [29] in the dialysis fluid, the high degree of clinical tolerance observed in the course of isolated ultrafiltration by Bergström [26] and interpreted as the effect of a limited osmotic shift and reduced dysequilibrium between extracellular and intracellular compartments were welcomed with extreme interest. One reason was that the number of elderly patients had progressively increased in all dialysis centers and the traditional short dialysis appeared inadequate for them because of vascular instability, predialysis hypertension, and metabolic acidosis. During the same period the experience of postdilution hemofiltration with the described high degree of clinical tolerance and hemodiafiltration with short session duration [27, 28] stimulated experimentation on new dialysis techniques capable of combining efficiency, clinical tolerance, and short treatment time.

Our recent experience with hemodiafiltration showed that the serum potassium could be easily managed due to better correction of acid-base status and independently of the limited amount of dialysis solution. In that period, it was also demonstrated that the maintainance of a stable blood pressure in the course of ultrafiltration was associated with increased production or high plasma concentration of catecholamines [30, 31, 32] and the maintenance of a high peripheral resistance [33].

Considering the advantages and disadvantages of a reduced dialysis frequency, the next step was to maintain approximately the same weekly duration (7/9 hours) with the following schedule: 2 hours every second day or 3 hours 3 times per week, blood flow 250 ml/min, dialysate flow 600 ml/min in recirculation, or 200–250 ml/min in single pass with a total amount of solution of 40 litres [34, 35, 36]. This trial, called ultra-short dialysis, was also performed utilizing different membranes to evaluate the consequences of high flux on clinical tolerance. Figure 1–3 summarizes the relationship between weight loss in regular dialysis treatment (above) and high flux recirculation (2–3 hours) compared with low flow single pass (below).

A detailed analysis of hemodynamic parameters measured with a Swan-Ganz flow-directed thermodilution catheter was performed by the experienced group of Hampl [33, 35] (figure 1–4). The cardiovascular indices of three groups of patients treated with conventional dialysis, hemofiltration, and recirculation dialysis with 20 liters of solution and dialysate buffering with bicarbonate were compared. In the first group, the cardiovascular parameters were unstable and characterized by symptomatic hypotension, high heart rate (+24%), and a limited increase of vascular resistance (+7%). On the contrary, patients treated with short-time recirculation cuprophan dialysis underwent only minor changes in blood pressure and heart rate, despite very high ultrafiltration with reduction of plasma volume (−15%). In parallel, the peripheral vascular resistance increases remarkably in hemofiltration as well as recirculation dialysis (19% versus 20%). In this trial only 2 out of 15 patients were withdrawn after 2–3 months because of malaise: during recirculation treatment both patients increased their body weight by 2%, and the traditional clinical 'markers' of adequacy of treatment, such as motor nerve conduction velocity, hematocrit, and body weight, remained stable.

The main conclusions from this experiment were the following:

1. Duration of the dialysis session can be further reduced to 2–3 hours thanks to high UF without deterioration in vascular stability.

2. Bicarbonate reduces the need of acetate, thus limiting its role in vascular destabilization.

3. It thus follows that the main advantage of hemofiltration in maintaining vascular stability cannot be related to the removal of larger solutes, but rather to the maintainance of better intravascular osmolality [32].

10

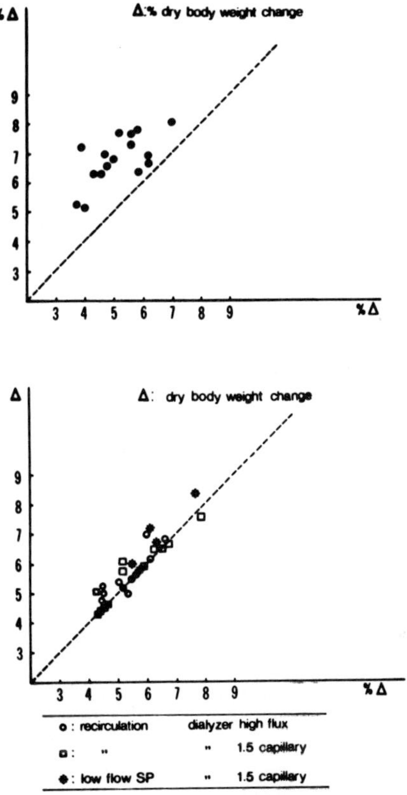


*Figure 1–3. Above*: Attempted versus achieved weight loss in patients on regular dialysis treatment. The dotted line indicates theoretical desired linear weight loss. The closed circles indicate the moment of interruption of treatment because of symptomatic disturbances. In every case the patient became symptomatic after varying and unpredictable amounts of fluid were removed. *Below*: Attempted versus achieved weight loss in patients on low volume dialysis with bicarbonate buffering (20 litres). In patients on low volume dialysis performed with different modalities (20 litres) and bicarbonate buffering, weight loss appears predictable and linear.

4. As a corollary to the previous statements, it seems that the major osmotically active factor is sodium.

A dialysis session of 2–3 hours obtained by either recirculating 20 or 40 litres of dialysate (simulation of standard hemofiltration) or with a dialysate flow of 200 ml/min (simulating low flow dialysis), in both cases with the addition of bicarbonate, appeared to be important technical advance, despite the fact that the limited volume of the dialysate also reduced the number of dialysis candidates to those with relatively low urea generation rate. This treatment limits the so called 'dialysis unphysiology' and allows better intravascular stability. In practice elderly patients often belong to this group, and recirculation bicarbonate dialysis is presently a routine treatment in several dialysis units [37].

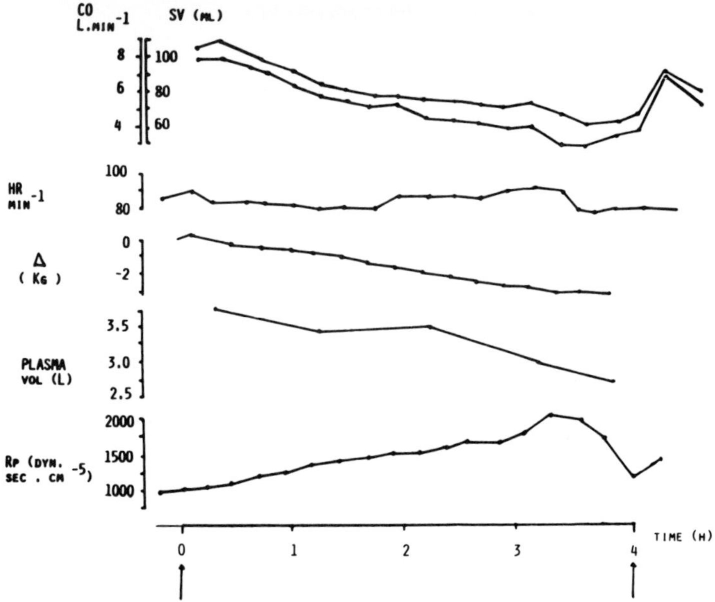


*Figure 1–4.* Hemodialysis with 20 L recirculation and $HCO_3$ Buffering (venous). Hemodynamic parameters (CO = cardiac output, HR = heart rate = ultrafiltration, Rp = peripheral resistances) with 20 litres recirculation dialysis and bicarbonate buffering. Despite uninterrupted, high ultrafiltration (see plasma volume) peripheral resistances increase during seven-eighths of treatment.

## Hypertonic hemodiafiltration

Traditional short dialysis with cuprophane dialyzers cannot be considered an optimal treatment because of inadequate control of vascular stability and insufficient correction of acid-base status. However, this treatment has been generally accepted as routine due to the proven advantage of sufficient removal of solutes of small molecular weight.

The factors that may improve clinical tolerance are presently unknown. The association of a higher sodium concentration in the dialysate, a relatively stable serum osmolality, limited shift of potassium during dialysis, mostly related to adequate acid-base correction, cannot be easily achieved with standard short dialysis. Presently, thanks to better membrane engineering and a correct approach to fluid balance, potentially higher dialysis efficiency seems compatible with increased clinical tolerance and without the former problems such as the dysequilibrium syndrome.

The importance of sodium in maintaining vascular stability has also been reappraised in hemofiltration. In fact, Quellhorst has observed that in either hemodialysis or in hemofiltration, the increase of sodium concentration in the dialysate and/or infusate from 130 to 150 mEq/l improved clinical tolerance [38].

12

The depressant role of acetate on cardiovascular activity has been stressed by many authors. However, in a previous study, despite the simultaneous use of 40 mEq of acetate in the dialysate, intravenous infusion of bicarbonate was followed by a significant increase of the dialysis tolerance [32]. Consequently, we conclude that the favorable role of complete correction of the acid-base status overcomes the acetate's depressant action on the cardiovascular system.

These considerations, together with the previous clinical trials performed in our center with different dialysis modalities prompted us to start a new experiment: 'hypertonic hemodiafiltration' [39, 40]. This consists in a simultaneous hypertonic (550 mOsm/kg), low volume (7.2 litres of replacing solution) short-time (180 min.) hemofiltration session and hypotonic hemodialysis (282 mOsm/kg).

In order to avoid high end-dialysis serum sodium, the sodium concentration of the main hemodiafiltration solution (solution A) is reduced in the last 30 minutes of treatment and substituted with glucose (solution B) (table 1–2).

The duration of the last part of treatment may vary ±10 minutes if needed (depending on thirst, hypertension, hypotension).

The use of an IV hypertonic infusion of sodium salts is motivated by the following: (1) it allows easy modulation of sodium infusion; (2) it offers a more reliable serum sodium concentration; (3) it allows a rapid change of the reinfusion bag in the last 30 minutes, thus avoiding a high end-dialysis serum sodium; (4) it corrects instantaneously unpredictable intradialytic hypotensive episodes by increasing the volume of the IV infusion.

Moreover, the simultaneous association of dialysis treatment allows easy separation of bicarbonate and calcium chloride and, through the reduction of the necessary volume of hemofiltration solution, increases the ratio of solute removal versus treatment cost.

*Table 1–2.* Hypertonic hemodiafiltration

| | Dialysis Solution (mEq/l) | A — Initial Reinfusate (mEq/l) | B — Final Reinfusate (mEq/l) |
|---|---|---|---|
| Na | 130 | 250 | 75 |
| K | 2.2 | — | — |
| Mg | 1.6 | — | — |
| Ca | 4.4 | — | — |
| Cl | 111 | 175 | — |
| Acctate | 27.1 | — | — |
| Bicarbonate | — | 75 | 75 |
| Glucose (g/l) | 1 | — | 50 |
| | (5.6 mOsm) | | (280 mOsm) |
| Osmolality (mOsm/kg) | 282 | 500 | 430 |

Composition of basic dialysis solution, hypertonic sodium solution for IV reinfusion (sol. A) and hypotonic sodium-hypertonic glucose solution (sol. B) for IV reinfusion.

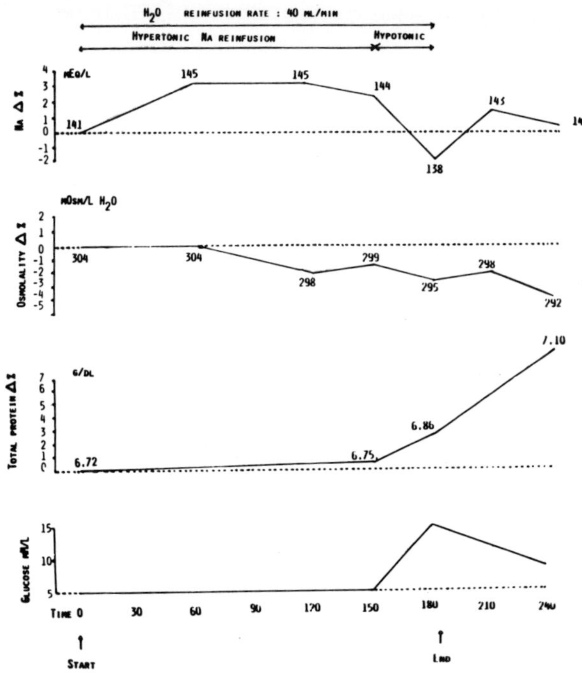



*Figure 1–5.* Hypertonic Hemodialfiltration. Biochemical changes (serum sodium, osmolality, total protein, and glucose) during hypertonic hemodiafiltration (180′). During the last 30′ of treatment (150′–180′), solution B sostituted solution A (see table 1–2).

Figure 1–5 describes the balance of serum sodium, osmolality, serum proteins, and glucose during hypertonic hemodiafiltration. The use of hypertonic sodium solution, followed by hypotonic reinfusate, does not change serum sodium concentration significantly; the addition of glucose in the last 30 minutes of treatment maintains a stable osmolality.

With regard to clinical tolerance, the significant increase of net ultrafiltration and the limited change of interdialysis body weight, despite a transient rise in sodium concentration, confirms that this treatment can be undertaken with few symptoms. When all the physiochemical and metabolic assumptions connected to the tolerance-related variables are respected, the following conclusions can be drawn:

1. An ultrafiltration rate of 25 ml/min appears well tolerated by the patient.

2. Urea and creatinine clearances greater than to 180 ml/min are not associated with vascular unstability or dysequilibrium syndrome.

3. No relationship between removal of uremic solutes and dialysis intolerance or dysequilibrium syndrome has been demonstrated.

14

## Present trend and future expectation

In the course of a recent workshop presented during the 1986 Congress of EDTA-European Renal Association in Budapest, the relationship between beta-2 microglobulin (B-2M) and amyloidosis has been analyzed in detail. Amyloid deposition are almost totally composed of B-2M [41]. The production of B-2M seems to be directly related to dialysis membranes: cuprophan favors an increase in serum concentration of B-2M, whereas with PAN membranes removal is greater than the accumulation [42].

It has also been observed that highly permeable membranes favor removal of B-2M as well as urine output of greater than 1,000 ml; in the meantime it has been underlined that blood exposure to dialysis membranes is always associated to a B-2M concentration greater than normal, independently of the quality of the material utilized: in peritoneal dialysis patients, on the contrary, serum B-2M has the same concentration as controls [43]. These observations suggest that different membranes present different levels of bioincompatibility as documented by the generalized high concentration of B-2M in all of the cases studied. Furthermore, the duration of blood exposure to the dialysis membrane can also be critical and can indirectly support the finding of a high incidence of carpal tunnel syndrome in patients treated with long dialysis schedules [21]. On the other hand, it has also been observed that CTS is not always caused by beta-2 associated amyloid [44, 45]: that implies that other dialysis-related factors, beside membranes, may trigger a dialysis disease.

Preliminary conclusions suggest that the use of highly permeable membranes other than cuprophan, for treatment sessions as short as clinically indicated, are advisable. As a consequence substitutive treatment should not be prolonged more than the needed time to remove efficiently small molecules. The urea generation model (see chapter 9) is, at present, the most appropriate parameter to quantify dialysis duration.

Clearly treatment time reduction to approximate 3 hours per session can be achieved without difficulty, provided a precise compliance to two major problems: (1) a stable hemodynamic status during the session and (2) a pharmacological type of control of solute removal.

In fact, the most negative consequence of a too-short session is the reduction of safety margins able to protect the patient from the unpredictable treatment failures, such as blood flow reduction, A-V fistula recirculation; finally it must be clearly stressed that clinical observation strongly discourages a treatment time less than 3 hours in the normal dialysis population, mainly represented by elderly patients.

Dialysis time reduction can be achieved either by potentiating diffusion or by combining convection, or by a combination of both. Considering the growing number of fragile patients and the need for prevention of arrythmias and acute hypotension, the use of bicarbonate-containing solutions distributed by the convection mode is presently the most appropriate means of achieving optimal hemodynamic stability. However, at present, standard postdilution hemofiltration can be performed in 3 hours only if blood flow is exceptionally high (500–600 ml/min). Clearly this fact represents an insurmountable limit for the majority of patients. On the other hand, the use of diffusion or a combination of diffusion and convection presents a main inconvenience: the need for large volumes of sterile solvent which is in open contradiction with the present trend toward high flux membranes: a new potential risk of infections in immunosuppressed patient; furthermore any possibility of precisely measuring uremic solutes in the dialysate ultrafiltered (pharmacological approach) will be frustrated by the presence of a solution which is extremely dilute and difficult to collect. This is also in contrast with the need to individualize treatment, which becomes compulsory if session times are to be reduced.

In recent years the feasibility of the in-line production of sterile pyrogen-free water has been demonstrated. An uninterrupted trial conducted in our center for over three years confirms that hemofiltration solutions can be produced in unlimited quantity at virtually no cost [45]. This result offers an important contribution to a rational formulation of future treatments. Considering the safety and the achieved low cost of hemofiltration solutions, postdilution hemofiltration can be implemented or completely substituted by Henderson's original predilution approach [46]. The most important advantages we have obtained refer to the patient's blood flow and volume requirements: the full use of predilution mode with present hemofilters allows the maintenance of the same treatment duration with significant reduction of blood flow. In practice the majority of patients can receive a treatment adequate to their solute distribution volume and urea generation rate (i.e., pharmacological type of therapy) in a session time not greater than 3 hours, a blood flow within 400 ml/min, and a volume of hemofiltrate of 50–60 litres.

Clearly a precise quantification of treatment is the appropriate and mandatory answer to the need for reducing session duration.


## References


1. Cambi, V., Dall'Aglio, P., Savazzi, G., Arisi, L. and Migone, L. (1972) Clinical assessment of haemodialysis patients with reduced small molecules removal. Proc. Europ. Dial. Transp. Ass. 9: 67.
2. Scribner, B.H. (1965) Discussion. Trans. Amer. Soc. Artif. Int. organs 11: 29.
3. Shaldon, S. (1966) Haemodialysis in chronic renal failure. Post Graduate Medical Journal (Supplement) 12/680. Kent: Kent Arms Printing Works Ltd.
4. Babb, A.L., Popovic, R.P., Christopher, T.G. and Scribner B.H. (1971) The genesis of the square meter-hour hypothesis. Trans. Am. Soc. Art. Int. org. 17: 91.
5. Christopher, T.G., Cambi, V., Haker, L.A., Hurst, P., Popovic, R.P., Babb, A.L. and Scribner, B.H. (1971) A study of haemodialysis with lowered dialysate flow rate. Proc. Am. Soc. Art. Int. Org. 17: 92.
6. Quadracci, L.I., Cambi, V., Christopher, T.G., Harker, L.A. and Striker, G.E. (1971) Assay of serum abnormalities in uremic and dialysis patients. Evidence for depletion of vital


16

substances in hemodialysis. Trans. Amer. Soc. Art. Org. 17: 96.

7. Cambi, V., Arisi, L., Bignardi, L., Bruschi, G., Rossi, E., Savazzi, G. and Migone, L. (1974) Short dialysis schedules: finally ready to become a routine? Proc. Europ. Dial. Transpl. Ass. XI: 112–120.

8. Cambi, V. (1976) Limits of dialysis technology. Proc. VI Int. Congr. of Nephrology, Karger, Basel, p. 624.

9. D'Amico, G., Petrella, E., Orlandini, G., Cambi, V., Savazzi, G., Migone, L., Castellani, A., Mioni, G. and Maiorca, R. (1976) Long term multicentric experience with short dialysis treatment. Proc. Int. Congr. of Nephrol., Karger, Basel, p. 629.

10. Cambi, V., Savazzi, G., Arisi, L., Buzio, C., Dall'Aglio, P., Rossi, E. and Migone, L. (1973) Dialysis schedules and peripheral neuropaty. Proc. Europ. Dial. Transpl. Ass. X: 271.

11. Mirahmadi, K.S., Kay, J.H., Miller, J.H., Gorman, J.T., Rosen, S.M. (1974) Clinical Evaluation of patients dialysed with double gambro 4 hours, three times per week. Proc. Eur. Dial. Transpl. Ass. 11: 121.

12. Nakagawa, S., Suenaga, M., Sasaki, S., Yoshiyama, N., Takeuchi, J., Kitaoka, T., Koshikawa, S. and Yamada, T. (1978) comparison of dialysis programmed on different molecular prescriptions: a preliminary study. Proc. Europ. Dial. Transp. Ass. 14: 167.

13. Shaldon, S., Deschodt, G., Beau, M.C., Ramperez, P. and Mion, C. (1978) The importance of serum osmotic changes in symptomatic hypotension during short dialysis. Proc. Clin. Dial. Transpl. Forum 8: 35.

14. Gotch, F.A., Sargent, J.A., Keen, H.L., Seid, H., Foster, R. (1973) Comparative treatment time with kill, gambro and cordis-dow kidney. Proc. Dialysis Transpl. Forum 3: 217.

15. Laurent, G., Calemard, E. and Charra, B. (1983) Long dialysis: a review of fifteen years experience in one centre 1968–1983. Proc. Europ. Dial. Transp. Ass. 20: 122.

16. Cambi, V., Garini, G., Savazzi, G., Arisi, L., David, S., Zanelli, P., Bono, F. and Gardini, F. (1983) Short dialysis. Proc. Europ. Dial. Transpl. Ass. 20: 111.

17. Friedman, E.A. and Lundin, A.P. (1982) Environmental and iatrogenic obstacles to long life on haemodialysis (editorial). New Eng. J. Med. 306: 167.

18. Leong, A.S.Y., Disney, A.P.S. and Gove, D.W. (1982) Spallation and migration of silicone from blood pump-tubing in patients on haemodialysis. New Eng. J. Med. 306: 135.

19. Bommer, J. and Ritz, E. (1985) Spallation of dialysis materials. Problems and perspectives. Nephron 39: 285.

20. Gutierrez, A., Alvestrand, A., Wahren, J. and Bergström, J. (1985) Blood-membrane interaction without dialysis indices increased protein catabolism in normal man. Proc. EDTA-ERA Workshop, Biocompatibility (Chairman, H. Klinkmann) p. 223.

21. Charra, B., Calemard, E., Uzan, M., Terrat, J.C., Vawel, T. and Laurent, G. (1984) Carpal tunnel syndrome, shoulder pain and amyloid deposits in long term hamodialyzed patients. Proc. Europ. Dial. Transpl. Ass. 21: 291.

22. Cambi, V., Nizzoli, M., paganelli, E., David, S. and Bono, F. (1986) Danger of an unnecessarily prolonged dialysis session: carpal tunnel syndrome. Artificial Organs 10: 178.

23. Teschan, P.E., Ginn, H.E., Bourne, J.R., Ward, J.W., Schaffer, J.D. (1983) A prospective study of reduced dialysis. ASAIO J. 6: 108.

24. Quellhorst, E., Rieger, J., Doht, B., Beckmann, H., Jacob, I., Kraft, B., Mietzsch, G. and Scheler F. (1976) Treatment of chronic uremia by an ultrafiltration kidney. First clinical experience. Proc. Europ. Dial. Transpl. Ass. 13: 314.

25. Henderson, L.W., Besarab, A., Michaels, A. and Bluemle, L.W., Jr. (1967) Blood purification by ultrafiltration and fluid replacement (diafiltration). Trans. Am. Soc. Artif. Int. Organs XII: 216.

26. Bergström, J., Asaba, H., Fürst, P., Oulès, R. (1977) Dialysis, ultrafiltration, and blood pressure. Proc. Europ. Dial. Transpl. Ass. 13.

27. Cambi, V., Arisi, L., Bignardi, L., Garini, G., Rossi, E. and Migone, L. (1977) Haemodiafiltration with reduced dialysis fluid. Opusc. Medica-Technica Lundensia XVII: 95.

28. Leber, H.W., Wizemann, V., Goubeaud, G. and Rawer, P. (1977) Hemodiafiltration, an

effective alternative to hemofiltration and conventional hemodialysis in the treatment of uremic patients. Opuscula Medica-Technica Lundensia XVII: 107.

29. Graefe, U., Milutinovich, J., Follette, W.C., Babb, A.L. and Scribner, B.H. (1977) Improved tolerance to rapid ultrafiltration with the use of bicarbonate in dialysis. Proc. Europ. Dial. Transp. Ass. 14: 153.

30. Wehle, B., Asaba, H., Castenfors, J., Fürst, P., Gunnarsson, B., Shaldon, S. and Bergström, J. (1979) Haemodynamic changes during sequential ultrafiltration and dialysis. Kidney Int. 15: 411.

31. Shaldon, S., Deschodt, G., Bean, M.C., Mion, H. and Mion, C. Vascular stability during high flux haemofiltration. Proc. Eur. Dial. Transpl. Ass. 16: 695.

32. Zucchelli, P., Catizone, L., Degli Esposti, E., Fusaroli, M., Ligabue, A. and Zuccalà, A. (1977) Influence of ultrafiltration on the plasma renin activity and the adrenergic system. Opuscula Medica Lundensia XVIII: 41.

33. Hampl, H., Praeper, H., Unger, V., Fischer, C.H., Resa, I. and Kessel, M. (1980) haemodynamic changes during haemodialysis, sequential ultrafiltration and haemofiltration. Kidney Int. (S) 27: 83.

34. Cambi, V., Hampl, H., Savazzi, G., Arisi, L., Bignardi, L., Rossi, E. and Migone, L. (1977) Una nuova metodologia dialitica: emodialisi ultrabreve a bassa efficienza. Attualità Nefr. Dial. 'Il Pensiero Scientifico' Ed., Roma, p. 407.

35. Cambi, V., Hampl, H., Savazzi, G., Arisi, L., Bignardi, L., Garini, G., Rossi, E., Praper, P., Kessel, M. and Migone, L. (1978) Principles and clinical application of ultra-short dialysis. Trans. Amer. Soc. Art. Int. Org. 24: 443.

36. Cambi, V., Arisi, L., Biasini, A., Bono, F., David, S., Savazzi, G. and Migone, L. (1980) Improvement of the intradialytic tolerance with low volume dialysis and bicarbonate buffering of the dialysate. Kidney Int. (S) 27: 207.

37. Castellani, A., et al., Lusvarghi, E., et al., Salv adeo, A. et al. and Petrecca, E. et al. (1980) La dialisi ultrabreve ricircolata con bicarbonato. Proc. Mitteleuropean Meeting of Nephrology and Dialysis 2: 15.

38. Quellhorst, E., Schuenemann, B., Hildebrand, U. and Falda Z. (1980) Response of the vascular system to different modifications of haemofiltration and haemodialysis. Proc. Europ. Dial. Transp. Ass. 17: 197.

39. Cambi, V., Buzio, C., Arisi, L., Calderini, C., David, S., Manari, A., Bono, F. and Zanelli, P. (1981) Vascular stability and middle molecules removal in hypertonic haemodiafiltration. Proc. Europ. Dial. Transpl. Ass. 18: 681.

40. Cambi, V., Arisi, L., Bono, F., Calderini, C., David, S., Manari, A. and Zanelli, P. (1980) Emodiafiltrazione ipertonica. Attualità Nefrol. Dial. 'Il Pensiero Scientifico' Ed. Roma, p. 119.

41. McClure, J.C., Ackrill, P. and Bartley, C. (1986) Deposition of beta-2 microglobulin in long-term haemodialysis patients. XXIII Congress EDTA-ERA p. 138 (Abstract).

42. Vandenbroucke, J.M. and Van Ypersele de Strihou, C. (1986) Relationship between membrane characteristics and dialysis induced changes. XXIII Congress EDTA-ERA p. 156 (Abstract).

43. Foret, M., Milongo, R., Meftahi, H., Dechelette, E., Hachache, T., Kuentz, F., Renversetz, J.C. and Cordonnier, D. (1986) XXII Congress EDTA-ERA p. 123 (Abstract).

44. Bommer, J., Seelig, H.P., Seelig, R. and Ritz, E. (1986) Beta-2 microglobulin levels in haemodialysed patients. XXIII Congress EDTA-ERA p. 111 (Abstract).

45. Cambi, V., David, S., Buzio, C., Arisi, L., Ferrari, M.E., Barani, R. and Quaretti, P. (1985) Emofiltrazione on-line: risultati a distanza. Aggiornamenti nefrologici Magna Grecia 3° Corso, p. 301, Edit. Bios.

46. David, S. and Cambi, V. (1986) Real time evaluation of high efficiency predilution haemofiltration and nitrogen balance (in press).

# 2. Short dialysis: a single center study

Vincenzo Cambi, Roberto Menta, Fabio Bono, Maria Elena Ferrari, and
Alessandro Castiglioni

Hemodialysis treatment of chronic renal failure was introduced in our department in 1964. In 1971, we began treating a number of patients with short dialysis, and since 1972, all hemodialysis treatment in our center has been short dialysis (SD). The results of treatment of 278 patients in chronic renal failure on SD from January 1, 1974, to December 31, 1984, are presented here.

Numerous reports deal with the rate of survival and diseases contracted by uremic patients on dialysis treatment, but they seldom take the modalities of dialysis into proper consideration. Moreover, there are often differences among the various groups examined, and patients are frequently subjected to different dialysis treatments as part of the overall approach to the treatment of chronic renal failure. It is thus difficult to examine the true long-term efficacy and safety of any single type of treatment. In fact, many case series present patients who pass from hemodialysis (HD) to intermittent peritoneal dialysis (IPD) or from substitutive treatment to transplantation. For SD, in particular, only limited observations regarding long-term survival exist, and reports dealing with survival beyond 10 years are extremely rare.

Moreover, variations in types of social services and health insurance programs in different countries condition data and distribution of the dialysis population in terms of treatment preference. In our dialysis unit, all uremic subjects regardless of age, as well as patients with malignant neoplasms (except for those of rapid evolution), undergo substitutive treatment.

The data reported here come from one of the most wide-scale trials of a single modality of dialysis therapy; a description of the epidemiological characteristics of this population can be utilized for comparison with other data in chiefly epidemiological terms.

It should be emphasized that the patients presented here underwent SD: most of them 3 times a week, with each single dialysis session lasting 4 hours regardless of size; only a small number of patients were treated 3 hours every other day. The quality of life of the patients undergoing SD was not taken into consideration in this study.

*Vincenzo Cambi (editor) Professor of Nephrology*
*© 1987 Martinus Nijhoff Publishing, Boston. ISBN 0-89838-858-9. Printed in The United States.*

## Patients and methods

The clinical data regarding 278 patients who underwent SD from January 1, 1974, to December 31, 1984, were examined. Exclusion from or inclusion in the study was based on the following criteria: (1) only those patients judged to be chronic were included; (2) patients with acute renal failure (ARF) or patients with chronic renal failure (CRF) who underwent less than 3 months of dialysis treatment were excluded; (3) patients transferred to or from other dialysis units during this period were excluded; (4) patients who underwent transplantation, patients who were treated with different dialysis modalities, and patients who returned to hemodialysis treatment after transplantation were excluded.

The overall survival rate of the entire population was calculated at the end of the observation period. The cause of CRF, age at the start of treatment, length of treatment at the end of the study or death, and cause of death were noted for each patient. The data were furnished as averages of the surviving and deceased populations and divided on the basis of sex.

The population (278 patients) was divided into 3 age groups at the start dialysis treatment: 0–29 years, 30–59 years, 60+ years. A comparison of the relative percents in each group was then made between the surviving and deceased patients.

During the entire period considered, hemodialysis was carried out according to the following modalities: 4h $\times$ 3/M$^2$/W (a small group of patients was treated for 3 hours every second day = 10.5 hours weekly); the dialysate was composed of Na 140 mEq/l; K 1–3 mEq/l; Ca 4 mEq/l; Mg 1 mEq/l; Cl 106–108 mEq/l; acetate 40 mEq/l; and glucose 1 g/L.

All patients underwent monthly SMA 18 and hemocytometric evaluation. Body weight, blood pressure, and heart frequency were measured before and after each dialysis session by the paramedical staff. The iPTH of each patient was checked twice a year.

All date were codified and stored in a Data Control 6006 computer. Calculations for each value considered were carried out on an average of every 3 months.

Predialysis body weight of the total population of surviving and deceased patients was evaluated. We established the postdialysis weight of the II trimester of treatment as the ideal body weight.

For each surviving patient, the predialysis systolic and mean pressures were studied during the entire treatment period and at the end of the study. The II trimester BP, too, was taken as a reference value. The percent of hypertensive patients 6 months before the start of treatment was compared to the percent of hypertensive patients at the end of the observation period. The percent of patients on antihypertensive therapy at the beginning and at the end of the study was also considered.

The percent of patients who underwent parathyroidectomy (PTX), with particular reference to preoperative and postoperative calcemia was studied.

Almost all patients were treated with aluminum hydroxide and/or vitamin D analogs. The number of pericardiotomies carried out on the population and the average duration of presurgical and postsurgical treatment were then considered. Frequency of the carpal tunnel syndrome was documented.

The characteristics of the population on dialysis from January 1, 1974, to December 31, 1984, were analyzed separately: in this particular subgroup, the effects of longer term short dialysis were studied.

The results, presented as averages and standard deviation, were evaluated with either the $X^2$ test or the student's t-test for paired data, depending on appropriateness [1]. Only results with significance greater than 0.05 are reported.

## Results

Of the 278 patients studied, 214 (76%) were alive at the end of the observation period; 64 (24%) had died. The population increased annually at a constant rate, with the user population remaining stable for the entire 11-year period considered. An average of 28 patients began dialysis each year, equal to 70 per million from a regional population of 400,000 inhabitants.

The population studied consisted of 161 (58%) males and 117 (42%) females: at the end of the period, 121 (75%) males were living and 40 (25%) had died; 93 females were living (79%) and 24 (21%) had died (figure 2–1).

The average age at the start of HD in the 278 patients was 54.2 ± 7.3, and the average length of treatment was 60 ± 6.3 months. The deceased patients were significantly older at the start of dialysis than the surviving patients (58.1 ± 7.5 versus 50.9 ± 10.4) (p < 0.05). The average age of the surviving males at the start of SD was greater than that of the surviving females (52.8 ± 6.3 versus 49.3 ± 7.6), but the difference is not statistically significant. On the contrary, the difference in initial average age between surviving and deceased males (52.8 ± 6.3 versus 58.9 ± 7.4, p < 0.05) and surviving and deceased females is statistically significant (49.3 ± 7.6 versus 56.5 ± 7.6, p < 0.005) (table 2–1).

The average duration of dialysis treatment between the surviving and deceased population is significantly different (72 ± 9.7 versus 41.4 ± 6.4 months; p < 0.001). The difference in duration of SD treatment between the surviving and deceased female population (96.1 ± 7.7 versus 38.5 ± 6.5; p < 0.001) is also significant, as well as the difference in treatment duration between the male and female surviving populations (96.1 ± 7.7 versus 46.7 ± 7.5; p < 0.01). The difference between surviving and deceased males was not statistically significant (p = n.s.). These results are reported in table 2–1. There were no differences between males and females, surviving or deceased, regarding the causes of CRF (table 2–2).

The importance of age as the chief factor influencing survival comes to light

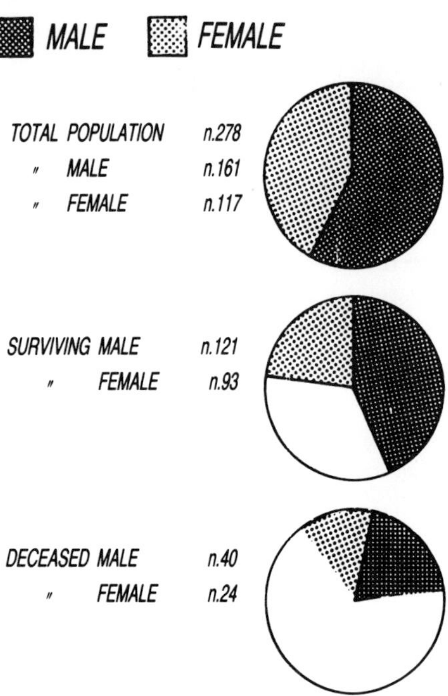


*Figure 2–1.* Population under study. Population under study: total population n. 278: 161 (58%) males, 117 (42%) females. Surviving males 121 (75%); decreased males 40 (25%); surviving females 93 (79%); decreased females 24 (21%).

when the surviving and deceased patients are divided into age groups (figure 2–2). The patients were divided into 3 groups — group 1: 0–29 years old; group 2: 30–59 years old; group 3: 60+ years old. The difference in death rate was statistically significant between groups. Statistical significance was greater between groups 2 and 3 ($p < 0.05$) than between groups 1 and 3, presumably because of the smaller number of patients in group 1. In fact, the majority of patients beginning SD treatment were in the 30–59 age group (56%), with a 39% death rate; on the contrary, in the 60+ group of patients beginning SD, 53.2% died and 32.8% were living at the end of the study.

Body weight studies on the surviving and deceased populations show that the percent drop in theoretical ideal weight (i.e., dry weight after the first trimester of treatment) was an average of 5% for the surviving population and 10% for the deceased population: this difference is of negligible significance.

Long-term blood pressure studies were also made. Although average BP values tended to decrease over time, the difference in systolic and mean predialysis BP between surviving and deceased populations (148 ± 12.9 versus 144 ± 12 and 104 ± 10.2 versus 102.6 ± 10.1 mmHg) was not significant. Thus neither weight nor BP could be considered decisive factors in determining survival.

Short dialysis nevertheless controls hypertension very efficiently: when

*Table 2–1.* Characteristic of the population and results on the basic of age and sex

| | Mean Age at the Beginning of SD (Years) | n | % | Mean Age at the End of the Study or at Death (Years) | Mean Duration of SD (Months) |
|---|---|---|---|---|---|
| Total population | 54.02 ± 7.3 | 278 | 100 | 59.1 ± 8.5 | 60.0 ± 6.3 |
| Surviving | 50.9 ± 10.4 <br> p < 0.05 | 214 | 76 | 57.0 ± 9.1 | 72.1 ± 9.7 <br> p < 0.001* |
| Surviving males | 52.8 ± 6.3 <br> p < 0.05** | 121 | 75 | 56.5 ± 8.7 | 46.7 ± 7.5 <br> p < 0.01** |
| Surviving females | 49.3 ± 7.6 <br> p < 0.005*** | 93 | 79 | 58.4 ± 7.9 | 96.1 ± 7.7*** <br> p < 0.01** |
| Deceased | 58.1 ± 7.5 <br> p < 0.05 | 64 | 24 | 61.5 ± 7.8 | 41.4 ± 6.4 <br> p < 0.001* |
| Deceased males | 58.9 ± 7.4 <br> p < 0.05** | 40 | 25 | 62.3 ± 6.9 | 42.9 ± 6.2 <br> p = n.s. |
| Deceased females | 56.5 ± 7.6 <br> p < 0.005*** | 24 | 21 | 59.9 ± 7.6 | 38.5 ± 6.5 <br> p < 0.001*** |

Characteristics and results of treatment among dialysis population: in table 2–1 is shown the mean age at the beginning of short dialysis (SD) for total population (54.02 ± 7.3 years); the mean age at the start of the treatment of surviving patients (50.9 ± 10.4 years) and deceased patients (58.1 ± 7.5 years): the difference is statistically significative (p < 0.05*). There was statistically significance, too (p < 0.05), when we compared the mean age of the deceased males (58.9 ± 7.4 years) versus the mean age of surviving male (52.8 ± 6.3 years) as well as between surviving females (49.3 ± 7.6 years) versus deceased females (56.5 ± 7.6 years) (p < 0.005).

There was statistically significance in difference between the mean age of surviving females (49.3 ± 7.6 years) versus surviving males (52.8 ± 6.3 years) (p < 0.05).

Differences in duration of treatment between surviving and deceased populations (*p < 0.001) and between surving males and surviving females (**p < 0.01) were statistically significant, too.

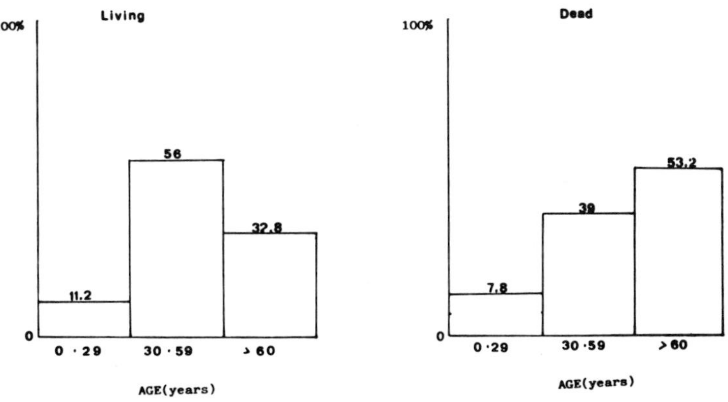


*Figure 2–2.* Comparison between surviving and deceased patients on the Basis of age. The death rate of patients entering hemodialysis at 60 years of age was higher (p < 0.05) than the death rate of patients entering dialysis at 30–59 years; the latter was higher (p < 0.01), than that of patients entering dialysis at 0–29 years of age.

*Table 2–2.* Primary renal disease in total population under study

| Primary Renal Disease | Surviving N° | Population % | Surviving N° | Males % | Surviving N° | Females % | Deceased N° | Pts. % | Deceased N° | Males % | Deceased N° | Females % |
|---|---|---|---|---|---|---|---|---|---|---|---|---|
| Aetiology uncertain | 53 | 24.8 | 31 | 25.6 | 22 | 24 | 13 | 20.3 | 7 | 17.5 | 6 | 25 |
| Biopsied glomerulopathy | 30 | 14 | 16 | 13.2 | 14 | 15 | 6 | 9.3 | 5 | 12.5 | 1 | 4.2 |
| Not biopsied glomerulopathy | 22 | 10.3 | 17 | 14 | 5 | 5 | 5 | 7.8 | 4 | 10 | 1 | 4.2 |
| Renovascular disease due to hypertension | 20 | 9.3 | 13 | 10.7 | 7 | 7.5 | 4 | 6.2 | 3 | 7.5 | 1 | 4.2 |
| Interstitial nephritis | 19 | 8.9 | 10 | 8 | 9 | 9.7 | 11 | 17 | 8 | 20 | 3 | 12.5 |
| Policystic kidney | 15 | 7 | 4 | 3 | 11 | 12 | 8 | 12.5 | 3 | 7.5 | 5 | 20.8 |
| Urolithiasis | 12 | 5.1 | 5 | 4 | 7 | 7.5 | 4 | 6.2 | 1 | 2.5 | 3 | 12.5 |
| Tubercolosis | 7 | 3.2 | 4 | 3 | 3 | 3 | — | — | — | — | — | — |
| Nephroangiosclerosis | 7 | 3.2 | 5 | 4 | 2 | 2 | — | — | — | — | — | — |
| Analgesic nephropathy | 5 | 2.3 | — | — | 5 | 5 | — | — | — | — | — | — |
| Diabetes (type II) | 4 | 2 | 4 | 3.3 | — | — | — | — | — | — | — | — |
| Obstructive nephropathy | 3 | 1.5 | 2 | 1.6 | 1 | 1 | — | — | — | — | — | — |
| Alport syndrome | 3 | 1 | 3 | 2.4 | — | — | — | — | — | — | — | — |
| Kidney tumor | 2 | 1 | 2 | 1.6 | — | — | — | — | — | — | — | — |
| Lupus erythematosus | 2 | 1 | — | — | 2 | 2 | — | — | — | — | — | — |
| Myeloma | — | — | — | — | — | — | 3 | 4.7 | 3 | 7.5 | — | — |
| Miscellanea | 10 | 5 | 5 | 4 | 5 | 5 | 10 | 5.6 | 6 | 15 | 4 | 17 |

Causes of chronic renal failure in males and females. There was no statistically significant difference between male and females surviving and deceased populations.

observation was limited to the surviving population, it was noted that 169 patients (79%) presented elevated BP values 6 months before entering dialysis treatment, and that 149 (70% of the total population) were on antihypertensive therapy. At the end of the study, only 60 patients (28% of the total population) were taking antihypertensive drugs. If the patients taking only nifedipine, used chiefly in the treatment of myocardial ischemia (6.5% of the total population), were excluded, the percent of patients in treatment falls to 21.5% of the total population (46 patients — table 2–3).

The incidence of PTX in the total population was 5.4%: 4.6% of the surviving population and 7.8% (5 patients) of the deceased group. In the surviving population, the average age at the time of surgery was $49.5 \pm 7$ years. The average length of postoperative treatment was $43.8 \pm 6.6$ months (as of December 31, 1984). The decision for surgery was based on the following clinical and laboratory criteria: bone pain, pruritus unmodified by a low phosphorus diet and/or the administration of phosphorus chelates and/or vitamin D analogues, hypertension, weight loss, muscle weakness, persistent elevated alkaline phosphatase, elevated iPTH, hypercalcemia, and hyperphosphatemia. The patients who underwent surgery gained weight and presented improved subjective symptomatology; preoperative and postoperative BP values were not significantly modified ($150.7 \pm 12.3$ versus $138.8 \pm 11.8$ p.n.s.). On the contrary, iPTH and alkaline phosphatase were significantly reduced. No correlation was found between the length of dialysis treatment and the progression of hyperparathyroidism (table 2–4).

*Table 2–3.* Causes of death in population under study

| Main Cause of Death | N | % |
|---|---|---|
| Myocardial ischemia and infarction | 14 | 21.8 |
| Cerebrovascular accident | 12 | 18.7 |
| Not determined | 8 | 12.5 |
| Cardiac arrest | 6 | 9.4 |
| Cardiac failure | 5 | 7.8 |
| Septicemia | 4 | 6.2 |
| Malignant disease not induced by Immunosuppressive therapy | 3 | 4.7 |
| Pulmonary infection (bacterial) | 2 | 3.2 |
| Dementia | 1 | 1.6 |
| Unknown | 1 | 1.6 |
| Suicide | 1 | 1.6 |
| Cirrhosis — not viral | 1 | 1.6 |
| Scleroderma | 1 | 1.6 |
| Hemorrhagic pericarditis | 1 | 1.6 |
| Hyperkalemia | 1 | 1.6 |
| Hypertensive cardiac failure | 1 | 1.6 |
| Hemorrhage | 1 | 1.6 |
| Pulmonary embolus | 1 | 1.6 |

Causes of death are listed on the right: about 40% of the deaths were due to cardiovascular disease or stroke.

*Table 2–4.* Efficiency of short dialysis in the correction of hypertension

|  | N° | % |
| --- | --- | --- |
| Total surviving population | 214 | 100 |
| Hypertension before SD | 169 | 79 |
| Hypertension + therapy before SD | 149 | 70* |
| Hypertension after SD | 60 | 28 |
| Hypertension + therapy after | 46 | 21.5* |
| Nifedipine alone | 14 | 6.5 |

Seventy percent of the total population was under antihypertensive therapy before entering short dialysis; only 21.5% was in pharmacological treatment at the end of the study (p < 0.001).

Sixteen pericardiectomies were carried out during the study period: 9 in males and 7 in females, equal to 5.8% of the total population. Sixty-nine percent of these operations were carried out from 1974 to 1979, and 31% were carried out during the 1979–84 period. Fifty-six percent of this surgery took place in the first trimester of treatment. The average age of patients at surgery was $51.2 \pm 7.1$ years, range 16–75, while the average age of these patients at the start of treatment was $49.3 \pm 7$ years. The average length of treatment before surgery was $20.5 \pm 4.5$ months, range 1–107 months. Thirteen patients recovered; 3 died within 3 months after surgery from metabolic complications. Pericardiotomy was carried out when intensification of dialysis during pericarditis did not improve objective symptomatology or when clinical conditions indicated suspected tamponade phenomena.

Five patients (1.8%) underwent surgery for carpal tunnel syndrome (CTS). Diagnosis was based on clinical symptoms, motor nerve conduction velocity (MNCV), and biopsy. At surgery, the presence of median nerve compression was verified in every case.

As previously described [11], the need for surgery for CTS in our population, with no regard for the temporal limits of this study, increased from 0.38% during the first 7 years to 36.3% after 14–20 years of treatment. The overall duration of dialysis sessions was 9,487 hours in the patients who underwent surgery versus 7,407 hours in patients who did not (p < 0.001). There was a highly significant correlation between duration of dialysis session and manifestations linked to the appearance of the clinical syndrome.

The appearance of the syndrome is strictly and perhaps decisively correlated to the dialysis method adopted. Short dialysis has had particularly positive effects regarding this syndrome with respect to long dialysis.

In 1974, 35 patients, 22 males (67%) and 13 females (33%), entered SD. The average age at which dialysis treatment was begun in this subgroup was $44.2 \pm 6.6$ years. On December 31, 1984, 20 patients were alive and 15 had died (55.5% versus 44.5%). The average age of the surviving patients at the start of treatment was $38.7 \pm 6.2$ years; the average age of the deceased patients entering dialysis was $52.7 \pm 7.2$ years. The age difference was statistically significant (p < 0.05) (table 2–5 and figure 2–3).

26

*Table 2–5.* Main clinical and laboratory parameters pre-PTX and post-PTX in 15 patients on short dialysis therapy

|  | Pre-PTX | Post-PTX | p |
| --- | --- | --- | --- |
| Systolic BP (mmHG) | 150.7 ± 12.3 | 138.8 ± 11.8 | n.s. |
| Symptoms: bone pain | +++ | ± | |
|      itching | +++ | + | |
|      muscle weakness | ++ | + | |
|      bw loss | ++ | — | |
| Ca (mg/dl) | 10.6 ± 1.1 | 9.8 ± 1.2 | n.s. |
| P (mg/dl) | 5.7 ± 1.4 | 5.3 ± 1.5 | n.s. |
| iPTH (ng/ml) | 7.4 ± 2.7 | 1.4 ± 1.1 | <0.001 |
| Alkaline phosphatase (U/I) | 247 ± 14 | 124 ± 81 | <0.001 |

Values are mean ± standard deviation.

Table 2–5 showed improvement of symptomatology and significant improvement of iPTH (p < 0.001) and alkaline phosphatase.

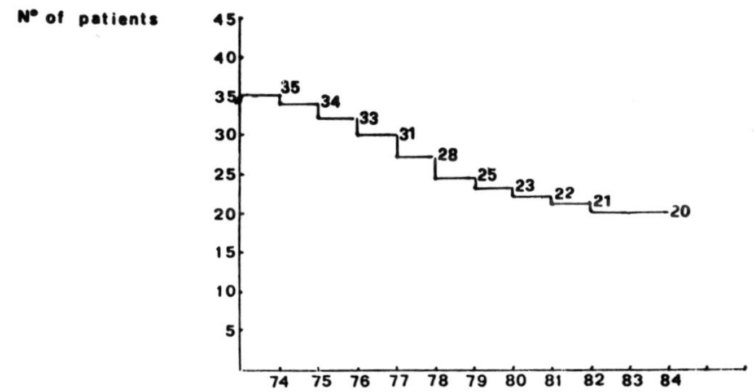


*Figure 2–3.* Curve indicating survival of patients who entered short dialysis in 1974. Eleven-year survival rate: 55.5%. Thirty-five patients began short dialysis; 20 were alive as of December 31, 1984.

The average length of dialysis treatment for surviving patients at the end of the study was 126 ± 11.6 months; for the deceased patients, it was 35 ± 5.9 months.

Five patients underwent PTX, two underwent pericardiotomy for dialysis paricarditis. Eight patients were hypertensive before starting treatment and afterwards became normotensive or hypotensive; 5 patients who were hypertensive before treatment remained hypertensive; the other 7, who had normal BP values before treatment, tend, at present, to be hypotensive. The causes of chronic renal failure correspond to what is found in the literature. Evaluation of the claimed long-term survival rate in polycystic kidney disease requires a larger population than what is encountered in a single unit: thus, we did not consider this problem.

The average age of patients beginning SD at our unit in 1984 was 57.0 ± 7.5 years and was significantly higher (p < 0.005) than the average age of patients who began SD in 1974 (44.2 ± 6 years).


## Discussion

An 11-year study permits evaluation of the biological characteristics of a dialysis population which is as thorough and conclusive as possible. Overall survival of the population was 76% (table 2–1): this is in accordance with data found in the literature. The survival rate of patients in dialysis for more than 10 years was 55.5% (table 2–5); this value is notably higher than that reported in the literature.

The data reported by Wing and associates in 1977 [2] regard survival rates for patients on home dialysis, that is, a selected group of patients whose general condition was markedly better than that of patients on hospital dialysis. The latter group, in fact, presumably has more clinical problems. The survival rate of patients on hospital dialysis presented by Wing is 38.5% [2]. Neff and associates [3] report an even lower 10-year survival rate: 18%. Charra and coworkers [4], however, report an 80% 10-year survival rate for patients undergoing 'traditional' dialysis (24–30 hours/week). Thus, treatment carried out 24–30 hours/week would seem to guarantee much longer survival. Nevertheless, in our opinion, the age at which dialysis is initiated plays a decisive role in survival. Charra's patients, in fact, entered hemodialysis at an average age of 34.4 ± 9.3 years. When we evaluated 10-year survival in a group of our SD patients, comparable in terms of primary kidney disease and age at the start of dialysis (34 ± 5.8 years) with those of Charra and coworkers, the 11-year survival rate was 85%. Rather than treatment modality, what seemed to be strictly linked to survival was the age at which dialysis was begun, as well as more careful and restrictive evaluation of patients to be subjected to extracorporeal treatment.

In recent years, the general profile of the population undergoing hemodialysis has changed. The population entering dialysis has progressively aged together with aging of the HD population itself. Our data indicate that in 1974, the average age of patients entering SD was 44.2 ± 6.6 years, while data for 1984 present an average 'entrance' age of 57.0 ± 7.5 years (p < 0.005). Age is thus the primary factor influencing survival; percents relative to age groups of surviving and deceased patients confirm this opinion (figure 2–2).

Body weight does not significantly influence long-term survival, although it can be the telltale sign of concomitant underlying pathological phenomena, insufficient treatment, or scarce attention paid to dietary or therapeutic regimins, which in themselves can become further risk factors. In our study, weight loss was greater in the deceased group than in the surviving group:

although this was not statistically significant, it points out the difficulty in evaluating the substantial weight losses seen in the deceased population which presumably indicated intercurrent acute pathologies.

Blood pressure, as well, did not seem to be a determining factor in long-term survival. In fact, no significant differences between the surviving and deceased groups were noted; moreover, as time passed, there was a progressive drop in systolic and mean predialysis BP. Control of BP could be an important factor in the younger population, while in older patients its role as a risk factor is more limited.

Further light could be shed on this matter by a controlled study of a large group of patients with nephroangiosclerosis in order to verify whether or not vascular and cardiac pathologies are the major cause of death in this group. However, the polyfactorial genesis of arteriosclerosis involves many parameters already compromised by uremia: lipid, glucose, and hormonal metabolism. Death rates due to cardiac or vascular disease in patients on dialysis are reported in the literature as 64.7% for patients on hospital dialysis and 67.7% for patients on home dialysis [2]. The overall death rate for cardiac and vascular disease in our patients was about 40% (table 2–3).

Among the causes of CRF influencing survival, only diabetes, which is less frequent in our case group than in American studies [5], differs significantly.

The percent of parathyroidectomies reported in the literature [6] varies from 0.8% during the first two years of treatment to 16% after 10 years. The overall rate in our population was 5.4%, with an average presurgery treatment time of about 4 years. The parathyroidectomy rate in surviving patients was 4.6%; in the deceased group it was 7.8%: the difference between the two populations is scarcely significant. The virtual absence of osteomalacia in our patients should be pointed out, although extensive histological confirmation from the entire population or sample groups is not available. However, the parallel absence of dialysis dementia when compared to the incidence reported in the literature [7] suggest that our unit is quite fortunate regarding water contamination, even taking into consideration the fact that aluminum hydroxide therapy for hyperphosphatemia is given to virtually all patients. Moreover, there is a higher concentration of Ca in the dialysis fluid [8] as well as widescale and aggressive vitamin D analog therapy. In any case, in our patients, parathyroidectomy reduced levels of iPTH (from 7.4 to 1.4 ng/ml) and alkaline phosphatase (from 247 to 124 U/l) significantly (p < 0.001) (table 2–4). We did not observe the significant correlation between treatment length and degree of hyprparathyroidism reported by other authors [9].

Sixteen pericardiotomies (9 in men, 7 in women) were carried out, with an incidence of 5.8%, which is midway between reported values of 8.4% for HD and 4.3% for IPD [10]. As already pointed out in the literature, there has been a decrease of pericarditis in dialysis patients. Our data indicate that 69% of the paricardiotomies were carried out during the first 5 years, and the other 31% were carried out over the next 6 years. Moreover, only one case of

*Table 2-6.* Survival rate and age of patients who began short dialysis in 1974

|                                | N  | %    | Mean age (Years) |
|--------------------------------|----|------|------------------|
| Total number                   | 35 | 100  |                  |
| Surviving in 1984              | 20 | 55.5 | 38.7 ± 6.2*      |
| Deceased before the end of 1984| 15 | 44.5 | 57.7 ± 7.2*      |

Thirty-five patients started SD in 1974; in 1984 20 (55.5%) were alive. The mean age at the start of SD of the surviving patients was 38.7 ± 6.2 years; the mean age at the start of SD for deceased patients was 57.7 ± 7.2 years. The difference between the two groups is statistically significant ($p < 0.005$).

hemorrhagic pericarditis was observed. These data lead to the conclusion that pericarditis occurs infrequently during short dialysis.

Data regarding the carpal tunnel syndrome are highly significant [11]. The shorter dialysis session is highly correlated to the low incidence of this syndrome in the entire population. Its pathogenesis is undoubtedly polyfactorial: venous stasis, chronic inflammation, exposition to stimuli from the dialysis membrane all combine to determine the final outcome. It should be emphasized as well that amyloid was not found in any of our histological examinations.

Survival beyond 10 years was studied in the patient group which had entered dialysis in 1974 (table 2-6). Analysis of this subgroup confirmed in a general way what has been reported for the entire population: that age at the beginning of dialysis is the crucial factor in determining long-term survival. In this subgroup, moreover, the length of SD is significantly correlated to the need for parathyroidectomy.

Blood pressure would seem to be a factor that accelerates the evolution of CRF to uremia, but not an essential factor in determining survival of a patient on hemodialysis. By reducing volemia, hemodialysis itself brings about lower peripheral resistance, and other presently unknown factors seem to influence long-term myocardial contractile efficiency [12]. The tendency to hypotension is moreover a constant always verified after prolonged dialysis treatment.

The fact that the population on SD is growing older raises certain questions regarding, most of all, the future of SD: given the increasing rate of renal transplantation, the age limits which are progressively moving up with consequently fewer limits to application, the diffusion of effective immunosuppressive therapies, it may be logically assumed that transplantation will become even more widespread. Substitutive therapies too are being perfected with the aim of reducing dialysis time to 2 hours, and new forms of treatment, such as hemofiltration and hemodiafiltration, are being integrated into substitutive therapies. In any case, it is of paramount importance to bear in mind the greater average age of patients on short dialysis.

# References

1. Colton, T. (1974) Statistics in Medicine. Boston: Little Brown and Co.
2. Wing, A.J., Brunner, F.P., Brynger, H., Chantler, C., Donckerwolcke, R.A., Gurland, H.J. and Jacobs, C. (1977) Combined report on regular dialysis and transplantation in Europe VIII, EDTA Proc. 15: 4–76.
3. Neff, M.S., Eiser, A.R., Slifkin, R.F., Baum, M., Baez, A., Gupta, S. and Amarga, E. (1983) Patients surviving 10 years of hemodialysis. Am. J. Med. 74: 996–1004.
4. Charra, B., Calemar, E., Cuche, M. and Laurent, G. (1983) Control of hypertension and prolonged survival on maintenance HD. Nephron 33: 96–99.
5. Kjellstrand, C.M., Whitely, K., Comty, C.M. and Shapiro, F.L. (1983) Dialysis in patients with diabetes mellitus. Diabetic Nephropathy 2: 5–17.
6. Kramer, P., Broyer, M., Brunner, F.P., Brynger, H., Challah, S., Oulés, R., Rizzoni, G., Selwood, N.M., Wing, A.J. and Balas, E.A. (1984) Annual report. EDTA Proc. 21: 2–68.
7. Alfrey, A.C., Gary, M.D., Le Grendre, G.R. and Kaehny, W.D. (1976) The dialysis encephalopathy syndrome. N. Engl. J. Med. 294: 184–188.
8. Goldsmith, R.S., Furszyfer, J., Johnson, W.T., Fournier, A.E. and Arnaud, C.D. (1971) Control of secondary hyperparathyroidism during long term hemodialysis. Am. J. Med. 50: 692–699.
9. Chan, Y.L., Furlong, T.J., Cornish, J.C. and Posen, S. (1985) Dialysis osteodistrophy. Medicine 64: 296–309.
10. Renfrew, R., Buselmeir, J.T., Kjellstrand, C.M. (1980) Pericarditis and renal failure. Ann. Rev. Med. 31: 345–360.
11. Cambi, V., Nizzoli, M., Paganelli, E., David, S. and Bono, F. (1986) The danger of an unnecessarily prolonged dialysis session: the carpal tunnel syndrome. Int. J. Art. Org. (in press).
12. Lawrence, W.H. and Misro, P. (1975) Cardiactive substances leached from a commercial hemodialysis set. N. Eng. J. Med. 292: 1356.

# 3. Hemodialysis strategies in European countries

Antony J. Wing, Felix P. Brunner, and Sabri Challah

The European Dialysis and Transplant Association (EDTA) Registry has collected information on hemodialysis strategies since the early 1970s. Regular annual reports from 1971 [1] to the most recent [2] contain descriptions of dialysis strategies and related technologies.

From 1970 data formed part of the computerized record compiled from annual returns updated on individual patient questionnaires. Core data are provided by the dated treatment sequence which records each patient's movements between the treatment modalities comprising renal replacement therapy (RRT). The numbers of patients who commenced hemodialysis in any year or who were on hemodialysis at December 31 of any year are computed from this data file. A subsection of the patient questionnaire is allocated for patients who were on hemodialysis (HD) or hemofiltration (HF) at any time during the year of report and since 1973 has asked:

1. How many times per week was this patient treated with HD or HF?
2. How many hours per week was this patient treated with HD or HF?
3. Which type of hemodialyzer or hemofilter was most frequently used for this patient?

Until 1976 we asked whether the patient was dialyzed at night, evening, or daytime. The body weight of all patients has been requested since 1976.

This chapter reports analyses based on these data, tracing the evolution of hemodialysis strategies in Europe to the pattern of the present practice. The effect of different groups of dialyzers and of the patients' weight on choice of dialysis frequency and duration is described, and variation between the practice in different countries is documented. We have therefore concentrated on a factual description of the demography of hemodialysis strategies. Massive Registry data provide a secure basis for such reporting.

However, comparison of the results achieved by different dialysis strategies cannot be built on such a data base. Years ago, we published comparison of survival in patients treated twice weekly with those treated 3 times weekly [3] but now regard this as misleading because of unknown factors which may have biased selection of patients for different strategies and which

*Vincenzo Cambi (editor) Professor of Nephrology*
© *1987 Martinus Nijhoff Publishing, Boston. ISBN 0-89838-858-9. Printed in The United States.*

may have a beneficial or adverse effect on survival. We have developed a possible approach to this problem by the retrospective selection of matched controls [4], but this should not be regarded as a satisfactory substitute for prospective randomization. A randomized controlled trial is the proper instrument for obtaining an answer to questions comparing the efficacy of different methods of treatment.

**Evolution of Dialysis Strategies**

The duration of dialysis has become progressively shorter since the earliest years for which data are available. Shortening of total weekly dialysis hours has been accompanied by the widespread adoption of thrice weekly dialysis. One of the earliest changes was phasing out of overnight hemodialysis used for the very lengthy schedules which characterized maintenance hemodialysis in the early 1970s. The most important factor in reducing dialysis hours was the introduction of the arteriovenous fistula [5] which brought with it pumped hemodialysis and thus ensured good blood flows throughout the period of treatment. The manufacture of reliably efficient dialyzers, commercial interests, and reimbursement arrangements probably also accelerated this evolution which found its theoretical justification in the square meter-hour hypothesis [6]. The period of most rapid change in practice was 1974–1978.

*Time of dialysis*

Comparison of the returns for the last four years over which the Registry collected information on timing of hemodialysis [7] showed that overnight dialysis was steadily decreasing in hospitals and, although there was a slight increase in proportions treated during the evening (finishing before midnight), over three-quarters of European hospital hemodialysis patients were treated in the daytime by 1976. Evening and overnight hemodialysis lingered on for an ever-dwindling proportion of patients in Israel, the United Kingdom, Spain, the Netherlands, and France. Among the smaller number of patients treated in the home, evening hemodialysis was becoming increasingly popular at the expense of overnight schedules (figure 3–1).

*Frequency of dialysis*

As early as 1973, over 80% of home dialysis patients had thrice weekly hemodialysis. Patients dialyzed in hospitals had a greater likelihood of twice weekly dialysis, little over 30% of them receiving treatment 3 times a week. However, the difference between hospital and home practice narrowed rapidly over the next few years, and by 1976, two-thirds of hospital patients had thrice weekly dialysis [8]. This trend has continued up until the most recent data (see below).

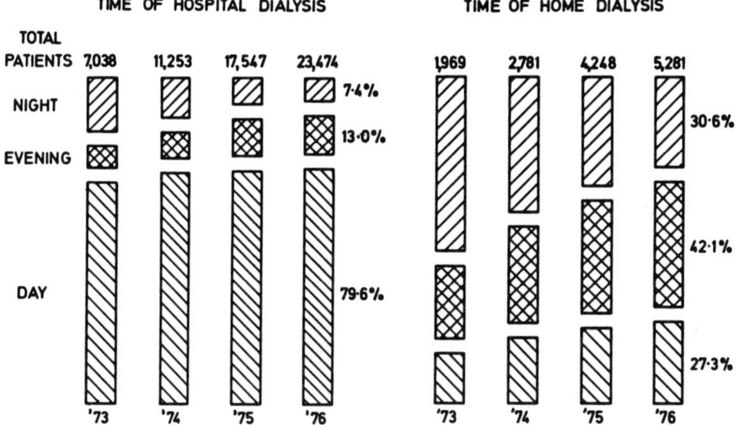


*Figure 3–1.* Analysis of the timing of hospital and home hemodialysis in Europe, 1973–76, showing the percentages of patients treated overnight, in the evening, and by day.

## Duration of dialysis

In 1973, 39% of hospital hemodialysis patients were dialyzed for between 18 and 23 hours per week, and 21% spent more than 23 hours on treatment. Among patients treated at home, these proportions were 27% and 62%, respectively [9]. By 1976, only 9% of hospital patients received 19 hours or more dialysis each week, although 44% of home-treated patients were still on these long schedules [8]. In 1976 the most popular duration was between 14 and 18 hours per week for both hospital (61% of patients) and home (42% of patients). Three years later, the greatest proportion of patients was on 12–13 hours per week [10], suggesting that 3 4-hour dialyses had become the norm in many centers.

## Choice of hemodialyzer

The period of 1975–1984 has witnessed the virtual abandonment of the Kiil type of dialyzer, the beginning in decline of disposable parallel flow dialyser, progressive erosion of the market held by coil dialyzers, and the burgeoning success of capillary (hollow fiber) dialyzers (figure 3–2). In 1984, capillary dialyzers were reported as the type most frequently used for over two-thirds of all hemodialysis patients. Since the performances of the 4 groups of dialyzers are comparable, it seems likely that these changes owe more to convenience in usage and to economic reasons than to any search for higher efficiency in order to minimize the duration of dialysis.

We noted in 1976 that although the number of weekly hours of dialysis was influenced by the surface area of the dialyzer used, the proportion of patients dialyzed for 10–13 hours had increased for all groups of dialyzers [8]. In 1979

35

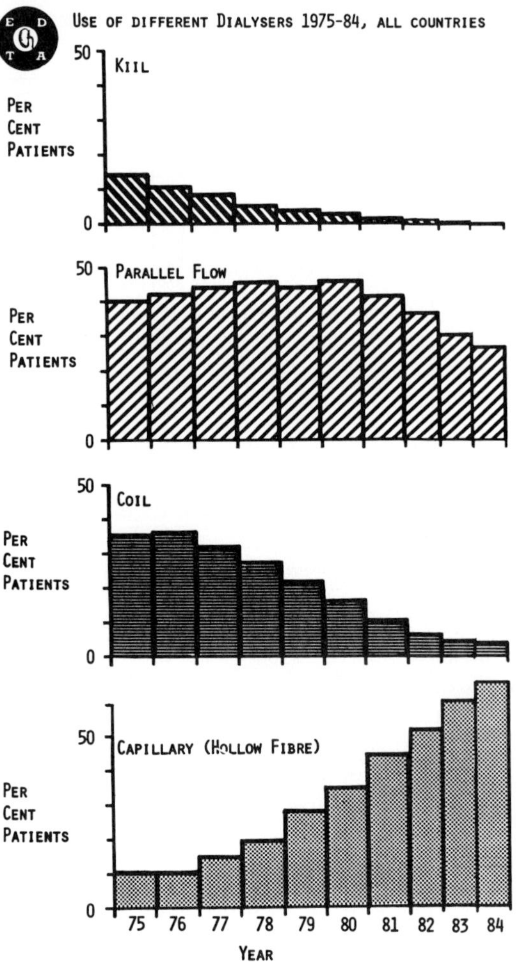


*Figure 3–2.* Proportions of patients for whom the four groups of dialyzers were reported as the ones most frequently used in each of the years 1975–84.

[10] the influence of dialyzer surface area on duration of hemodialysis was detectable only among patients on home hemodialysis (figure 3–3). Thus the picture emerges from these pooled data of standard dialysis strategies more likely to dictate the choice of dialyser than to be influenced by it.

*Body weight*

The introduction in 1976 of a question asking the patient's body weight was expected to provide a further dimension of another individual variable likely to modify dialysis strategies. However, the proportions of patients receiving various durations of dialysis per week did not show very striking differences in

36

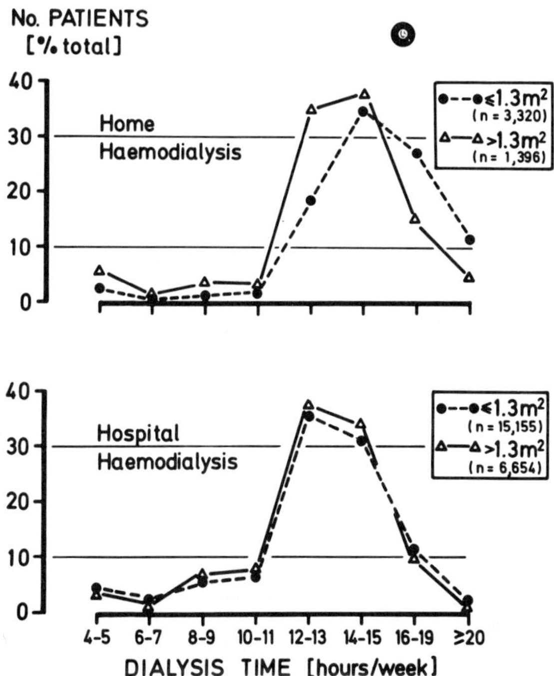



*Figure 3–3.* Distribution of dialysis time schedules in home and hospital hemodialysis patients in relation to dialyzer membrane surface area. Patients were grouped into those using dialyzers with a surface area of ≤ 1.3 m² and those with > 1.3 m².

relation to their body weight. Distributions of patients weighing 50.0–59.9 Kg and those weighing 60.0–69.9 Kg between the various durations of dialysis were very similar. When patients weighing 40.0–49.9 were compared with those weighing 70.0–79.9 Kg, a trend did emerge for the heavier patients to be given more dialysis [8].

When narrower time brackets were used to dissect the dialysis schedules in 1977, a relationship between body weight and dialysis time was demonstrated when extremes of weight were compared, 1–39 Kg versus 90–129 Kg. Thus 38.5% of the lighter patients received 12–13 hours but only 18.9% of the heavier.

Analysis of dialysis time using dialysers of surface area ≤ 1.3 m² against body weight was performed on 1979 data (figure 3–4). We had expected to find that the proportions of high weight patients would be larger on the long dialysis schedules and that there would be relatively large percentages of low weight patients on short time schedules. However, as figure 3–4 shows, dialysis time was barely adjusted in accordance with body weight. Differences which we had found in 1977 were no longer predictable. Furthermore, only 267 out of 872 patients who weighed over 80 Kg were treated with large surface area dialyzers [10].

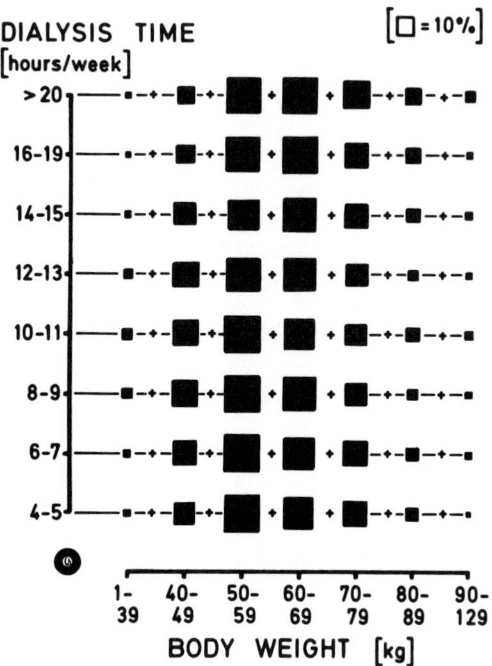


*Figure 3–4.* Percentage of 11,872 hospital hemodialysis patients treated on different time schedules with a dialyzer surface area of ≤ 1.3 m² in relation to body weight. The number of patients treated with the same time schedule is defined as 100%, and the proportions of patients in the different weight groups are illustrated by squares: the larger the square, the higher the percentage of patients.

## *Residual renal function*

A survey was conducted in 1980 to find out what proportion of centers routinely monitored residual renal function [11]. Measurement was carried out for all patients in 70% of 299 hospital hemodialysis centers and the most popular methods were determination of urinary volume (82% of centers) and creatinine clearance using the day before dialysis (58%) or whole interdialytic period (30%).

Analysis of dialysis time schedules in relation to residual urinary volume (recorded on the individual patient questionnaire for one year only) was performed on 1979 data (figure 3–5). The percentage of patients with a urine volume over 1,000 ml was found to be higher among patients on short dialysis times, whereas in anephric patients there was an opposite tendency. The mean increase in dialysis time in anuric patients compared to those with a high urine output was just over 2 hours per week [10]. If dialysis schedules are modified in the light of residual renal function then it is necessary to monitor the patient's renal function because this shows a tendency to diminish progressively in prolonged RRT (figure 3–6).

38

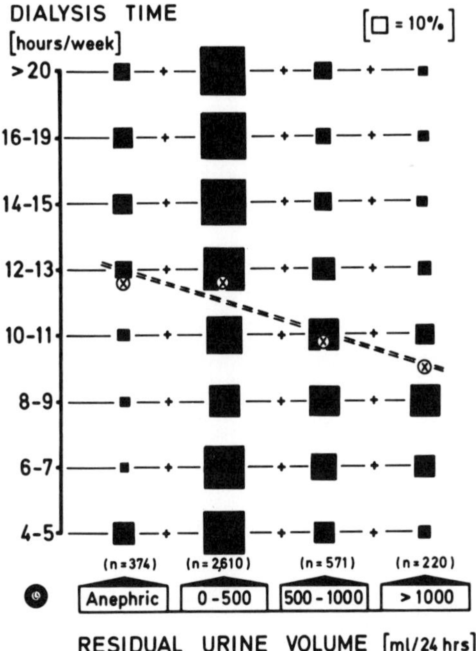


*Figure 3–5.* Dialysis time per week in relation to residual urine volume. The number of patients treated on the same dialysis time schedule is defined as 100%, and the proportion of patients and the different categories of residual daily urine volume are illustrated by the size of the squares.

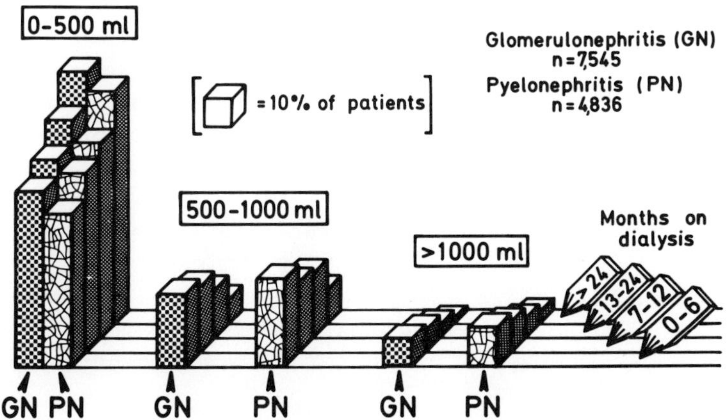


*Figure 3–6.* Residual daily urine volume in relation to time on dialysis in patients whose renal diagnosis was glomerulonephritis or pyelonephritis.

## Dialysis strategies in 1984

*Average European Schedules*

In each of the tables and figures in this section the proportional distribution of patients according to their duration of dialysis in 1984 is divided as follows: 1–9 hours, 10–13 hours, 14–18 hours, 19–24 hours, and 25 or more hours of hemodialysis per week.

The first table shows the relationship between frequency and duration of hospital hemodialysis (table 3–1), and figure 3–7 illustrates the proportional distribution of hemodialysis per week in those treated 2 times and 3 times per week, both on hospital and home hemodialysis. In 1984, 85% of hospital hemodialysis was given on a 3 times schedule with 65% of patients receiving a total of 10–13 hours, indicating that 3 dialyses of 4 hours each appears to be the standard treatment regimen in the majority of European centers. If this is considered to represent short dialysis then we must conclude that short dialysis is far from the exceptional prescription for a minority of patients; it is now the norm in Europe.

Those dialyzed 3 times per week mostly received between 10 and 16 hours per week, and those dialyzed 2 times per week mostly received between 7 and 13 hours. For many patients, twice weekly schedule consists of 2 sessions of 4 hours, since 44% of those in this strategy received 1–9 hours of treatment. It thus appears that in many centers work routines have been constructed around 4-hour sessions of hemodialysis, and that when a reduction in weekly dialysis is considered reasonable, then the frequency of treatment is reduced from 3 times to 2 times per week. A small number of patients had only one hemodialysis per week, and it is thought that a proportion of these patients were on peritoneal dialysis as background therapy since this is known to be combined with occasional hemodialysis for a small proportion of patients, of whom there were 131 reported in 1984 [2], mostly large men for whom CAPD regimens provide inadequate treatment. A similar small number of patients received four hemodialyses per week and 58% of these received between 14–18 hours treatment, again suggesting that treatment sessions consisting of 4 hours of hemodialysis were considered the most convenient.

*Table 3–1.* Proportional distribution of patients according to hours of hemodialysis per week and according to frequency of hospital hemodialysis: data for total Registry for 1984

| Dialyses per Week | Patients (N) | Hours Hosp. HD per Week (% Patients) | | | | |
|---|---|---|---|---|---|---|
| | | 1–9 | 10–13 | 14–18 | 19–24 | 25+ |
| 1 | 556 | 96.4 | 2.2 | 0.4 | 0.5 | 0.5 |
| 2 | 8,629 | 43.6 | 45.5 | 10.3 | 0.6 | <0.1 |
| 3 | 58,210 | 8.0 | 64.9 | 26.6 | 0.5 | 0.1 |
| 4 | 689 | 2.6 | 33.2 | 58.2 | 5.8 | 0.1 |

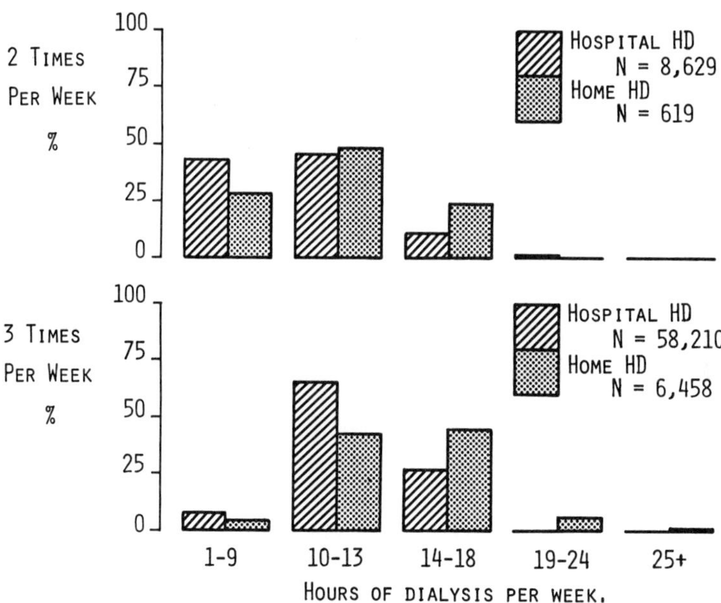


*Figure 3–7.* Proportional distribution of patients according to hours of hemodialysis per week in hospital and home hemodialysis, total Registry 1984.

The length of treatment sessions is not so constrained at home, and it is notable that greater proportions of home patients received longer durations than in hospital hemodialysis (figure 3–7). Schedules were influenced by the main groups of dialyzers (table 3–2). The dwindling number of patients treated on nondisposable parallel flow dialyzers (Kiil type) had a high proportion (80%) who received 19 or more hours per week. Coil dialyzers were also associated with selection of longer dialysis hours, 59% of patients on coils receiving between 14 and 18 hours of treatment. The proportional distribution of patients according to dialysis hours was remarkably similar for disposable parallel flow and capillary dialyzers, with 64% receiving 10–13 hours and 27% receiving 14–18 hours in each group. Hemofilters also had

*Table 3–2.* Proportional distribution of patients according to hours of hemodialysis per week in patients dialyzed 3 times per week according to group of dialyzer, 1984

| Dialyser Group | Patients (N) | Hours Hemodialysis/Week (% Pats.) | | | | |
|---|---|---|---|---|---|---|
| | | 1–9 | 10–13 | 14–18 | 19–24 | 25+ |
| Nondisposable parallel flow | 302 | 0.3 | 5.3 | 14.6 | 72.5 | 7.3 |
| Disposable parallel flow | 17,125 | 6.6 | 64.3 | 27.2 | 1.6 | 0.4 |
| Coil | 1,676 | 4.7 | 35.4 | 59.1 | 0.8 | 0.1 |
| Hollow fiber — Capillary | 42,359 | 8.0 | 63.8 | 27.7 | 0.3 | 0.1 |
| Hemofilters | 1,411 | 16.1 | 64.3 | 19.1 | 0.4 | 0.1 |

41

64% of patients treated for 10–13 hours but a higher proportion (16%) treated for 1–9 hours than was found for any other of the groups of dialyzers.

*Schedules in individual countries*

Hemodialysis programs are stamped with distinctive national characteristics. For the first time, we are publishing a full breakdown of the proportional distribution of patients according to the number of hours of hospital hemodialysis per week in each of the individual countries reporting to the EDTA Registry (table 3–3). The size of reported hospital hemodialysis programs varies from over 15,000 patients in the Federal Republic of Germany to a mere handful of patients in Lebanon. It is apparent that the pattern of practice in the large Western European countries, Belgium, the Federal Republic of Germany, France, Italy, Spain, and the United Kingdom has a strong impact on the average European schedules reported above. This pattern is reinforced by practice in Scandinavian countries and in Switzerland. Larger numbers of patients were treated 2 times rather than 3 times in Czechoslovakia, Egypt, the Netherlands, and Turkey. In Eastern European countries where coil dialyzers are employed to a considerable extent, schedules are longer, and in Czechoslovakia, Hungary, and Poland (and also in Lebanon) over 70% of thrice weekly dialyzed patients received 14–18 hours of treatment. Yugoslavia and the Democratic Republic of Germany had intermediate patterns of dialysis schedules.

Home hemodialysis is no longer practiced widely in Europe, and so we have included only the five largest Western European countries in table 3–4 which shows the same proportional distribution of dialysis schedules among patients dialyzed at home even in 1984. The longer schedules available at home are displayed and in both the Federal Republic of Germany (FRG) and the United Kingdom (UK), 70% of patients on thrice weekly home hemodialysis received 14 or more hours per week.

Five large Western European countries — France, FRG, Italy, Spain, and the UK — have sufficient numbers of patients to make it possible to assess the effects of patients' weight on choice of HD schedules. Firstly, we note that the distribution of patients' weights is remarkably similar in these countries (table 3–5) and therefore the populations are comparable with respect to weight. The analysis presented in table 3–5 includes patients on treatment in 1984 but excludes those who started treatment in 1984 in order to discard patients whose weight was suboptimal because of illness prior to commencement of RRT. Secondly, selection of dialyzers is not the same in these five countries (figure 3–8). Hollow fiber dialyzers predominated, being used for over 70% of patients in France, FRG, and Spain; in Italy 53% and in UK 42% of patients used disposable parallel flow dialyzers; nondisposable parallel flow dialyzers (Kiil type) have almost disappeared, but France reported 2.5% and UK 2% of patients using this type of dialyzer.

Table 3–6 shows the effect of weight on choice of 2 times versus 3 times

42

*Table 3–3.* Proportional distribution of patients according to total and average hours of hospital hemodialysis per week in 2 and 3 times treatment according to country, 1984

| Country | 2 Times per Week | | | | | | 3 Times per Week | | | | | |
| --- | --- | --- | --- | --- | --- | --- | --- | --- | --- | --- | --- | --- |
| | | Hours Hospital HD/Week (% pats) | | | | Av. hrs./ week | | Hours Hospital HD/Week (% pats) | | | | Av. hrs./ Week |
| | N | 1–9 | 10–13 | 14–18 | 19+ | | N | 1–9 | 10–13 | 14–18 | 19+ | |
| Algeria | 12 | 8 | 50 | 42 | 0 | 10 | 61 | 5 | 82 | 13 | 0 | 11 |
| Austria | 169 | 70 | 12 | 18 | 0 | 8 | 1,200 | 14 | 57 | 29 | <1 | 11 |
| Belgium | 147 | 83 | 6 | 11 | 0 | 7 | 2,117 | 16 | 76 | 8 | <1 | 11 |
| Bulgaria | 205 | 57 | 43 | 0 | 0 | 8 | 582 | 2 | 86 | 12 | 0 | 11 |
| Cyprus | 50 | 100 | 0 | 0 | 0 | 7 | 58 | 3 | 95 | 2 | 0 | 11 |
| Czechoslovakia | 606 | 6 | 45 | 48 | 0 | 12 | 315 | 10 | 15 | 75 | 1 | 14 |
| Denmark | 109 | 79 | 20 | 1 | 0 | 7 | 303 | 32 | 61 | 7 | <1 | 10 |
| Egypt | 726 | 15 | 85 | 0 | 0 | 10 | 140 | 1 | 74 | 25 | 0 | 12 |
| Fed. Rep. Germany | 609 | 79 | 18 | 2 | <1 | 7 | 14,386 | 11 | 49 | 40 | <1 | 12 |
| Finland | 40 | 75 | 25 | 0 | 0 | 8 | 289 | 2 | 88 | 11 | 0 | 11 |
| France | 1,328 | 38 | 37 | 21 | 4 | 10 | 7,873 | 8 | 63 | 25 | 3 | 12 |
| German Dem. Rep. | 191 | 54 | 46 | 0 | 0 | 8 | 1,454 | 5 | 55 | 40 | <1 | 12 |
| Greece | 96 | 68 | 32 | 0 | 0 | 8 | 1,129 | 2 | 79 | 19 | 0 | 11 |
| Hungary | 84 | 5 | 94 | 1 | 0 | 9 | 309 | <1 | 27 | 72 | 0 | 13 |
| Iceland | 6 | 0 | 17 | 83 | 0 | 13 | 16 | 6 | 94 | 0 | 0 | 10 |
| Ireland | 22 | 5 | 95 | 0 | 0 | 9 | 187 | 0 | 57 | 43 | 0 | 12 |
| Israel | 102 | 65 | 35 | 0 | 0 | 8 | 798 | 11 | 79 | 10 | 0 | 11 |
| Italy | 404 | 81 | 10 | 9 | 0 | 8 | 10,616 | 6 | 82 | 12 | <1 | 11 |
| Lebanon | 2 | 0 | 50 | 50 | 0 | 14 | 9 | 0 | 22 | 78 | 0 | 16 |
| Libya | 25 | 16 | 84 | 0 | 0 | 9 | 26 | 4 | 46 | 50 | 0 | 12 |
| Luxembourg | 6 | 50 | 50 | 0 | 0 | 8 | 90 | 2 | 80 | 18 | 0 | 11 |
| Netherlands | 1,134 | 33 | 64 | 3 | 0 | 9 | 570 | 11 | 74 | 14 | <1 | 11 |
| Norway | 91 | 82 | 18 | 0 | 0 | 7 | 245 | 46 | 159 | 40 | 0 | 11 |
| Poland | 148 | 10 | 78 | 11 | 0 | 11 | 820 | 1 | 11 | 87 | 1 | 15 |
| Portugal | 64 | 95 | 5 | 0 | 0 | 7 | 1,438 | 2 | 86 | 12 | 0 | 11 |
| Spain | 182 | 66 | 26 | 8 | 0 | 8 | 7,919 | 4 | 79 | 16 | <1 | 11 |
| Sweden | 181 | 71 | 26 | 3 | 0 | 9 | 521 | 17 | 73 | 9 | <1 | 10 |
| Switzerland | 358 | 72 | 27 | <1 | 0 | 7 | 575 | 29 | 55 | 16 | <1 | 10 |
| Tunisia | 41 | 49 | 51 | 0 | 0 | 8 | 177 | 3 | 81 | 16 | 0 | 11 |
| Turkey | 230 | 54 | 39 | 7 | 0 | 9 | 189 | 2 | 66 | 32 | 0 | 13 |
| United Kingdom | 705 | 31 | 52 | 17 | 0 | 10 | 1,544 | 8 | 50 | 39 | 3 | 13 |
| Yugoslavia | 556 | 22 | 76 | 1 | 0 | 9 | 2,227 | 5 | 45 | 50 | <1 | 12 |

*Table 3–4.* Proportional distribution of patients according to total and average hours of home hemodialysis per week and average hours per week in 2 times and 3 times treatment in 5 large western European countries, 1984

| Country | 2 Times per Week | | | | | | 3 Times per Week | | | | | |
| --- | --- | --- | --- | --- | --- | --- | --- | --- | --- | --- | --- | --- |
| | | Hours Home HD/Week (% pats) | | | | Av. Hours/ Week | | Hours Home HD/Week (% pats) | | | | Av. Hours/ Week |
| | N | 1–9 | 10–13 | 14–18 | 19+ | | N | 1–9 | 10–13 | 14–18 | 19+ | |
| France | 100 | 34 | 46 | 18 | 2 | 10 | 1,674 | 7 | 46 | 32 | 15 | 13 |
| Fed. Rep. Germany | 15 | 60 | 33 | 7 | 0 | 8 | 1,547 | 7 | 24 | 65 | 5 | 13 |
| Italy | 18 | 89 | 6 | 6 | 0 | 7 | 780 | 2 | 73 | 25 | 0 | 12 |
| Spain | 9 | 56 | 44 | 0 | 0 | 9 | 341 | 1 | 74 | 25 | 0 | 12 |
| United Kingdom | 378 | 16 | 49 | 34 | 1 | 11 | 1,523 | 2 | 29 | 60 | 9 | 15 |

*Table 3–5.* Distribution of the weight of patients on hemodialysis in 1984 who started treatment before 1984 in 5 large western European countries

| Country | Patients (N) | Weight of Patients (Kg) | | | | | | | | | |
| --- | --- | --- | --- | --- | --- | --- | --- | --- | --- | --- | --- |
| | | <20 | 20–29 | 30–39 | 40–49 | 50–59 | 60–69 | 70–79 | 80–89 | 90–99 | 100+ |
| France | 8,446 | 0.5 | 0.8 | 3.0 | 16.0 | 31.8 | 28.0 | 14.0 | 4.3 | 1.2 | 0.5 |
| Fed. Rep. Germany | 11,795 | <0.1 | 0.2 | 1.3 | 10.3 | 28.0 | 31.2 | 19.9 | 6.9 | 1.6 | 0.6 |
| Italy | 9,881 | 0.1 | 0.3 | 2.0 | 14.6 | 31.5 | 31.3 | 14.2 | 4.4 | 1.0 | 0.6 |
| Spain | 6,629 | 0.3 | 0.6 | 1.5 | 12.7 | 30.8 | 32.6 | 15.5 | 4.7 | 0.9 | 0.3 |
| United Kingdom | 2,614 | 0.1 | 0.7 | 2.0 | 11.7 | 25.2 | 28.4 | 20.6 | 7.8 | 2.6 | 0.9 |

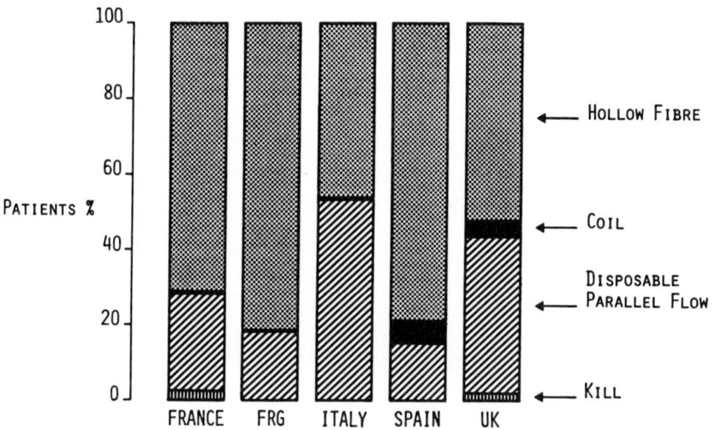


*Figure 3–8.* Selection of hemodialyzers in 5 large western European countries. Proportions are based on reports of dialyzer most frequently used for each patient in 1984.

hemodialysis strategies and figure 3–9 shows the influence of weight on weekly duration of hemodialysis in the five countries. Hospital and home hemodialysis patients have been included in both these analyses. Lighter patients (1–49 Kg) were slightly more likely to be treated twice weekly, and heavier patients (70 Kg and over) were more likely to be treated thrice weekly. Thus, in France, 13.4% of lighter patients had two dialyses per week, whereas only 8.2% of heavier ones had two dialyses per week; in FRG, these proportions were 4.1% and 1.7%, respectively (table 3–6). These adjustments were not so pronounced in the other countries. There were more marked international differences in the use of 2 times versus 3 times dialysis with 2 times dialysis offered to a very small proportion of Spanish and Italian patients, whereas one-quarter of British patients had twice weekly treatment.

International differences are again the most striking feature of analysis of the influence of weight on length of dialysis (figure 3–9). Among the small number of patients on twice weekly hemodialysis (upper panel) those in FRG, Italy, and Spain appear most likely to receive two 4-hour treatments. In France and the UK, a greater proportion were treated for 10–13 and 14–18 hours, suggesting that their two sessions might last between 5 and 9 hours each. When the patients weighing 40–49.9 Kg were compared with those weighing 70–79.9 Kg, it appears that adjustment for weight occurred more often in France and UK and to a lesser extent in the very small number of patients dialyzed twice weekly in Spain. Among the larger number of patients on thrice weekly hemodialysis (lower panel), the most frequent routine appears to be three 4-hour sessions, especially in Italy and Spain, and to a lesser extent in France. In FRG and UK, a greater proportion of patients were not on short dialysis and received upwards of 14 hours per week. Also, in these two countries, schedules were more frequently adjusted in the light of

*Table 3–6.* Proportions of patients dialyzed 2 times and 3 times per week according to weight in 5 large western European countries

| Country | Weight (Kg) | N | Dialyses per Week 2 Times (%) | 3 Times (%) |
|---|---|---|---|---|
| France | 1–49 | 1,703 | 13.4 | 86.1 |
| | 50–69 | 5,056 | 12.4 | 87.2 |
| | 70+ | 1,687 | 8.2 | 91.2 |
| Fed. Rep. Germany | 1–49 | 1,400 | 4.1 | 94.0 |
| | 50–69 | 6,976 | 2.8 | 97.1 |
| | 70+ | 3,419 | 1.7 | 94.9 |
| Italy | 1–49 | 1,684 | 3.7 | 93.0 |
| | 50–69 | 6,201 | 2.8 | 94.7 |
| | 70+ | 1,996 | 2.5 | 94.0 |
| Spain | 1–49 | 1,008 | 1.9 | 97.1 |
| | 50–69 | 4,204 | 1.9 | 97.4 |
| | 70+ | 1,417 | 1.4 | 98.0 |
| United Kingdom | 1–49 | 377 | 23.6 | 74.3 |
| | 50–69 | 1,402 | 27.1 | 71.5 |
| | 70+ | 835 | 22.4 | 77.5 |

Percentages add up to less than 100% because of the small numbers of patients dialyzed for frequencies less or more than 2 or 3 times per week.

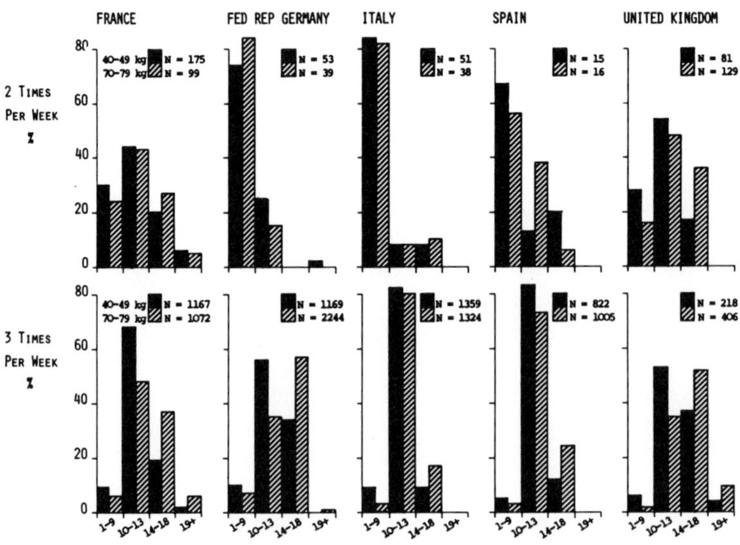


*Figure 3–9.* Proportional distribution of patients according to weekly duration of hemodialysis (hospital and home) in 5 European countries. Patients who weighed 40–49.9 Kg are compared with those who weighed 70–79.9 Kg and the numbers of patients in each of these cohorts is shown in each panel. Upper row of panels is patients dialyzed 2 times, and lower row, those dialyzed 3 times per week.

46

the patients' weight, distribution of heavier (70–79.9 Kg) patients being shifted to the right in comparison to lighter (40–49.9 Kg) patients, so that the most frequently used strategy for the heavier patients lay in the range 14–18 hours compared to 10–13 hours for the lighter patients. In the other three countries, 10–13 hours was the most popular strategy for patients of both weight ranges.

## Conclusions

Hemodialysis strategies in Europe have progressively shortened since the early 1970s. In 1984, the majority of patients were on thrice weekly hemodialysis mostly using between 10 and 16 hours of hemodialysis in each week. It appears that 4-hour sessions are found most convenient and that if the physician wishes to reduce dialysis hours, he may use twice weekly dialysis rather than adjusting the length of each treatment.

Changing choice of dialyzers has resulted in the virtual disappearance of Kiil type dialyzers and the eclipse of coil dialyzers. In their place, disposable parallel flow dialyzers and, especially in recent years, hollow fiber dialyzers, have helped toward the adoption of shorter dialysis schedules. In those countries still using coil dialyzers to any extent, schedules are longer, and longer dialysis was also used for patients on home treatment where they are not constrained by the needs of other patients and by economic factors.

International comparisons show differences in hemodialysis schedules which are only subject to slight modification in the light of patients' weights. The differences in schedules are not accounted for by the patient populations having any difference in weight distribution. In the absence of any scientific rationale for the choice of different lengths of dialysis, we can only attribute these observations to national fashions.

Commercial interests, reimbursement protocols, and staffing convenience have probably all played a part in reaching the present profile of hemodialysis which is dominated by 4 hourly treatment sessions. Since the reasons for choice of different dialysis schedules are obscure, selection of patients for the different strategies is likely to include unrecognized confounding factors which would invalidate any comparison of results achieved, for instance by evaluation of patient survival or level of rehabilitation. Therefore, we have not made any attempt to use the EDTA Registry data base to engineer any such comparison.

## Acknowledgements

Figures 3–3 through 3–6 have previously been published in the Proceedings of EDTA-ERA, and the permission of the editor to use them again is acknowledged.

The work of the Registry was supported by grants from the governments or national societies of nephrology of Austria, Belgium, Bulgaria, Cyprus, Czechoslovakia, Denmark, Egypt, the Federal Republic of Germany, France, the Germany Democratic Republic, Greece, Iceland, Ireland, Israel, Luxembourg, the Netherlands, Norway, Sweden, Switzerland, and the United Kingdom.

Grants were also made by Asahi Medical GmbH, B. Braun Melsungen AG, Bellco S.p.A., Cobe Laboratories, Inc., CD Medical International, Ltd., Enka AG, Fresenius AG, Gambro AB, Hospal Ltd., Sorin Biomedica S.p.A., and Travenol Laboratories Ltd.

We acknowledge the cooperation of UK Transplant Service, Bristol, United Kingdom.

We thank those doctors and their staff who have completed questionnaires Without their collaboration, this chapter could not have been prepared.

## References


1. Brunner, F.P., Gurland, H.J., Harlen, H., Scharer, Kaud Parsons, F.M. (1972) Combined report on regular dialysis and transplantation in Europe, II, 1971. Proc. EDTA IX: 3–34.
2. Brunner, F.P., Broyer, M., Brynger H., Challah, S., Fassbinder, W., Oules, R., Rizzoni, G., Selwood, N.H. and Wing, A.J. (1985) Combined report on regular dialysis and transplantation in Europe, XV. Proc. EDTA-ERA 22: 3–53.
3. Brunner, F.P., Brynger, H., Chantler, C., Donckerwolcke, R.A., Hathway, R.A., Jacobs, C., Selwood, N.H. and Wing, A.J. (1979) Combined report on regular dialysis and transplantation in Europe, IX. Proc. EDTA 16: 2–73.
4. Kramer, P., Broyer, M., Brunner, F.P., Brynger, H., Challah, S., Oules, R., Rizzoni, G., Selwood, N.H., Wing, A.J. and Balas, E.A. (1984) Combined report on regular dialysis and transplantation in Europe, XIV. Proc. EDTA-ERA 21: 2–65.
5. Brescia, M.J., Cimino, J.E., Appel, K. and Hurwich, B.J. (1966) Chronic haemodialysis using venipuncture and a surgically created arteriovenous fistula. N. Engl. J. Med. 275: 1089.
6. Babb, A.L., Popovich, R.P. Christopher, T.G. and Scribner, B.H. (1971) The genesis of the square meter — hour hypothesis. Trans. Am. Soc. Artif. Intern. Organs 17: 81.
7. Wing, A.J., Brunner, F.P., Brynger, H., Chantler, C., Donckerwolcke, R.A., Gurland, H.J., Jacobs, C. and Selwood, N.H. (1978) Dialysis strategies and techniques in Europe and the United Kingdom. In *Dialysis Review*, A.M. Davison (ed.). Pitman Medical, pp. 59–71.
8. Jacobs, C., Brunner, F P., Chantler, C., Donckerwolcke, R.A., Gurland, H.J., Hathway, R.A., Selwood, N.H. and Wing, A.J. (1977) Combined report on regular dialysis and transplantation in Europe, VII. Proc. EDTA 14: 3–69.
9. Brunner, F.P., Giesecke, B., Gurland, H.J., Jacobs, C., Parsons, F.M., Scharer, K., Seyffart, G., Spies, G. and Wing, A.J. (1975) Combined report on regular dialysis and transplantation in Europe, V. Proc. EDTA 12: 3–64.
10. Brynger, H., Brunner, F. P., Chantler, C., Broyer, M., Brunner, F.P., Brynger, H., Jacobs, C., Kramer, P., Selwood, N.H. and Wing, A.J. (1980) Combined report on regular dialysis and transplantation in Europe, X. Proc. EDTA 17: 2–86.
11. Broyer, M., Brunner, F. P., Brynger, H., Donckerwolcke, R.A., Jacobs, C., Kramer, P., Selwood, N.H. and Wing, A.J. (1982) Combined report on regular dialysis and transplantation in Europe, XII. Proc. EDTA 19; 2–59.

# 4. Middle molecule hypothesis and short dialysis

Carlo Buzio and Roberta Barani

Uremia is characterized by the retention of numerous substances normally metabolized or excreted by the kidneys. Its pathogenesis has thus always been strongly linked to the concept of the toxicity of abnormal or abnormally increased substances.

It was long held that substances of a low molecular weight such as urea, creatinine, uric acid, etc., were responsible for the uremic syndrome, and that their plasma concentrations could express the adequacy of dialysis treatment. However, it was not always possible to correlate the signs and symptoms of uremia with plasma levels of low molecular weight substances in patients in chronic renal failure undergoing both conservative and dialysis treatment. In 1965, Scribner [1] hypothesized that 'large' substances (with a molecular weight > 300 D), inefficiently removed by standard hemodialysis might play an etiopathogenetic role in uremic morbidity and chiefly in peripheral neuropathy. Two clinical observations sustained Scribner's hypothesis: Jebsen and associates [2] reported that the prevention of neuropathy was related more to adequate dialysis time than to urea and creatinine values. Tenckoff and associates [3, 4] reported that patients in peritoneal dialysis did not suffer from peripheral neuropathy despite high serum urea and creatinine values. In 1971, the Seattle group formulated a theory based on the toxicity of substances with a high molecular weight [5]. This theory, called the 'square meter/hour' hypothesis, indicated, among other things, that the surface area of the dialyzer and dialysis time played a more important role than the rate of blood and dialysate flow in removing molecules with a high molecular weight. It furnished a logical, though theoretical, explanation for the reported clinical observations. The square meter/hour hypothesis attributed the absence of peripheral neuropathy to the greater removal of high molecular weight molecules, brought about by the larger dialysis surface for patients in peritoneal dialysis and by the longer dialysis time for patients in hemodialysis. In 1972, the same group modified the previous hypothesis and called it the 'middle molecule hypothesis' [6]. The middle molecule hypothesis contended that substances with a molecular weight between 300 and 1,500–2,000 D (the so-called middle molecules or 'MM') were responsible for the uremic syndrome.

*Vincenzo Cambi (editor) Professor of Nephrology*
© *1987 Martinus Nijhoff Publishing, Boston. ISBN 0-89838-858-9. Printed in The United States.*

The presence of these substances, their accumulation in the blood of uremic patients, and finally their toxicity had to be demonstrated in order to confirm this hypothesis. Numerous chromatographic techniques were utilized to separate and isolate the MM. Numerous in vitro tests were carried out to establish if and what biological activity these substances were involved in. New dialysis strategies were applied, and new dialysis membranes were manufactured to evaluate clinically the effects of the variations in MM plasma concentrations of patients in hemodialysis treatment.


**Biological and clinical aspects of the middle molecules**


Chromatographic studies have demonstrated with certainty that substances with molecular weight (mw) between 300 and 1500 are accumulated in the serum of uremic patients. The peaks corresponding to the MM become evident only when creatinine clearance is less than 11 ml/m' [7, 8] or 15 ml/m' [9]. Renal failure can cause increased serum levels either by decreasing urinary excretion or renal catabolism or by increasing the production of MM. It is also possible that renal failure stimulates the synthesis of substances not present in normal subjects, though proof is lacking. However, not all MM are specific to uremia: there is an increased MM serum concentration in patients affected by psoriasis, hepatic coma, malnutrition, or burns in the absence of renal failure [10–13].

MM intracellular synthesis has been demonstrated: various tissues — muscle, liver, kidney, and brain — incubated in vitro release MM in the culture medium. However, the MM produced by the various tissues are perceptibly different [14]; it thus seems evident that each tissue produces its own characteristic MM. MM have also been isolated in urine, erythrocytes, and cerebrospinal fluid as well as in plasma and serum. Erythrocytes seem to have a higher MM concentration than plasma [15, 16] and are considered as MM transporters [14, 16]. Urinary and serum MM are apparently similar in the same subject, and urinary MM concentrations are correlated to serum concentrations [7, 15, 17–21]. Urinary excretion of MM varies greatly from subject to subject; thus, if we assume that excretion rate equals generation rate, we can deduce that MM production varies from one subject to another [7, 8, 17].

In order to evaluate renal control of MM serum concentrations, the clearances of different MM fractions were correlated to inulin or creatinine clearance. Some authors [7, 8] have demonstrated that MM are not reabsorbed by the tubules but are actively secreted by them. Other authors [20, 22–24] instead contend that numerous MM are secreted, then also reabsorbed and presumably catabolized by the tubular cells.

Numerous techniques are used to separate and isolate MM, and almost every research group has developed its own separation techniques [25–40]. Difficulties in comparing results have been the chief cause of slow progress in

50

our understanding of the clinical significance of MM. The use of deproteinization membranes with different cut-offs, or with the same cut-off but with different ultrafiltration techniques, modifies MM recovery both quantitatively and qualitatively. Different columns, different buffers, and recordings at different wave lengths makes comparison difficult. It is thus often impossible to establish whether apparently corresponding fractions isolated by different laboratories contain the same substances or not. Although serious attempts have been made [41–43] to compare different separation techniques, they have only resulted in confirming that the problem exists. It should also be emphasized that the graphs obtained from the serum of various subjects using the same technique evidences quantitative and qualitative differences from one subject to another [8, 15, 17, 19]. These differences are found between one normal subject and another, as well as between one uremic patient and another even when renal failure is exactly the same. They are attributed to different MM generation rates in different subjects examined [8, 17, 44]. However, there are no studies which evaluate long-term MM modification in the same subject or demonstrate the influence of meals and the hour of MM sampling.

Other factors such as diet and metabolic state can condition individual variations of MM concentrations [45]. The correlations between MM plasma concentrations and urea plasma concentrations [20, 46] as well as dietary protein intake [9, 20, 39, 45–48], and moreover the demonstration that peptides resistant to proteolytic enzymes are formed by dietary proteins [49], attest to the dietetic origin, at least in part, of MM, and emphasize the importance of diet in determining plasma MM concentrations. Accentuated endogenous catabolism such as what is seen in malnourished subjects or burn patients can determine increased MM synthesis [12]. Thus, it could also be possible that MM increases found in complications of uremia are derived from the associated increased catabolism.

There is a statistically significant correlation between some complications of renal failure (vomiting, edema, pericarditis, infections, peripheral neuropathy) and MM [9, 45, 50–52]. The plasma concentration of some MM increases concurrently with the complication and then returns, when the episode is over, to the range of complication-free patients. This correlation is not seen between complications and plasma concentrations of urea and creatinine [9, 45]. Whether or not the increase in MM is the cause or consequence of clinical complications, or simply and epiphenomenon is not known. Moreover, it should be emphasized that independent of the demonstrated correlation between uremic complications and single MM fractions, there is a notable overlap in MM plasma levels between symptom-free and symptomatic patients.

A complicating factor is that numerous drugs have been detected at the same wave length used to identify MM. Some of these — aminophylline, furosemide, beta-blockers, methyldopa, allopurinol, hydralazine, which are often used in chronic renal failure, have elution volumes from Sephadex and ion exchange resin identical to MM-containing fractions [15, 53].

**In vitro toxicity**

Several studies have attempted to identify the in vitro biological activities of substances with mw between 300 and 2,000. MM isolated from the serum, plasma, and urine of uremic patients in conservative and substitutive treatment were tested on different tissue, cell, and enzymatic substrates (table 4–1). These studies conclude that MM could be responsible, wholly or in part, for clinical complications of uremic patients. In vitro toxic effects of the MM, such as inhibition of motor nerve conduction, lymphocyte blastogenesis, hemoglobin synthesis, glucose and triglyceride utilization, platelet aggregation are well correlated to peripheral neuropathy, sensitivity to infection, anemia, glucose intolerence, hypertriglyceridemia, and hemorrhagic diasthesis seen in the uremic patient.

*Immunodeficiency*

Patients in chronic renal failure present a cell-mediated immunodeficiency [108]: skin allograft survival is significantly prolonged [109–111], cutaneous reactions to various antigens are depressed [112–115], the total number of white cells is reduced [114, 116–118], and the serum of uremic patients inhibits or reduces in vitro macrophage migration [112] and lymphocyte proliferation [114, 119–121].

Since uremic lymphocyte reactivity to mitogens or to allogenic cells was normal when cultured in the presence of normal serum [114, 118, 120, 122], it was assumed that substances capable of influencing the normal immune response were present in uremic blood. As shown in table 4–1, numerous authors have performed tests to establish whether or not the immunodeficiency of the uremic subject can be considered an effect of increased MM plasma concentrations. The most common test measures inhibition of thymidine incorporation into lymphocyte DNA induced by different mitogens [12, 34, 44, 61, 63–65, 67, 118]. It is possible to isolate from uremic plasma, serum, urine, and dialysate, factors in the middle-mw range able to inhibit normal lymphocyte reactivity. The MM would not inhibit cell proliferation by directly damaging the cells [59, 63], but would rather strongly inhibit DNA synthesis [34, 59, 63, 64].

It has recently been demonstrated that a heptapeptide isolated in the dialysate and its des-HIS fragment inhibits cell proliferation induced by antigenic viral stimuli, while the heptapeptide fragment alone inhibits lymphocyte response to the Pokewed mitogen [55].

Leukocyte migration in vitro also seems to be inhibited by MM substances [60, 100]. It is supposed that the MM inhibit migration of unseparated leukocytes either by decreasing the electrostatic surface charge or by blocking cell-to-cell transmission of substances involved in migration regulation [60]. In the presence of MM, unseparated white blood cells were shown to adhere to one another, forming cellular clumps [60].

*Table 4–1*. Toxic effects of middle molecules

| Reference | Molecular Weight | Biological Activity In Vitro | In Vivo | Biological Activity Hemodialysis Effect | Middle Molecule Permeability | |
|---|---|---|---|---|---|---|
| Abiko [54] | 860 | Inhibition of E-Rosette formation | | | Dialysable | |
| Rola [55] | 860 | Inhibition of lymphocyte proliferation by Pokeweed<br>Inhibition of lymphocyte citotoxic activity by high concentration<br>Stimulation of lymphocyte citotoxic activity by low concentration | | | | |
| Abiko [56] | 376 | Inhibitory effects on same neurones | | | Dialysable | |
| Abiko [57] | 376 | Inhibition of LDH activity | | | Dialysable | |
| Abiko [58] | 761 | Inhibition of E-Rosette formation | | | Dialysable | |
| Hanicki [59] | 1,500–5,000 | Inhibition of lymphocyte proliferation by PHA<br>Inhibition of unstimulated lymphocyte proliferation | | Decrease | Dialysable | (Cuprophane) |
| Cichoki [60] | 1,200–5,000 | Inhibition of leukocyte migration | | | Dialysable | (Cuprophane) |
| Touraine [61]<br>Gay ]12]<br>Hurst [62] | 1,200 | Inhibition of lymphocyte proliferation by PHA | | Decrease | Dialysable | (Cuprophane) |
| Navarro [63] | ? | Inhibition ot iymphocyte proliferation by allogeneic cells<br>Inhibition of proliferation of tumural (varius tumurous) cells by allogeneic cells) | | No Change | | (Cuprophane) |

*Table 4–1.  (Continued)*

| Reference | Molecular Weight | Biological Activity In Vitro | In Vivo | Biological Activity Hemodialysis Effect | Middle Molecule Permeability |
|---|---|---|---|---|---|
| Navarro [34] Traeger [64] | ? | Inhibition of lymphocyte proliferation by PHA, Pokeweed, Concanavalin A Inhibition of lymphocyte proliferation by allogeneic cells | Inhibition of graft-versus-host reaction in irradiated mice Prolong rejection time of skin allograft in rats No modification antibody production in rats | | |
| Ota [65] | ? | Influence on osmotic fragility of red blood cells Inhibition of lymphocyte proliferation by PHA | | | Dialysable (Polymethylme-thacrylate) |
| Lutz [105] " [49] | 1,200–1,500 | Inhibition of lipoproteinlipase activity | | | Poorly dialysable |
| Milutinovich [106] | ? | Inhibition of insulin binding to erytherocytes | | | |
| Braguer [107] | | Inhibition regeneration of the axon of nerve cells No inhibition of proliferation tumoral and fibroblastic cells | | | Poorly dialysable |
| Delaporte [66] | | Inhibition of proliferation tumoral and fibroblastic cells | | Normalize | |
| Bergström [67] " [44] | 1,000–2,000 | Inhibition of lymphocyte proliferation by PHA Inhibition of lymphocyte proliferation by allogeneic cells | | | |

| | | | | | |
|---|---|---|---|---|---|
| Man [68] | 1,500–1,800 | Toxicity for fibroblastic cells | Decrease | Dialysable | (Polyacrylonitrile) |
| Funck-Brentano [69] | | | | Poorly dialysable | (Cuprophane) |
| | 350–370 | | | | |
| | 250–280 | | | | |
| Man [70] | 1,300–1,500 | Toxicity for fibroblastic cells | | Dialysable | (Polyacrylonitrile) |
| Funk-Brentano [47] | | | | Poorly dialysable | (Cuprophane) |
| Cloix [71] | 1,000–1,500 | Inhibition of adenylate cyclase activity by PTH in bovine renal cortex | | | |
| Man [51] | 1,187 | Inhibition of amplitude response to stimulation of frog sural nerve | Decrease | Dialysable Poor dialysable | (Polyacrylonitrile) (Cuprophane) |
| Funck-Brentano [26] | 1,289 | | | | |
| Le Moel [72] | 300–400 | Inhibition of amplitude response to stimulation of frog sural nerve | | Dialysable | (Polyacrylonitrile) |
| Boudet [73] | | | | | |
| Cueille [18] | 526–568 | Inhibition of amplitude response to stimulation of frog sural nerve | | Poorly dialysable | (Cuprophane) |
| ″   [31] | | | | | |
| Odeberg [74] | | | | | |
| Odeberg [74] | | Inhibition of iodination capacity of normal granulocytes | | | |
| Ringoir [38] | 113–1,029 | Inhibition of phagocytosis | | Not dialysable | (Polyacrylonitrile) |
| Dzurik [35] | 1,000–1,500 | Inhibition of glucose utilization in rat diaphragm, brain, kidney, cortex slices | No Change | Not dialysable | |
| ″   [75] | | | | | |
| | | Inhibition of glucose utilization in human erythrocytes | No Change | Not dialysable | |
| Tison [76] | ~1,000 | Inhibition of platelet glucose utilization | | | |
| Dzurik [77] | | Inhibition of glucose utilization in rat diaphragm | | | |
| ″   [78] | | | | | |
| Gajdos [79] | 1,000–5,000 | Inhibition of glucose utilization in erythrocytes | | | |

*Table 4–1.* *(Continued)*

| Reference | Molecular Weight | Biological Activity In Vitro | In Vivo | Biological Activity Hemodialysis Effect | Middle Molecule Permeability | |
|---|---|---|---|---|---|---|
| Lindsay [80] | | Inhibition of platelet aggregation | | | Dialysable | |
| Gallice [81] Rinaudo [82] | | Inhibition of platelet aggregation | | | | |
| Rinaudo [83] ”   [82] | | Inhibition of oxidative phosphorylation in mitochondria | | | | |
| Bernard [84] Rinaudo [82] | | Cardiotoxicity on embryonic chick heart | | | Dialysable | (Cellulose Acetate) |
| Mabuchi [85] | ? | Inhibition of platelet aggregation | | | Dialysable | (Cuprophane) |
| Leber [36] ”   [86] ”   [87] | 500–1,500 1,200–1,400 ”   ” | Inhibition of hemoglobin synthesis | | | | |
| Goubeaud [88] | 1,000–1,400 | | | | | |
| Goubeaud [88] Leber [36] | 1,000–1,400 500–1,500 | Inhibition of porphobilinogen synthesis | | | | |
| Leber [36] | 500–1,500 | Inhibition of glucose utilization in erythrocytes | | Decrease | Dialysable | (Polyacrylonitrile) |
| Leber [87] ”   [36] | 500–1,500 | Increase oxidative hemolysis rate | | Decrease | Dialysable | (Polyacrylonitrile) |
| Gutman [89] | 1,000–10,000 2,000–5,000 | Inhibition of thymidine incorporation in rabbit and dog bone marrow Inhibition of Fe incorporation in to heme | | Decrease | Dialysable | |
| Rege [90] Moriyama [91] ”   [91] | ~2,300 2,000–5,000 | Inhibition of Fe incorporation in to heme | | | | |

| Reference | Concentration | Effect | | Change | Dialysability | Membrane |
|---|---|---|---|---|---|---|
| Brunner [92]<br>" [93]<br>" [40] | | Inhibition of thymidine incorporation in rat bone marrow and HeLa cells | | | Dialysable | (Polyacrylonitrile)<br>(Cuprophane) |
| Bourgoigne [94]<br>" [95] | <1,000 | Inhibition of transepithelial sodium transport in the frog skin and in the toad bladder<br>Inhibition of p-aminohyppurate uptake by rabbit kidney cortical slices | | Decrease | Dialysable | |
| Burgoigne [96]<br>" [95] | 500–1,000 | | Increase sodium excretion rate and fractional sodium excretion in rats | | | |
| Kinniburgh [97] | 1,000–2,000 | Inhibition of phenytoin-protein binding | | | | |
| Menyhart [98]<br>Grof [99] | 1,300–1,500 | | Toxicity (minimal lethal dose) in mice | | Poorly or not dialysable | (Cuprophane) |
| Dall'Aglio [100] | 800–10,000 | Inhibition of leukocyte migration | | | | |
| Ehrlich [101] | 700–1,200 | Inhibition of fibroblastic cell poliferation | | | Dialysable | |
| Pogglitsch [102] | | | Reduction in blood pressure and cardiotoxic effects in rat | | Dialysable | (Cuprophane) |
| Lutz [103] | 1,300–1,800<br>500–1,500 | Inhibition of LDH | | Decrease | Dialysable | (Cuprophane) |
| Lutz [104]<br>" [49] | 1,200–1,500 | Inhibition of insulin binding to cell receptors | | | Poorly dialysable | |

MM isolated from the dialysate inhibit E. Rosette formation in vitro [54, 58], while MM isolated from serum do not have this effect [34, 118]. These conflicting results can probably be attributed to difficult test standardization. Various separation methods applied to different biological fluids could also isolate different MM with opposite effects.

The injection of MM delays the rejection of skin allografts in rats, but it does not modify their antibody production [34, 64]. A significant inhibition of graft-versus-host reaction occurs when allogenic splenic lymphocyte suspension incubated with middle molecular fractions is injected inter-peritoneally to irradiated mice [34, 64].

In vivo phagocytic activity of normal human blood is inhibited by the MM [38]. Uremic serum influences granulocyte function by inhibiting the granulocyte enzymes involved in the killing of ingested microorganisms [74]. This inhibition has been localized in two serum fractions: one contains a nondialysable high mw substance, the other contains a dialysable middle mw substance [74].

These data lead to the contention that MM play an important role in determining the immunodeficiency seen in uremic patients. Many authors [30, 34, 59, 60, 63–65, 100, 123] maintain that these MM are peptides. The aminoacid sequence of a MM inhibiting rosetta formation [54] and lympho-cyte proliferation [55], as well as the aminoacid composition of another that inhibits lymphocyte proliferation [44, 65, 67], have been established. Although there is disagreement [124], proof is available that some of these peptides are at least partially dialysable [38, 54, 58, 59, 60, 65, 66, 125].

*Anemia*

Anemia is a constant complication of patients in chronic renal failure. The principal cause of anemia is reduced erythropoietin production. Other factors determining anemia include iron deficiency, bleeding, and increased red cell hemolysis rate.

It has also been demonstrated that substances able to inhibit erythropoiesis in vivo [126, 127] and in vitro [128, 129] are present in uremic serum. In the reticulocytes of uremic patients, decreased porphyrin synthesis for reduced delta-amino-levulinic acid dehydrogenase activity (which catalyzes the con-version of delta-amino-levulinic acid to porphobilinogen) as well as decreased porphobilinogen desaminase (which permits further metabolism of porpho-bilinogen to uroporphyrinogen) has been demonstrated [130]. Moreover, uremic blood shows increased oxidative hemolysis with respect to blood of normal subjects [131]: this might be responsible for the shortened erythrocyte half-life in uremic patients.

Hemoglobin synthesis seems influenced in various phases by substances in the MM weight range. They depress heme synthesis by inhibition of iron incorporation into the heme [89–91, 132], porphyrin synthesis by inhibition of the dehydrogenase delta-amino — levulinic dehydrase enzymatic activity

[36, 88], and hemoglobin synthesis by inhibiting the incorporation of amino acids into the globin [86]. Moreover, MM depress marrow DNA synthesis in dogs [89], rats [92, 93], and rabbits [89] by inhibiting the incorporation of thymidine in the marrow cells. Finally, MM reduce normal red cell resistance to oxidative hemolysis by affecting on the SH-groups of the erythrocyte membrane [36, 87] and increasing red cell fragility to osmotic stress [65].

Toxic factors related to oxidative hemolysis [87], osmotic hemolysis [65], inhibition of marrow DNA synthesis [92], and iron incorporation [89] are at least partially dialysable [36, 87, 89, 92], and have been detected in the ultrafiltrate [65], dialysate [88], and hemofiltrate [92]. Hemodialysis treatment reduces the plasma concentration of substances inhibiting DNA-synthesis and iron incorporation [89] and reduces erythrocyte sensitivity to oxidative damage [36, 87].

*Peripheral neuropathy*

Peripheral neuropathy is a frequent complication of uremia. Dialysable substances are at least in part responsible for this condition: in fact, neuropathy improves with hemodialysis treatment, and inadequate hemodialysis favors the appearance of uremic neuropathy [2]. After the clinical trials of Thenckhoff [3, 4], Scribner assumed a direct correlation between neuropathy and substances with mw between 300 and 5,000.

Funk-Bretano and his group [26, 51] evaluated, in vitro, the neurotoxic effects of the MM with the frog sural nerve test. Testing the effects of ultrafiltrates (obtained from high MM-permeable membranes) of plasma from normal subjects and from patients in hemodialysis with and without neuropathy, they demonstrated that only the ultrafiltrate of plasma from patients in dialysis with severe neuropathy is neurotoxic [26, 51]. The same authors then separated a fraction containing numerous substances of different chemical nature, carbohydrates, and peptides in the middle mw range from the plasma of hemodialysis patients with severe neuropathy [18, 26, 51, 73] and from the urine of normal subjects which has an in vitro neurotoxic effect [73, 18]. Among these substances, a peptide with a mw of 1,187–1,289 [26, 51] and an acid polyol with a carbohydrate structure [31, 52, 72] were isolated. Further studies have confirmed the neurotoxic effect of the fraction to a glycuro-conjugate [18, 31]; its molecular weight, according to the methods used in defining it, is 568 [18, 41, 73] or 537 [31] or between 300 and 400 [72]. Other authors [56] have isolated, in the ultrafiltrate, a peptide which has an inhibitory effect on the neurons of the dorsal horn of the spinal cord [133].

The test for MM neurotoxicity demonstrates only that the MM reduce the response to an electric stimulus of an isolated nerve and not that they determine histological alterations of the nerve fibers. There is as yet no demonstration that the MM are able to damage nerve cells and induce the subsequent demyelination of the axons which causes the reduced nerve conduction velocity and electromyographic alterations characteristic of uremic neuropathy. Moreover, the accumulation of numerous substances which are not MM, vitamin and protein deficits, as well as metabolic alterations specific to uremia (a recent review of the subject will be found in 134) are involved in the pathogenesis of uremic polyneuropathy.


*Abnormal carbohydrate metabolism*

Altered carbohydrate metabolism is frequently found in uremic patients [135–137] and is manifested clinically as glucose intolerance. Carbohydrate intolerance in uremia is probably secondary to diminished cell sensitivity to insulin, as is demonstrated by the exaggerated insulin response to a glucose load, by hyperinsulinemia after fasting, and by the reduced glycemia drop after administration of exogenous insulin [124, 137–142]. The diminished sensitivity to insulin of peripheral tissues might depend on a defect in the binding of insulin to its receptors, on a postreceptoral deficit or on both.

Uremic serum is able to determine an in vitro inhibition of glucose utilization in slices of rat diaphragm [35, 77, 78, 143], brain [35, 101, 129], liver [144] renal cortex [35], and in human red cells [36, 79] and platelets [76]. It has also been demonstrated that uremic serum decreases insulin binding to normal and uremic erythrocytes [145] and inhibits lactate-dehydrogenase activity [146–148].

MM inhibit insulin binding to its cellular receptors [104, 106] by forming MM-insulin complexes [104]; they also inhibit glucose transmembrane transport and enzyme activity in carbohydrate metabolism such as phosphofructokinase [143] and lactic dehydrogenase [103, 149].

Only after long-term dialysis treatment will the altered carbohydrate metabolism of chronic renal failure improve [150], together with reduced serum concentration of peptides correlated to glycolysis inhibition [151]. A single dialysis session will not modify the inhibitory activity of uremic serum, and dialysis extraction of substances which inhibit glucose trans-membrane transport, and phosphofructokinase is very low [75]. The MM which prevent insulin from binding to its cell receptors are also dialyzed with difficulty [104]. Lactic dehydrogenase inhibitors, in particular those of isoenzyme LD5, are instead removed by dialysis [103, 149].


*Coagulopathy*

The coagulation defect found in uremic patients has many causes. Altered platelet function plays the most important role in the bleeding of uremic patients. In subjects in chronic renal failure in conservative and hemodialysis treatment, abnormal platelet adhesiveness [152, 153], diminished platelet aggregation [80, 81, 85, 154], and a reduced P. F. 3 [155–159] have been

60

demonstrated. The possible role played by the MM has been studied by Lundsay and associates [80] and Gallice and associates. [81] They isolated substances with mw in the middle molecule range from human serum able to inhibit in vitro platelet aggregation.

Dialysis treatment corrects the qualitative defects of the platelets [152, 155, 160]. The degree of improvement of platelet function depends on the efficiency of dialysis and on dialysis time. Lengthened time or increased frequency of hemodialytic treatment [152, 161], but above all peritoneal dialysis [152, 160, 162], improve platelet aggregation significantly.

*Other toxic effects correlated to the MM*

Uremic serum inhibits multiplication in vitro of tumor and fibroblastic cells [63, 66]. Serum from patients in dialysis, however, no longer has this inhibitory effect [66]. The polyacrylonitrile dialysate of serum from neuropathic uremic patients and of urine from normal subjects [47, 70] as well as the hemofiltrate [101] are cytotoxic to fibroblasts [47, 68]. This effect is attributed to the MM [47, 68, 70] which inhibit the incorporation of thymidine into DNA [101]. While some authors [63] sustain that the MM themselves are able to inhibit proliferation of various tumoral cells, others [66] affirm that the presence of plasma macromolecules together with MM is required for the appearance of these properties.

Middle molecules isolated from normal urine inhibit bovine renal adenylate cyclase activity stimulated by various factors: one of them is parathormone [71].

Lipoprotein lipase regulates triglyceride assimilation in adipose tissue and influences the rate at which these lipids are removed from the plasma. Basic peptides in the MM mw range can depress the metabolic activity of lipoprotein lipase, forming complexes with the lipoproteins themselves or reducing lipoprotein lipase synthesis in adipose cells [105].

Middle molecules at concentrations higher than those found in uremic serum cause cardiac arrest and/or rhythm and frequency alterations in embryonic chicken hearts [84]. A peptide isolated in the ultrafiltrate and administered to rats caused a reduction in blood pressure at low dosages, and cardiotoxic effects at high dosages [102].

Uremic plasma in toto has a toxic effect on cellular respiration by decoupling oxidative phosphorylation in the mitochondria [163–165]. In the same way, MM isolated from normal urine and from the serum of uremic patients determine a loss of mitochondrial respiration [83].

The binding of drugs and other substances with plasma proteins is altered in uremia [166–169]. This might be due to hypoprotidemia, to alterations in protein structure and to competitive or noncompetitive inhibition [170–172]. There is proof that peptides with molecular weights between 1,000 and 2,000 can inhibit pharmaco-protein binding by means of a competitive or noncompetitive mechanism [97].

*Limits of in vitro tests* The variety of separation and isolation techniques has created some confusion about whether the different demonstrated biological activities can be attributed to the same fraction isolated with different methodologies or to fractions that are truly different. The discriminating factor might be the mw attributed to the single fractions; however, mw range is so wide that only in rare cases can we establish with certainty that two different activities are referred to two different fractions. When different toxic effects point to substances with overlapping mw, it is impossible to establish if the same substance has different toxic effects or if these effects are the expression of different toxic substances. Moreover, the nontoxic effect of a fraction can be attributed to its true nontoxicity or to the presence of substances with antithetic action.

Almost all authors attribute the demonstrated biologic effect to peptides because the tested fractions contain substances of a protein nature. Nevertheless, this does not exclude the possibility that other substances eluated together with the peptides are toxic. Moreover, the toxicity noted could be in some cases referrable to substances with both a low (<200) and high (>2,000) mw showing the same toxic effects as those of the MM (table 4–2).

In vitro test results may be conditioned by factors unrelated to the MM [173]. In fact, in vitro tests are extremely sensitive to a number of variables such as pH, ionic charge, osmolality; they vary greatly from one fraction to another, even when isolated with very similar elution volumes. Enzyme-dependent in vitro tests are also influenced by traces of metals, and higher quantities of metals have been found in uremic than in normal fractions.

It is thus necessary either to improve MM separation and isolation techniques or to define their chemical characteristics. In fact, only by testing pure single synthesized MM on the different substrates can we determine to which of these a particular toxic effect can be attributed. With this in mind, some authors have demonstrated the toxicity of fractions containing apparently pure MM and corresponding synthesized MM. The same toxicity was observed in both [31, 54–58, 72].

Nevertheless, two fundamental criticisms of in vitro studies should be made: first, the exclusion of factors (acidosis, ionic alterations, exclusion of possibly antagonistic substances) which may determine or inhibit MM toxicity in vivo, and secondly, the short exposure time of the substrates which precludes evaluation of possible adaptation phenomena which might come about in vivo as a result of chronic exposure.


**Toxicity in vivo**

The hypothesis of MM toxicity originated from observation of patients in dialysis treatment: this led to the supposition that MM toxicity could be unequivocally demonstrated in the clinical setting. On the contrary, despite

*Table 4–2.* Toxic effects that substances with mw <300 D and >2,000 D have in common with middle molecules

| Biological activity in Vitro of Middle Molecules | Urea | Creatinine | Guanidine Succinic Acid | Methyl guanidine | Guanidine | Phenoles | AMP Cyclic | Alyphatic Amines | Indoles | Oxalic Acid | >2.000 |
|---|---|---|---|---|---|---|---|---|---|---|---|
| Inhibition of LDH activity | | | | | | | | | | | 176 |
| Inhibition of lymphocyte proliferation by PHA and allogenic cells | 174 | | 61 64 114 118 | 61 114 118 175 | | 61 114 118 175 | | | | | 61 114 118 178 |
| Inhibition of unstimulated limphocyte proliferation | | | 64 175 179 | 64 175 179 | | 175 | | | | | |
| Inhibition of fibroblastic cell proliferation | | | | | | | | | | | 66 |
| Inhibition of amplitude response to stimulation of frog sural nerve | | | 180 | | | 181 | | | | | |
| Inhibition of granulocyte function | | | | | | 182 | | | 182 | | 43 74 183 184 |
| Inhibition of glucose utilization in rat diaphragm, brain, kidney cortex slices | 150 185 | 150 | | | | | | | | | |
| Inhibition of glucose utilization | 150 | 76 | 76 | | | | 76 | | | | |

*Table 4–2.  (Continued)*

| Biological activity in Vitro of Middle Molecules | Urea | Creatinine | Guanidine Succinic Acid | Methyl guanidine | Guanidine | Phenoles | AMP Cyclic | Alyphatic Amines | Indoles | Oxalic Acid | >2.000 |
|---|---|---|---|---|---|---|---|---|---|---|---|
| in human erytrocytes and platelet | | 150 | | | | 186 | | | | | |
| Inhibition of platelet aggregation | 187 | 152 | 157 188 | | | 128 157 189 190 | | | | | |
| Inhibition of oxidative phosphorilation in mitochondria | 191 | | | | 194 | 193 | 192 | 191 | | | |
| Cardiotoxicity on embryonic chicken heart | 195 | | | | | | | | | | |
| Inhibition of hemoglobin synthesis | | | 86 | 86 | | | | | | | |
| Increase oxidative hemolysis rate | | | | | 196 | | | | | | |

64

all efforts, research has furnished conflicting data and created such confusion that even today (almost 20 years after the formulation of the MM toxicity hypothesis) the true clinical meaning of the middle molecules is still under discussion.

*The square meter/hour hypothesis*

As stated in the introduction, clinical observation of dialyzed patients led to the hypothesis that molecules with molecular weights between 300 and 5,000 ('large' molecules) were more responsible for uremic complications (and neuropathy in particular) than molecules with a mw below 300 [1]. This hypothesis could be tested directly by measuring substances with low and high molecular weight in the serum and correlating their concentrations with clinical symptomatology, or indirectly by modifying dialysis schedules to determine substantial variations in plasma concentrations of the 'small' and 'large' molecules, and then evaluating the clinical consequences.

Scribner and his group chose the indirect method due to the technical impossibility of observing the accumulation of large molecules in patients in dialysis treatment. This choice necessitated the development of mathematical models to indicate variations in dialysate and blood flow rate, dialyzer surface area, and dialysis time that would modify serum concentrations of small or large molecules (the square meter/hour hypothesis) [5].

In vitro dialysis, carried out with substances of known weights (between 60 and 5,200) substantiated the mathematical hypothesis according to which clearance of low mw molecules depended more on dialysate flow rate than on dialyzer surface and dialysis time, and that the clearance of large molecules depended on the dialyzer surface area and dialysis time more than on dialysate flow rate [5, 197].

In order to evaluate this hypothesis in vivo and propose it as a clinical guide, dialysis schedules were carried out using mathematical models which increased serum concentrations of large molecules and left small molecules unaltered, or else increased small molecule concentration and left the large molecules unchanged [5, 6]. The first clinical trials, carried out with a low dialysate flow (to increase predialysis values of low mw molecules and maintain plasma concentrations of large molecules), demonstrated that urea, creatinine, and uric acid values increased as foreseen by the square meter/hour hypothesis [197, 198]. This led to the supposition that the mathematical hypothesis and the results of in vitro dialysis were valid in vivo for the large molecules as well. Less sure results were obtained using large surface area dialyzers and a reduced dialysis time (so as to increase prediaysis concentrations of small molecules and maintain plasma concentrations of large molecules) [201]. This dialysis schedule applied to only 3 patients (for 12, 7, and 5 weeks, respectively), brought about delayed urea increase in 1 patient and its decrease in another; serum creatinine showed unexplainable variations in 1 case, but serum uric acid remained unchanged in all 3. While the positive clinical results obtained with the two schedules demonstrated the nontoxicity of low mw molecules, they did not demonstrate the toxicity of large molecules: instead, they supported the hypothesis that a reduced extraction of dialysable substances brings about the correction of a deficiency syndrome, responsible for at least some complications of uremia, such as altered platelet function [197, 198, 201]. The hypothesis that reduced dialysis extraction of low mw molecules might be clinically beneficial has been taken into consideration by various authors [47, 70, 199, 202–204].

*The middle molecule hypothesis*

The attribution of toxicity to substances with mw between 300 and 1,500–2,000 (middle molecules), and therefore to dialyzer clearance at least partially dependent on the dialysate flow rate (middle molecule hypothesis) [6,205] stemmed from clinical studies using low dialysate flow rate (100 ml/m') that increased plasma concentrations of small molecules [197–200] (table 4–3), large surface area dialyzers (3 m$^2$) almost impermeable to molecules with mw above 2,000 (larger molecules) [197, 201] (table 4–4) and high efficiency small surface area dialyzers (0.4–0.44 m$^2$) [6, 205, 206] that removed more small than middle and larger molecules (table 4–5). These studies suggested that toxins have a molecular weight between 300 and 1,500–2,000. In fact, motor nerve conduction velocity (MNCV) remained constant or improved in patients who accumulated small and larger and not middle molecules. MNCV worsened, sometimes to the point of clinical neuropathy, in patients with increased middle and larger molecules and acceptable small molecule concentrations.

Unfortunately, isolated changes in MNCV as well as the significance of small molecules are meaningless without information on patient nutrition and protein catabolic rate.

Subsequent studies in which hemodialysis treatments modified serum concentration ratios between middle and small molecules in favor of the small (table 4–6) or the middle molecules (table 4–7) furnished elements both for and against the hypothesis of MM toxicity. These conflicting data led some authors to affirm that the severity of uremia at the start of hemodialysis treatment and patient compliance to dietary recommendations condition the evolution, at least of neuropathy, more than do theoretical MM levels [213–215].

*Dialysis indexes*

The requirement for easy and certain comparison of clinical results in patients on different dialysis schedules in different dialysis units in relation to the variations induced in predialysis MM concentrations, as well as the demonstrated necessity to consider other variables (aside from dialysis

*Table 4–3.*

| References | Patients | Dialyzers | | Dialyzers | Follow-up Time (Months) | Middle Molecules | Small Molecules | Laboratory and Clinical Fundings |
|---|---|---|---|---|---|---|---|---|
| Graham Christopher (1971) [198] | 4 | Standard Kiil<br>Qb 200<br>Qd 100<br>A   1<br>T   27–30 | vs | Standard Kiil<br>Qb 200<br>Qd 500<br>A   1<br>T   27–30 | 3–12 | = | ↑ | Nomalized platelet function<br>= ↑ MNCV<br>=   Ht<br>=   Ca |
| Milutinovic (1971) [197] | 6 | Standard Kiil<br>Qb 200<br>Qd 100<br>A   1<br>T   27–30 | vs | Standard Kiil<br>Qb 200<br>Qd 500<br>A   1<br>T   27–30 | 3–10 | = | ↑ | Normalized platelet function<br>= ↑ MNCV<br>↑ P<br>↑ Well being |
| Cambi (1972) [199] | 8 | Ultra-Flo 100<br>Qb 180<br>Qd 100<br>A   1<br>T   24–33 | vs | Standard Kiil<br>Qb 200<br>Qd 500<br>A   1<br>T   27 | 12 | = | ↑ | ↓ = Bleeding time<br>↓ = MNCV<br>=   Ht<br>=   Body weight |
| Rattazzi (1974) [200] | 39 | Standard Kiil<br>Qd 200<br>A   1<br>T   18–30 | vs | Standard Kiil<br>Qd 500<br>A   1<br>T   18–30 | 3 | = | = | =   Bleeding time<br>=   Platelet function<br>=   MNCV<br>=   Ht<br>=   Ca = P<br>=   Cholesterol<br>=   Triglycerides<br>=   Alk. Phosphatase<br>=   PTH |

Middle molecules unchanged, Small molecules increased.
Area-time product constant.
Low dialysate flow rate.
The constant product of dialyzer surface area and dialysis time (constant area × constant time) does not modify middle molecule serum concentrations.
Decreased dialysate flow rate (Qd 100 ml/min) determines an increase in small molecule serum concentrations. A Qd of 200 ml/min does not modify small molecules concentrations.
Qb and Qd: blood and dialysate flows respectively expressed in ml/m'.
A:     dialyzer surface area in m$^2$.
T:     weekly treatment time in hours.
↑ :     increase in the parameter.
↓ :     decrease in the parameter.
=:     unchanged parameter.
↑ =: modest, nonuniform increase.
↓ =: modest, nonuniform decrease.

*Table 4–4.*

| References | Patients | Dialyzers | | Dialyzers | Follow-up Time (Months) | Middle Molecules | Small Molecules | Laboratory and Clinical Findings |
|---|---|---|---|---|---|---|---|---|
| Rosenzweig (1971) [201] | 3 | 3 Dow HFAK<br>Qb 200<br>Qd 500<br>A 3<br>T 6–8 | versus | Dow HFAK<br>Qb 200<br>Qd 500<br>A 1<br>T 18–24 | 1–3 | = | ↑ = | ↑ Platelet function<br>= ↑ MNCV<br>= Body Weight<br>↑ Well being |

Middle molecules unchanged, small molecules increased.
Area-time product constant.
Dialysate flow rate constant.
The constant product of dialyzer surface area and dialysis time (increased area × decreased time) does not modify middle molecule concentrations.
Decreased dialysis time determines increased serum concentrations of small molecules.
See table 4–3 for abbreviations.

*Table 4–5.*

| References | Patients | Dialyzers | | Dialyzers | Follow-up Time (Months) | Middle Molecules | Small Molecules | Laboratory and Clinical Findings |
|---|---|---|---|---|---|---|---|---|
| Ginn (1971) [206] | 10 | Mini Klung Cuprophan<br>Qb 200<br>Qd 500<br>A 0.44<br>T 20–21 | versus | Klung Cuprophan<br>Qb 200<br>Qd 500<br>A 2<br>T 14 | 6–19 | ↑ | ↑ = | ↓ MNCV<br>(clinical neuropathy) |
| Babb (1972) [6] Scribner (1973) [205] | 1 | Mini-Dialyzer<br>Qb 200<br>Qd 500<br>A 0.4<br>T 21 | versus | Mini-Dialyzer<br>Qb 200<br>Qd 500<br>A 0.4<br>T 27 | 1 | ↑ | ↑ = | ↓ MNCV |

Middle molecules increased, small molecules unchanged.
Area-time product decreased.
Dialysate flow rate constant.
The reduced product of dialyzer surface area and dialysis time (greatly decreased area × increased time) increases serum concentrations of middle molecules. Longer dialysis time maintaines small molecules serum concentrations more or less constant.
See table 4–3 for abbreviations.

*Table 4–6.*

| References | Patients | Dialyzers | | Follow-up Time (Months) | Middle Molecules | Small Molecules | Laboratory and Clinical Findings |
|---|---|---|---|---|---|---|---|
| Teehan (1974) [207] | 10 | 2 HFAK Mod 4<br>2 EX-21;2 EX-23<br>2 EX-29;2 UF2;<br>2 UF1. 5;2 Gambro 17$\mu$<br>Qb 200<br>Qd 350–500<br>A 2.4<br>T 12 | | 15.5 | = ↓ | = | ↓ MNCV |
| Mirahmadi (1974) [208] | 14 | 2 Gambro 13.5$\mu$<br>Qb 200<br>Qd 500<br>A 2<br>T 12 | versus Ex-01, Ex-03<br>Qb 200<br>Qd 500<br>A 1<br>T 15–18 | 6.7 | ↓ | = | ↑ HT<br>= MNCV<br>= Body weight<br>↑ Well being |
| Cambi (1973) [209] | 4 | 2 EX-03;UF 1.5<br>2 Gambro Lundia<br>Qb >250<br>Qd 500<br>A 1.7–2<br>T 10.5 | versus Coil<br><br>Qb >250<br>Qd 500<br>A 1<br>T 10.5 | 4 | ↓ | ↓ = | = MNCV |
| Hurst (1975) [62]<br>Lowrie (1976) [210] | 10 | Coil<br>Cuprophan<br>Qb 260<br>Qd 125<br>A 1.5<br>T 12 | versus Coil<br>Cuprophan<br>Qb 260<br>Qd 500<br>A 1<br>T 15 | 4 | = | ↑ | = Inhibited mitogenic response<br>  of normal lymphocytes<br>= Bleeding time<br>= MNCV<br>= Ca ↑ P<br>↓ Cholesterol<br>↓ T4 |
| | 10 | Coil<br>Cuprophan<br>Qb 260<br>Qd 310<br>A 1.5<br>T 15 | versus Coil<br>Cuprophan<br>Qb 260<br>Qd 500<br>A 1<br>T 15 | 4 | ↓ | = | = Inhibited mitogenic response<br>  of normal lymphocytes<br>= Bleeding time<br>↑ MNCV<br>= Ca = P<br>= Cholesterol<br>= T4 |

Dialysis schedules modifying the ratio between plasma concentration of middle and small molecules in favor of small molecules.
See table 4–3 for abbreviations.

*Table 4–7.*

| References | Patients | Dialyzers | | Dialyzers | Follow-up Time (Months) | Middle Molecules | Small Molecules | Laboratory and Clinical Findings |
|---|---|---|---|---|---|---|---|---|
| Teschan (1976) [211] | 4 | Cordis Dow Mod4 | versus | D4 Kiil Cuprophan | 5 | ↑ | = | = ↓ Neurobehaviour (EEG, choice reaction time) |
| Hurst (1975) [62] Lowrie (1976) [210] | 10 | Coil Cuprophan Qb 300 Qd 1500 A 0.64 T 15 | versus | Coil Cuprophan Qb 260 Qd 500 A 1 T 15 | 4 | ↑ | = | = Inhibited mitogenic response of normal lymphocytes<br>= Bleeding time<br>↑ MNCV<br>= Ca = P<br>= Cholesterol<br>= T4 |
| | 10 | Coil Cuprophan Qb 300 Qd 1500 A 1 T 14 | versus | Coil Cuprophan Qb 260 Qd 500 A 1 T 15 | 4 | = | ↓ | = Inhibited mitogenic response of normal lymphocytes<br>= Bleeding time<br>↑ MNCV<br>↑ Ca ↓ P<br>↓ Cholesterol<br>= T4 |
| Ben Ari (1976) [212] | 13 | 2 UF2 Qb 200 Qd 600 A 2 T 7–9 | versus | UF 145 Qb 200 Qd 300 A 1 T 14–18 | 2 | = | = ↓ | = Ht<br>= Well-being |

Dialysis schedules modifying the ratio between plasma concentrations of middle and small molecules in favor of middle molecules. See table 4–3 for abbreviations.

parameters) able to influence MM removal led to the formulation of the dialysis index [216].

The dialysis index is based on the following assumptions:

1. MM are toxic.

2. Vitamin $B_{12}$ (molecular weight: 1,355 D) is a realistic MM marker.

3. In vivo dialyzer clearance of all the different middle molecules is equal to that of vitamin $B_{12}$ quantified in vitro.

4. MM renal clearance is the same as the residual glomerular filtration rate.

5. MM generation rate is constant and proportional to body surface area.

6. MM distribution volume is equal to that of total body water.

7. Middle molecules have the same rate of passage across the cell wall and dialysis membranes.

8. A MM clearance (evaluated as vitamin $B_{12}$ clearance) of 30 liters per week is sufficient to maintain MM serum concentrations nontoxic.

The dialysis index takes different parameters into account: frequency of weekly dialysis (nd), duration in hours of each dialysis session (td), dialyzer MM (Vitamin $B_{12}$) clearance ($K_B$), residual renal filtration rate (ml/min) referred to one week (168 hours) ($K_k$), 'adequate' weekly MM clearance for a body surface of 1.73 $m^2$ (30 liters per week), and finally the body surface of the patient in question (S./1.73 $m^2$). The dialysis index (216) is calculated on the basis of the following equation:

$$DI = \frac{nd \cdot td \cdot K_B + K_k}{(30L/WK) \cdot (S/1.73)}$$

$K_B = K_{Bo} + m Q_u$ where $K_{Bo}$ is vitamin $B_{12}$ clearance without ultrafiltration, $m$ is the permeability coefficient, and $Q_u$ is the ultrafiltration rate (ml/min).

The ratio between weekly vitamin $B_{12}$ clearance of the dialysis schedule (adding the patient's residual glomerular filtration rate, if it exists) and the minimum weekly clearance (clearance = 30 liters per week) furnishes an index to establish the adequacy of dialysis in terms of MM removal. A ratio of 1 indicates adequate dialysis treatment, a ratio below or above 1 indicates inadequate or excessive dialysis respectively [204, 217].

Variations in predialysis MM serum concentrations brought about by different hemodialysis treatments (in many of the experiments aimed at establishing their clinical meaning) are determined by a dialysis index, even if the majority of the postulates on which it is based are certainly mistaken.

Undoubtly incorrect is the assumption that the MM generation rate is constant. Each MM probably has its own endogenous generation rate which can vary from patient to patient [39, 218]. Clinical condition [7, 8, 17, 53, 219] and protein intake [9, 20, 39, 45–48] are probably factors that regulate MM generation rate. The generation rate of some but not all MM [9, 45] correlates to that of urea (20, 46). Moreover, it is possible that metabolic adaptations in patients bring about unforeseen modifications in MM synthesis and catabolism. In fact, an increasing MM concentration could decrease MM synthesis or stimulate MM catabolism, just as a decrease could increase synthesis or decrease catabolism.

It is doubtful that the MM have easy access to the intracellular spaces. In most cases, middle molecule fractions are removed from the blood at the same rate as urea and creatinine [53], although the in vitro dialyzer clearance is lower for MM than for the other two substances. This would lead to the supposition that the MM distribution volume is smaller than that of urea and creatinine. Calculations indicate that this would equal the extracellular volume [53, 220, 221]. Moreover, it is possible that the distribution volume of the MM immediately available for exchange is small, but that the MM have a double intraextracellular distribution pool with a low transport coefficient between the two compartments [20, 22, 220, 222]. The second hypothesis is sustained by the rapid rebound in serum MM concentration that appears within 30 minutes after the end of dialysis [53].

The assumption that the renal MM clearance and residual renal clearance are equal is probably true. In fact, as renal function is progressively reduced, the ratio between MM clearance and glomerular filtrate approaches 1 [20, 22, 223].

Instead, it is erroneous to consider vitamin $B_{12}$ as a MM marker and to attribute an identical dialyzer clearance to the numerous MM with their different molecular weights and chemical structure, as well as to maintain that dialysis clearance is the same as that of vitamin $B_{12}$ measured in vitro. The mw of MM, when calculated on the basis of their clearance in calibrated dialyzers [53, 224, 225] or of their chemical structure [16, 18, 72, 226–228] is always variable and, moreover, lower than that of vitamin $B_{12}$.

It is doubtful that a weekly vitamin $B_{12}$ dialyzer clearance of 30 liters is indicative of a dialysis MM extraction able to safeguard the patient from uremic complications [204, 217]. Some clinical studies have led to the conclusion that a weekly vitamin $B_{12}$ clearance of 30 liters is an overestimation of dialysis necessity, at least in clinically stable hemodialyzed patients [217, 229–231].

Table 4–8 shows the correlations between different dialysis index values and clinical conditions. Clinical and laboratory improvement and worsening are discerned in patients with dialysis indexes of 1, above 1, and below 1. In short, it is impossible to determine from these studies whether or not uremia is correlated to plasma MM concentrations.

These discrepancies may arise principally because the dialysis index does not have an absolute value for different clinical conditions, and thus when the dialysis index is set at one, the actual patient need may be overestimated or underestimated [217, 229–231, 234]. If diet, metabolic, and clinical conditions are truly important in determining the MM generation rate, it is obviously difficult to establish a value for the dialysis index that would accurately foresee MM predialysis values in different patients or in the same patient at different times.

*Table 4–8.* Correlation between dialysis index and clinical condition

| References | Patients | Dialysis Index | | Dialysis Index | Follow-up Time (Months) | Laboratory and Clinical Findings |
|---|---|---|---|---|---|---|
| Graefe (1979) [229] | 23 | 0.6–1 | versus | 1–>1.2 | 20 | ↑ Vibration sensitivity<br>= MNCV<br>↑ Ht<br>= Ca |
| Raja (1978) [234] | 24 | 1.2 | | | 27 | (2/24) Pericarditis<br>(1/24) Blood transfusions<br>        No clinical neuropathy |
| | 18 | 1.37 | | | 29 | (3/18) Pruritus<br>(6/18) Blood transfusions<br>(3/18) Clinical neuropathy |
| | 18 | 1.23 | | | 36 | (5/18) Weakness<br>        No clinical neuropathy |
| | 9 | 0.78 | | | 33 | (2/9) Blood transfusions<br>        No clinical neuropathy |
| Milutinovic (1978) [232] | 10 | 1.19 (1–1.6) | versus | 0.76 (0.6–0.9) | 18 (7–40) | (1/10) Pericarditis<br>(1/10) Weakness<br>↓ (6/10)  = (4/10)   MNCV<br>= Ca  = P |
| | 8 | 0.76 (0.6–0.9) | versus | 1.24 (1–1.4) | 17 (6–32) | ↓ (7/10)   ↑ (1/10)   = (2/ 10)   Ht<br>↑ (4/8)  = (4/8)   MNCV<br>↑ (6/8)  = (2/8)   Ht<br>= Ca  = P |
| Milutinovic (1974) [217] | 15 | 1.53 (1–2.6) | versus | 0.94 (0.4–1.7) | 2–18 | ↓ (3/15)  = (12/15)   MNCV<br>(1/15) Clinical neuropathy<br>= ↑ (15/15) Well-being<br>= Ht |

| Teehan (1977) [231] | 14 | 1.32 (1.01–1.78) | | | 17 | ↑ (2/14)  ↓ (2/14)  = (10/14)  MNCV<br>(1/14) Pericarditis<br>(1/14) Clinical neuropathy<br>(2/14) Transfusions<br>= Ht<br>↑ P |
| | 5 | 0.96 (0.91–0.99) | | | 17 | ↓ (1/5)  = (4/5)  MNCV<br>(1/5) Clinical neuropathy<br>(2/5) Transfusions<br>= Ht<br>↑ P |
| Shaldon (1975) [230] | 12 | 1 ± 0.11 | | | 6 | = Ht<br>= MNCV<br>= Ca  = P |
| | 10 | 0.91 ± 0.08 | | | 6 | = Ht<br>= MNCV<br>= Ca  = P |
| Teschan (1983) [233] | 10 | 0.8 (0.5–1.6) | versus | 1 (0.8–2) | 6 | = Ht<br>= Ca  = P<br>= Body Weight<br>↓ Neurobehaviour (EEG, choice reaction time, clinical self-evaluation, continuous memory test) |

The Dialysis Index shows modifications of MM serum concentrations brought about by different hemodialysis treatments. See table 4–3 for abbreviations.

Middle molecule toxicity could also be demonstrated through reduction of plasma concentration by means of membranes highly permeable to these substances (table 4–9). Funk-Bretano and associates demonstrated that with the use of a polyacrylonitrile membrane, which has a vitamin $B_{12}$ dialysis efficiency at least double that of a cuprophane membrane (with equal dialyzer surface areas), weekly dialysis time can be reduced by half, without the appearance of neuropathy [47, 68, 203, 204]. Nevertheless these studies (in which vitamin $B_{12}$ was still used as a MM marker) did not demonstrate MM neurotoxicity, since total MM extraction was the same with both polyacrylonitrile and cuprophane [68, 204], and when the number of dialysis hours with a polyacrylonitrile membrane was increased, some patients presented reduced MNCV [70, 203].

## Short Dialysis

Short dialysis was introduced in an attempt to demonstrate MM toxicity: in theory, the drastic reduction in dialysis time would bring about a high predialysis MM concentration, while serum urea and creatinine increases would be partially controlled by high dialysate and blood flow. The unexpected positive clinical results of this hemodialysis treatment reported by Cambi [209, 235] and subsequently by other authors (table 4–10) seemed to contradict the hypothesis of MM toxicity. Nevertheless, the good clinical results obtained can be explained without invalidating the MM hypothesis.

The efficiency of short hemodialysis could be greater than expected if the toxic MM have a lower mw than the reference substance, vitamin $B_{12}$. The MM would thus be more responsive to diffusive forces than what has been supposed. Chromatographic measurements of MM plasma concentrations demonstrated that short hemodialysis leads to increased predialysis MM plasma concentrations with respect to standard Kiil dialysis, but also that this increase is, in reality, less than what would be presumed (table 4–11). The modest MM increase is attributed chiefly to the fact that despite reduced dialysis times, ultrafiltration in toto is unchanged [53, 68, 240–243].

Other factors influencing MM plasma concentrations during short dialysis, such as the slightly reduced MM generation rate [39] or the supposed improvement in nutritional state [230] due to reduced aminoacid and polypeptide dialysis losses, must still be carefully evaluated.

Long-term short hemodialysis seems to prevent further increases in plasma MM. In patients on short dialysis for 2–3 years, some middle molecule fractions remain unchanged while others decrease, although a significant reduction in the glomerular filtrate [218] has been documented. However, a significant increase in the MM pool concentration in patients in dialysis over 10 years (8 of whom were in short dialysis) in comparison to patients in short

*Table 4–9.* Dialysis with membranes highly permeable to MM

| References | Patients | Dialyzers | | Dialyzers | Follow-up Time (Months) | Middle Molecules | Small Molecules | Laboratory and Clinical Findings |
|---|---|---|---|---|---|---|---|---|
| Teschan (1976) [211] | 2 | D4 Kiil polycarbonate | versus | D4 Kiil Cuprophan | 8 | ↓ | = | = ↑ Neurobehaviour (EEG, choice reaction time) |
| Man (1973) [68] | 2 | Polyiacrilonitrile<br>A  1<br>T   15 | versus | Cuprophan<br>A   1<br>T   27 | 2 | = | ↑ | ↑  MNCV |
| Funck-Brentano (1972) [203] | 4 | Polyiacrilonitrile<br>A  1<br>T   10–15 | versus | Cuprophan<br>A   1<br>T   20–30 | 2–3 | = | ↑ | =  Platelet function<br>= ↓ MNCV<br>=  Ca   ↑ P<br>=  Ht<br>↑  Well-being |
| Man (1973) [204] | 5 | RP 1E;<br>Polyiacrilonitrile<br>Qb  150–200<br>Qd  100–130–260<br>A   0.9<br>T   15–19.5 | versus | RP 1D<br>Cuprophan<br>Qb  150<br>Qd  300<br>A   0.9<br>T   20–30 | 12 | = ↓ | ↑ | =  MNCV<br>↑  P<br>↑  Well-being |
| Man (1974) [70]<br>Funck-Brentano (1975) [202] | 3 | RP 6;<br>Polyiacrilonitrile<br>T  9 | versus | RP6<br>Cuprophan<br>T   27 | 6 | = | ↑ | ↑  MNCV |

See table 4–3 for abbreviations.

*Table 4–10.* Short dialysis

| References | Patients | Dialyzers | | Dialyzers | Follow-up Time (Months) | Middle Molecules | Small Molecules | Laboratory and Clinical Findings |
|---|---|---|---|---|---|---|---|---|
| Cambi (1972) [199] | 7 | Ultra-Flo 100<br>Qb 170<br>Qd 300–400<br>A 1<br>T 14 | | | >5 | ↑ | ↑ | ↑ Ht<br>↑ Body weight<br>↑ Well-being |
| Cambi (1973) [209] | 18 | Gambro Nova<br>Dasco SP75<br>UF 100; UF 2<br>Qb >250<br>Qd 500<br>A 1<br>T 10.5–12 | versus | Standard Kiil<br><br>Qb 200<br>Qd 500<br>A 1<br>T 27 | 8 | ↑ | ↑ | = MNCV<br>= ↑ Ht<br>↑ P |
| Cambi (1974) [235] | 40 | Coil<br>Qb >250<br>Qd 400–600<br>T 10.5–12 | versus | Standard Kiil<br>Qb 200<br>Qd 500<br>A 1<br>T 27 | 12 | ↑ | ↑ | = ↑ MNCV<br>↑ Ht<br>↑ P<br>↑ Well-being |
| | 53 | Coil<br>Qb ≥250<br>Qd 400–600<br>A 1<br>T 10.5–12 | | | 3–24 | | | = ↑ MNCV<br>↑ Ht<br>↑ Well-being |
| Cambi (1974) [244] | 28 | UF100; UF2<br>Cordis Dow Mod4<br>Dasco SP75<br>Gambro 13.5µ<br>T 10.5–12 | versus | Standard Kiil<br>Qb 200<br>Qd 500<br>A 1<br>T 27 | 12 | ↑ | ↑ | = ↑ MNCV<br>↑ P<br>↑ Ht |

| Reference | N | | | | | | | | |
|---|---|---|---|---|---|---|---|---|---|
| Cambi (1975) [237] | 115 | Coil | | | | | | | |
| | | Qb 300 | | | | | | | |
| | | Qd 400–500 | | | 6–36 | ↑ | ↑ | = | MNCV |
| | | A 1 | | | | | | = | P |
| | | T 10.5–12 | | | | | | = | Body weight |
| Maiorca (1974) [239] | 43 | Gambro Nova 13.5$\mu$ | | Standard Kiil | | | | | |
| | | Gambro Nova 17$\mu$ | | Qb 200 | | | | = | Bleeding time |
| | | Cordis Dow HFAK Mod4 | | Qd 500 | | | | = | MNCV |
| | | Qb 300 | versus | A 1 | | | | = | Ht |
| | | Qd 500 | | T 27 | >6 | ↑ | ↑ | = | Triglycerides |
| | | T 9–12 | | | | | | = | Body weight |
| | | | | | | | | ↑ | Well-being |
| Castellani (1975) [46] | 9 | Gambro Nova 13.5$\mu$ | | Standard Kiil | | | | | |
| | | T 12 | versus | T 27–30 | 6 | ↑ | ↑ | = | Ht |
| | | | | | | | | = | P |
| | | | | | | | | = | Body weight |
| Shaldon (1975) [237] | 10 | Gambro Nova 13.5$\mu$ | | | | | | | |
| | | Qb 200–250 | | | | | | | |
| | | Qd 500 | | | 6 | ↑ | ↑ | = | MNCV |
| | | A 1 | | | | | | = | Ht |
| | | T 15 | | | | | | = | Ca = P |
| | | | | | | | | = | Well-being |

Middle and small molecules increased.
Area-time product decreased.
Dialysate flow rate constant.
The product of dialyzer surface area and reduced dialysis time (constant area $\times$ very reduced time), increases MM serum concentrations. Reduced dialysis time, increased small molecules serum concentrations.
See table 4–3 for abbreviations.

*Table 4–11.* Short dialysis

| References | Patients | Dialyzers | Dialyzers | Follow-up Time (Months) | Middle Molecules | Small Molecules | Laboratory and Clinical Findings |
|---|---|---|---|---|---|---|---|
| Chapman (1980) [236] | 9 | Gambro 17$\mu$<br>CDAK 1.3;CDAK 1.8<br>Qb 160–200<br>T 9–14 | Gambro 17.1$\mu$<br>CDAK 1.3;CDAK 1.8<br>Qb 160–200<br>versus T 18–27 | 3 | $\uparrow$ = | $\uparrow$ | = Alkaline Phosphatase<br>$\uparrow$ P<br>= Ht<br>= Body weight<br>= Well-being |
| Valek (1980) [218] | 40 | Coil<br>Cuprophan<br>Qb 250<br>Qd 500<br>A 1<br>T 12 | | 24–36 | $\downarrow$ = | $\uparrow$ | Good metabolic state<br>= Body weight<br>= Well-being |
| Buzio (1980) [37] | 5 Pts. in HD for 5 yrs, compared to 10 Pts. in HD for 10 yrs | Coil<br>Qb >200<br>Qd 500<br>A 1<br>T 10.5–12 | | | $\uparrow$ | $\uparrow$ | = MNCV<br>= PTH<br>= Body weight<br>= Well-being |

Modifications in middle molecule serum concentrations evaluated by chromatography.
See table 4–3 for abbreviations.

dialysis for 5 years matched for age, BW, degree of neuropathy, residual renal function, hematocrit, and serum creatinine and urea, is also reported [37]. This result does not contradict the efficiency of short dialysis with respect to the MM. The increase should probably be correlated to dialysis age rather than to the type of hemodialysis treatment.


## Techniques for the separation, isolation, and chemical characterization of middle molecules

Numerous techniques are used to separate and isolate middle molecules, and almost every research group has developed its own separation techniques [25–40]. However, they are for the most part based on the following methodology: deproteinization of the sample, gel-filtration on a Sephadex column and chromatography on an ion exchange resin column. Table 4–12 illustrates the main steps of the method we used to separate and isolate middle molecules.


## Separation and isolation of middle molecules

### Deproteinization of samples

Serum and plasma samples must undergo deproteinization before further examination. In fact, some proteins bind strongly with the Sephadex used for

*Table 4.12.* The method used by our group to separate and isolate middle molecules

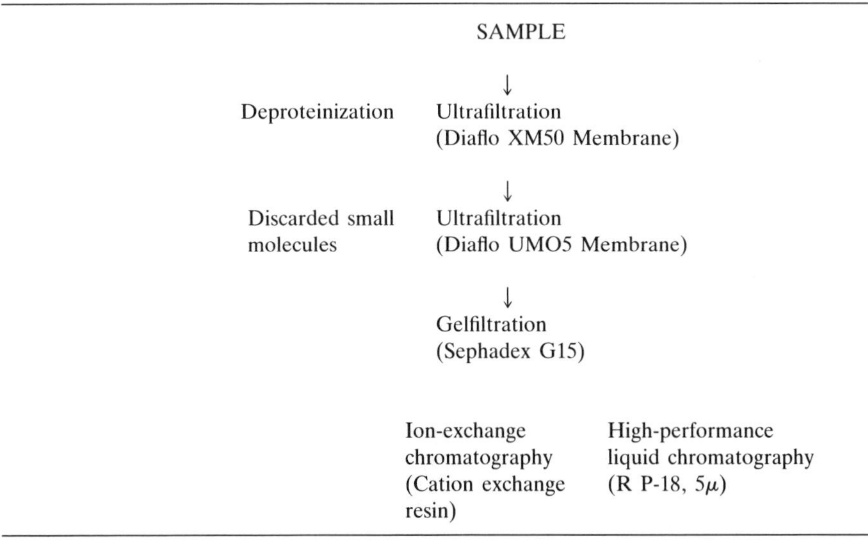

subsequent gel-filtration analyses. This causes a loss in the separating capacity of Sephadex and rapid 'clogging' of the column. Deproteinization with potent acids is not possible because the strong acidification of the sample modifies the Sephadex matrix and chemical structure of some middle molecules. Thus, deproteinization of the samples is for the most part performed by ultrafiltration using membranes with high theoretical cut-off. The most commonly used membranes include: Diaflo UM 10 (cut-off 10,000 D) [37, 89, 100, 244, 248], Diaflo XM 50 (cut-off 50,000 D) membranes [36, 37, 43, 86–88, 90, 184, 244, 248, 249] as well as Centriflo CF 50 (cut-off 50,000 D) [27, 28, 44, 67, 80–83, 85, 250–254], and Centriflo CF 25 (cut-off 25,000 D) [10, 15, 23, 24, 33, 39] membrane cones — all manufactured by Amicon — are most commonly used. Even though they have a high theoretical cut-off, these membranes retain varying percents of substances in the MM weight range. Retention of solutes is a function of their spatial configuration and molecular weight and can be strongly influenced by the pH of the solution in which the substances are dissolved as well as by adsorption phenomena.

Table 4–13 shows the percent retention of three of these membranes for substances with known molecular weights and for a pool of substances with a molecular weight lower than 1,500 isolated from human serum. Ultrafiltration with UM 10 and XM 50 membranes is carried out in 10 ml stirred Amicon cells under positive nitrogen pressure (3 Kg/cm$^2$) while ultrafiltration with CF 50 cones is performed by centrifugation at 3,000 rpm. In all cases, 5 ml of saline solution were added to 5 ml of the sample, and ultrafiltration was carried out until the residual volume was halved. Ultrafiltration was repeated three more times, each time with the addition of 5 ml of saline solution to obtain 20 ml of ultrafiltrate and 5 ml of residual material (244) at the end of the procedure.

*The problem of middle molecule recovery* The deproteinization technique most commonly used consists in ultrafiltration on CF 50 or CF 25 membranes carried out once without washing the residual material. This technique,

*Table 4–13.* Ultrafiltration on deproteinized membranes (Percent retention of substances with known mw)

| Test Substances | mw | % Retention | | |
| --- | --- | --- | --- | --- |
| | | UM10 | XM50 | CF50 |
| Creatinine | 116 | 2 | 1 | 9 |
| K-Iodide | 166 | 3 | 5 | 12 |
| Uric acid | 168 | 2 | 1 | 13 |
| Glutathion | 307 | 28 | 16 | 17 |
| Vit. B$_{12}$ | 1,355 | 59 | 12 | 15 |
| Blue dextran | 2,000,000 | 100 | 100 | 100 |
| Molecules from uremic serum | <1,500 | 33 | 17 | 29 |

Ultrafiltration was repeated 4 times before calculations were made.

preferred for its simplicity and rapidity, causes a remarkable loss of substances of middle molecular weight which, together with the proteins, are retained by the membrane.

The degree of recovery of middle molecular weight substances depends more on the number of ultrafiltrations than on the type of membrane. In the case of ultrafiltration on CF50 membranes, for example, the percent retention of substances with mw 1,500 reaches 64% after 20 minutes of centrifugation and 42% after 90 minutes of centrifugation [244]. Ultrafiltration is not necessary for urine or hemodialysate samples because of their poor protein content.

*Sephadex Column Gel-filtration Chromatography*

Different types of Sephadex columns — G 100, G 75, G 25, G 15, G 10 — are used by various authors [10, 12, 15, 18–21, 23–27, 29–40, 43, 44, 47, 51, 52, 56, 61, 63–67, 70–72, 74, 76, 79, 81–83, 86–99, 101, 105, 107, 123, 226, 228, 244, 247–251, 254–257] to separate substances from the deproteinized samples. Our opinion, shared by other authors, is that the G 15 Sephadex column is most satisfactory for the separation of MM.

The ideal eluant should prevent MM adsorption by the Sephadex matrix, evaporate easily, and thus be completely eliminated by lyophilization. A nonvolatile buffer may render the eluate useless for further analytical studies or biological tests.

The sample which has undergone G 15 Sephadex column chromatography contains all the substances ultrafiltered by the deproteinizing membrane. The graphs obtained include heavy molecules (mw between 2,000 and 50,000 D) and light molecules (mw below 300 D) together with MM (mw between 300 and 2,000 D).

Figure 4–1 illustrates two chromatograms obtained by Sephadex Chromatography of ultrafiltrate using an XM50 membrane: one from 5 ml of normal serum, the other from uremic serum. Middle molecules are eluated in correspondence to peaks 2 and 3, as seen by chromatographic comparison with test substances in the middle molecule weight range [245–247].

Other authors [15, 19, 26, 32, 34, 35, 38, 67, 86, 94] use the same type of Sephadex but different buffers — tris HC1, sodium acetate, ammonium acetate, potassium phosphate — and obviously obtain morphologically different graphs. Of the substances of known middle molecular weight, vitamin $B_{12}$ is considered a reliable middle molecule marker because of its representative weight. Its elution volume is assumed to be that of the MM.

*Advantages and limits of Sephadex G 15 Chromatography* Sephadex G 15 excludes substances with molecular weights above 1,500 and separates only those with molecular weights lower than 1,500. It is thus most likely that all substances with molecular weights between 50,000 (the theoretical cut-off of the deproteinizing XM50 membrane) and 1,500 are excluded from the

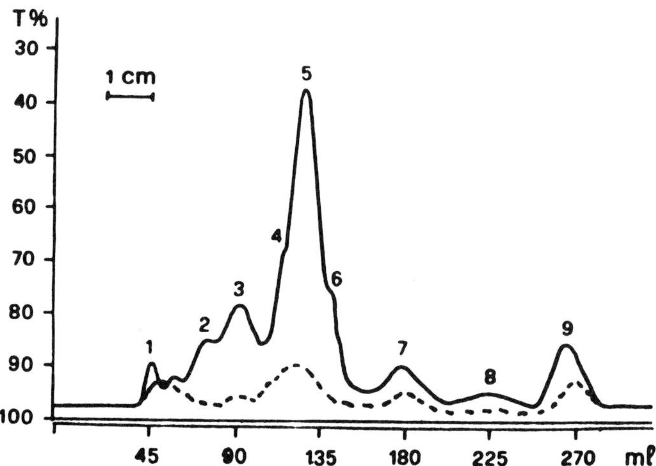


*Figure 4-1.* Chromatography of ultrafiltered normal (− − −) and uremic (________) serum from XM50 membrane. Column: Sephadex G 15, 26 × 500 mm. Flow rate: 0.75 ml/min. Temperature: ambient. Detector: 254 nm. Eluent: 0.02 M, $NH_4HCO_3$, pH 7.5. Sample: Deproteinized serum. Injection volume: 5 ml. Paper speed: 2 cm/hr.

Sephadex particles and are quickly eluted together in a single well-separated peak. Substances with molecular weights lower than 1,500 are retained in the gel matrix and subsequently eluted. Thus, the peaks (except for the first) of the chromatograms in figure 4-1 correspond to substances with mw lower than 1,500 eluted from the column with different retention times.

However, this resin limits analysis to the middle molecules with a molecular weight below 1,500 and excludes the MM with molecular weights between 1,500 and 2,000. Gel-filtration chromatography has another drawback: substances that have undergone chromatography are not always eluted with a buffer volume inversely proportional to their molecular weight [15, 18, 42, 72, 123, 244, 248, 257−260]. That is, certain substances are eluted with a buffer volume different from the volume expected on the basis of their molecular weight, due to physical-chemical absorption phenomena and ion exclusion.

If the substances tested had been eluted with a buffer volume inversely proportionate to their molecular weight, they would have been distributed in succession between the blue dextran (which is excluded by the Sephadex matrix) and the acetone (which completely penetrates the Sephadex matrix) with a Kav (elution volume corrected for the column volume used) which increases as the mw of the substances examined decreases. Figure 4-2 illustrates clearly that substances with a higher molecular weight can be eluted after substances with a lower mw and vice versa, as well as the fact that substances with different molecular weights can have equal elution volumes. For this reason, the 7C fraction of Furst and associates [19, 27, 250] and the neurotoxic fraction of Funck-Bretano and associates [26], to which a mw of 1,000−2,000 is attributed on the basis of elution volume, both contain

84

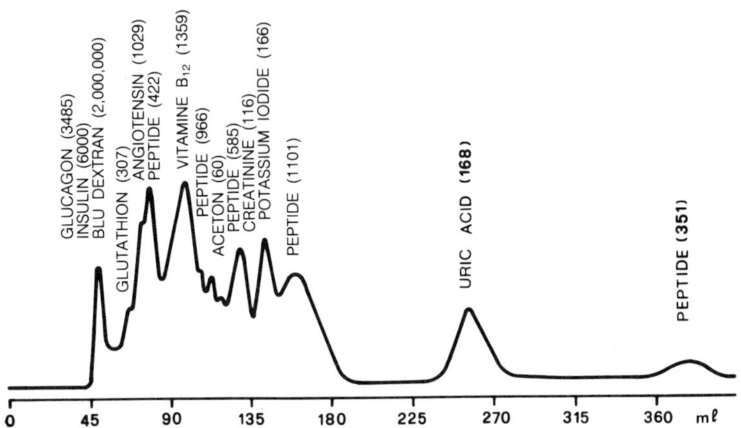



*Figure 4–2.* Eluation volume of the single test substances from Sephadex column (2.6 × 50 cm.). The eluant used is 0.02 M, NH$_4$HCO$_3$, pH 8, flow rate 0.75 ml/min. The eluate is recorded at a wave-length of 254 nm. The amino acid compositions of various peptides are reported in table 4–14.

substances which have a mw notably lower when analyzed chemically: 371 [226, 227] and about 500 [18, 31, 72], respectively. On the other hand, the possibility that MM are eluated in peak 1 must be taken into consideration.

There is no precise correlation between elution volumes and mw of substances even when G–25 gelfiltration [32, 123], Biogel P$_2$ [123], or high-pressure chromatography on TSK-gel 2000 SW [28] are used in place of gelchromatography on a Sephadex G 15 column.

One particular problem is the presence of free aminoacids in samples undergoing G 15 gel-filtration. Although their molecular weights are in the range of 75–204, the Kav of each aminoacid is extremely different (from 0.21 to 1.65); thus, some of them are eluated together with the small molecules and others with the middle molecules [20, 257]. Amino acid concentrations of the samples examined are not usually high enough to influence significantly the Sephadex chromatography graphs. Nevertheless, they should be kept in mind when concentrated samples or samples with high amino acid concentrations are examined, or when extremely sensitive separation and isolation techniques able to detect amino acids are used [256].

None of the fractions obtained by Sephadex gelchromatography can be considered to consist entirely of MM on the basis of Kav alone. Reports in which a clinically significant toxic effect is attributed to a fraction said to contain only MM should be regarded with extreme caution.

*The problem of molecules with a low molecular weight (below 3,00 D): use of the Diaflo UM 05 membrane*

Sephadex G 15 chromatographs of the ultrafiltrate from deproteinizing membranes are contaminated by substances with a molecular weight below

85

300 D which, by definition, are not middle molecules. As reported above, the separating capacities of Sephadex G 15 are such that the peaks corresponding to these substances and those corresponding to the MM are not identifiable with certainty in chromatograms on the basis of their elution volume. Substances with low molecular weights could be eluated with elution volumes so low that the corresponding peaks could be interpreted as consisting of MM, and the MM could eluate with an elution volume so high that the corresponding peaks could be interpreted as consisting of substances with low molecular weights. Moreover, two substances, one with a molecular weight above 300 and the other with a mw below 300 could eluate with the same elution volume in the same peak: the peak's height and morphology could thus be due to the mixing of the two substances [42, 244, 248, 257].

A Diaflo UM 05 membrane is used to avoid these problems and obtain a chromatogram consisting entirely of MM [25, 34, 37, 40, 58, 64, 89, 92, 93, 97, 244, 248, 259, 261]. The permeability of this membrane, with a theoretical cut-off of 500 D, was measured in tests using substances of known molecular weights [244, 248, 259]. With the exception of amino acids, the membrane provided for nearly total ultrafiltration of substances with a mw below 200 (less than 10% retention of these substances) as well as a percent retention of substances with mw above 300 which increased together with their mw. Although the correlation is not perfectly linear, it is certainly an improvement over the correlation between Kav and molecular weight of the same substances (table 4–14).

*Table 4–14.* Ultrafiltration of Diaflo UM05 membrane (percent retention with known mw.)

| Tested Substances | MW | Kav | % Ret Diaflo UM05 Membrane |
|---|---|---|---|
| Aminoacid solution | 75–204 | 0.21–1.65 | 7–29 |
| Acetone | 59 | 0.46 | 2 |
| Creatinine | 116 | 0.62 | 6 |
| Potassium iodide | 166 | 0.82 | 6 |
| Uric acid | 168 | 1.65 | 1 |
| Glutathion | 307 | 0.16 | 40 |
| PHE-TRY | 351 | 2.49 | 34 |
| LYS-PHE-LYS-2 ACETATE | 422 | 0.22 | 47 |
| TYR-D.ALA-GLY-PHE-D-LEU | 585 | 0.49 | 46 |
| PRO-GLN-GLN-PHE-GLY-LEU-MET-NH$_2$ | 966 | 0.42 | 49 |
| TRY-PRO-ARG-PRO-GLN-ILE-PRO-PRO | 1,101 | 0.87 | 52 |
| Angiotensin 1 | 1,200 | 0.21 | 59 |
| Vitamin B$_{12}$ | 1,355 | 0.32 | 82 |
| Glucagon | 3,485 | 0.0 | 100 |
| Insulin | 6,000 | 0.0 | 100 |
| Blue dextran | 2,000,000 | 0.0 | 100 |

Ultrafiltration was repeated 4 times before calculations were made. 8.5% aminoacid solution (Freamine III, Baxter): Ileu, Leu, Lys, Phe, Thr, Try, Val, Ala, Arg, His, Pro, Ser, Cysh.

Other authors have reached similar conclusions using different types of membranes (cellulose acetate or PSAC Millipore) [18, 31].

The percent retentions of the UM 05 membrane expressed in table 4–14 were calculated after 4 ultrafiltrations (as in the case of deproteinized membranes). The concentration of the test substances in each of the 4 ultrafiltrates demonstrated that substances with mw below 200 and those with mw above 300 are ultrafiltered in a characteristically different way. After each ultrafiltration, the concentration of substances with mw below 200 is halved, while the concentration of substances with high mw remains fairly constant [244, 248].

As shown in figure 4–3, the height of single peaks in the chromatograms of the UM 05 residual and ultrafiltered material depends on UM 05 membrane permeability to substances present in the corresponding peaks of the XM 50 chromatogram. If we compare the percent retention of the single peaks (table 4–15) with those of the test substances (table 4–14), we note that the low retention values (below 10%) of peaks 5, 8, and 9 indicate the presence of molecules with mw lower than 200, that the high retention index (above 50%) of peaks 2, 3, and 4 attests to the presence of substances with mw above 300

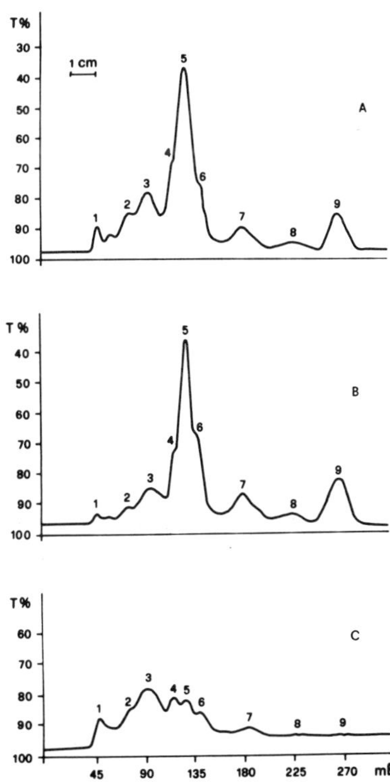


*Figure 4–3.* Chromatograms from gelfiltration of 5 ml uremic serum on Sephadex G15 column. (A) XM50 ultrafiltrate; (B) UM05 ultrafiltrate; (C) UM05 residual. UM05 ultrafiltrate and residual materials were obtained from ultrafiltration of XM50 ultrafiltrate.

87

*Table 4–15.*

| Peak No. | Residual Material Kav | Ultrafiltrate Kav | % Retention UM05 |
|---|---|---|---|
| 2 | 0.19 ± 0.03 | 0.19 ± 0.02 | 56 ± 8 |
| 3 | 0.32 ± 0.09 | 0.36 ± 0.08 | 55 ± 7 |
| 4 | 0.50 ± 0.03 | 0.50 ± 0.04 | 51 ± 6 |
| 5 | 0.60 ± 0.03 | 0.59 ± 0.03 | 5 ± 0.4 |
| 6 | 0.70 ± 0.05 | 0.68 ± 0.05 | 37 ± 6 |
| 7 | 0.89 ± 0.06 | 0.89 ± 0.09 | 17 ± 6 |
| 8 | 1.29 ± 0.03 | 1.33 ± 0.07 | 5 ± 0.1 |
| 9 | 1.55 ± 0.04 | 1.62 ± 0.08 | 3 ± 0.2 |

Residual and ultrafiltrated material peaks are identified on the basis of their respective Kavs. The percent retention of the UM05 Diaflo membrane for the single corresponding peaks is calculated. Evaluation was carried out on 15 uremic patients in hemodialysis.

(thus in the MM range), and finally that the intermediate retention range (37–17%) of peaks 6 and 7 leads to the speculation that substances with mw between 200 and 300 are present.

Chemical analysis confirms that small molecules such as urea and creatinine are eluated in peak 5 and that uric acid is eluated in peak 9.

Variations in the height of single peaks after each ultrafiltration make it possible to evaluate how the substances contained in single peaks are ultrafiltered across the UM 05 membrane. While the substances contained in peaks 5, 8, and 9 behave like test substances with mw below 200, and an almost linear reduction of their concentration at each ultrafiltration, the substances contained in peaks 2, 3, and 4 behave like test substances with mw above 300: in fact, their concentrations are similar in each of the four ultrafiltrations. Peaks 6 and 7 show a modest reduction which is consonant with their intermediate mw [244, 248, 259, 260].

*Advantages and limits of Diaflo UM 05 membranes* One advantage of UM 05 membranes is that the residual material of this membrane furnishes a chromatogram whose peaks are made up for the most part of MM. Moreover, as we have pointed out for deproteinizing membranes, ultrafiltration of the substances with a UM 05 membrane depends not only on their weight but also on their molecular configuration, on the pH of the solution in which they are dissolved and on adsorption phenomena: thus, we cannot be certain that all substances with a mw below 200 have a retention of below 10%. This is certainly the case for some amino acids. The UM 05 membrane in our experimental conditions retains 7% of some amino acids, but 39% of others, although all of them have a molecular weight below 204 D. The presence of amino acids in the samples is a serious problem when extremely sensitive separation and isolation methods are used or when the chemical composition of the single middle molecules is studied. Even though total elimination of amino acids would be ideal, their partial elimination from the samples is still an advantage. It should, however, be emphasized that some authors [123] maintain that the UM 05 membrane is nearly impermeable to amino acids. Results so different from ours are probably due to the different ultrafiltration methods used as well as the different pH of the solutions.

Data regarding UM 05 membrane permeability were obtained (except for the aminoacid solution) by subjecting each single substance to ultrafiltration. Thus, we cannot rule out that the same substance dissolved in serum or other organic fluids present percent retention values different from those we have reported.

One disadvantage is represented, instead, by the loss of MM when the UM 05 membrane is used. The loss is difficult to quantify because a lowering of the peak after UM 05 ultrafiltration may be in part due to MM passage across the membrane and in part to the elimination of substances with mw lower than 200 which eluate from the column together with the MM. This possibility could justify the relatively low percent retention values of substances contained in the peaks unquestionably representing MM.

*Ion exchange resin column chromatography*

The Sephadex G 15 eluate can be collected with a fraction collector. In this way, fractions thought to contain MM can be isolated and subjected to further analyses after they are lyophilized and resuspended. Ion exchange resin column chromatography is the most common analysis carried out to further separate substances contained in the fractions isolated by Sephadex G 15. This separation is based on the ionic charge and not the mw of the substances undergoing chromatography. The most commonly used ion exchange resins are Sephadex DEAE A 25 [10, 15, 18, 19, 21, 23, 24, 26, 27, 31, 33, 35, 39, 44, 51, 52, 63, 65, 67, 72, 77, 81, 88, 89, 101, 104, 105, 107, 226, 227, 250, 251, 254] and Dowex 50 [30, 32, 60, 98, 228, 262].

Figure 4–4 shows the graphs we obtained with ion exchange chromatography of Sephadex fractions 2 and 3. The eluate from this column was detected after ninhydrine reaction [37, 248].

*Advantages and Limits of Ion Exchange Chromatography* Our graphs demonstrate the presence of numerous ninhydrine-positive substances in fractions 2 and 3 isolated by gel-filtration (figure 4–4). Some of these (also present in normal subjects) are increased in patients with renal failure; others are seen only in uremic patients. Of the techniques in use, ours seems most able to separate and isolate peptide substances. Ninhydrine, in fact, is an elective colorant of the $NH_2$ terminal radicals and permits easy identification of peptide substances. This seems to be particularly important because the probability of a biological effect is much higher for peptides than for other substances. The chief limit of ion exchange chromatography, no matter what ion-exchange resin is used, is its modest resolution capacity. Moreover, our

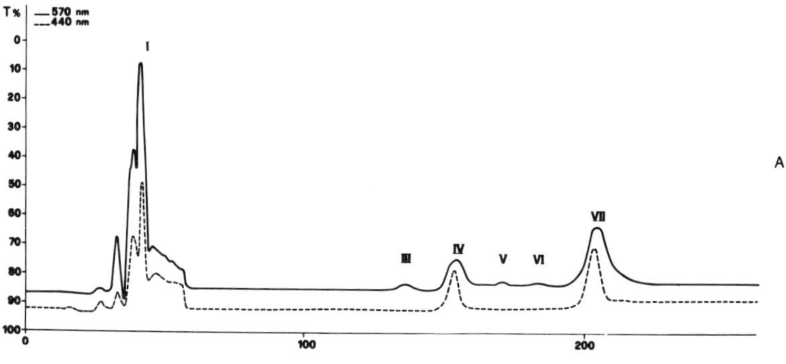
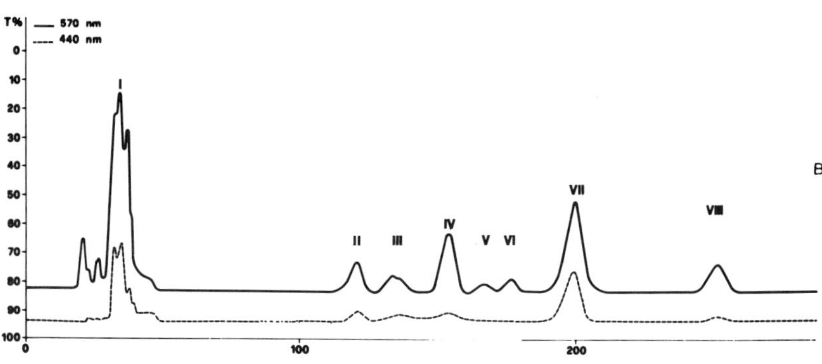
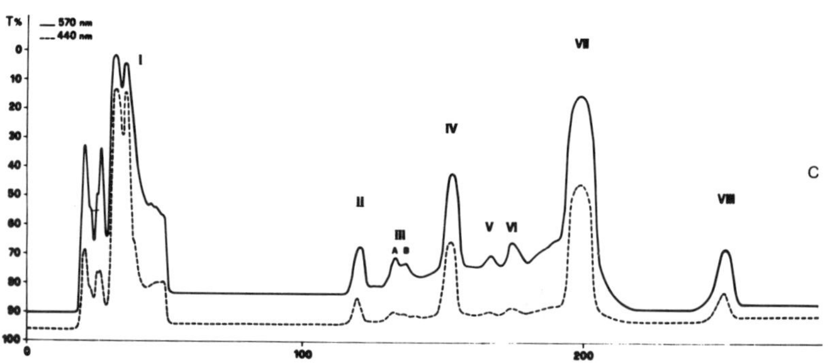

*Figure 4–4.* Ion exchange chromatography of G15 Sephadex Fractions 2 and 3. (A) Normal serum; (B) Uremic serum (conservative treatment); (C) Uremic serum (haemodialysis for 10 years). Column: 4% cross-linking cation exchange resin (M47 Beckman) $9 \times 580$ mm. Flow rate: 1 ml/min. Temperature: 50°C. Detector: 570–440 nm. Eluent: (A) 0.1 M Piridin Acetic Acid pH 3.5, (B) 2.0 M Piridin Acetic Acid pH 5.0. Program: Linear gradient from 0 to 100% B in 240 min. Sample: See text. Injection volume: 1 ml. Paper speed: 1 cm/m'.

90

technique presents some difficulties in execution and requires an aminoacid analyser.

*Other MM Separation and Isolation Techniques*

Numerous other techniques, substituting or combined with ion exchange chromatography, have been utilized to obtain better MM separation and purer MM. These techniques include paper electrophoresis [30, 104, 105, 226, 227], paper chromatography [18, 25, 31, 35, 56, 58, 72, 76, 104, 105, 228, 262], thin-layer chromatography [18, 26, 29, 31, 36, 51, 52, 72, 86–88, 102, 249], high-voltage electrophoresis [77, 102], high pressure liquid chromatography [28, 33, 85, 107, 123, 252, 253, 256, 257], isotacophoresis [21, 226, 227, 257], gas-chromatography [257], and mass spectrometry [258]. These studies have demonstrated that the number of MM present in the serum of normal and uremic subjects is much higher that what was supposed.

At present, in our laboratory, HPLC (high performance liquid chromatography) follows gel-filtration. Figure 4–5 includes two graphs obtained by reversed phase chromatography of normal serum and uremic serum. The fractions eluated from the sephadex G 15 column were lyophylized after removal of the fraction with mw above 1,500, corresponding to the first peak. They were then resuspended in distilled water to a volume of 5 ml, and HPLC was carried out. Other authors [256], utilizing columns with the same stationary phase but a different mobile phase, have separated up to 100 MM from the dialysis ultrafiltrate.

## Chemical characteristics of the middle molecules

Particular attention has been paid to MM of protein nature because it is known that fragments of proteins and protein hormones maintain the same biological activity as that of whole molecules, and because there is increased serum accumulation of these substances as kidney function diminishes.

Various authors report the aminoacid composition of peptides in the MM weight range [25, 26, 37, 44, 56, 58, 65, 67, 77, 95, 102, 104, 228, 248, 256]. Abiko and associates have defined the amino acid sequence of two peptides, one of 7 aminoacids and the other of 5: the first corresponds to a fragment of Beta-2-microglobulin [25], and the second to a fragment of fibrinogen [58]. Their research supports the hypothesis that intermediate catabolites of normal protein metabolism are accumulated in uremic patients.

Attention has recently been drawn to nonprotein substances which are eluated in the middle-molecular fraction. Two carbohydrates have been isolated by two groups and recognized as glycuro-conjugates [18, 41, 52, 72, 226, 227]. After isotacophoresis, these two glycuro-conjugates show the same thermal mobility, but are different on the basis of 254 nm UV detection.

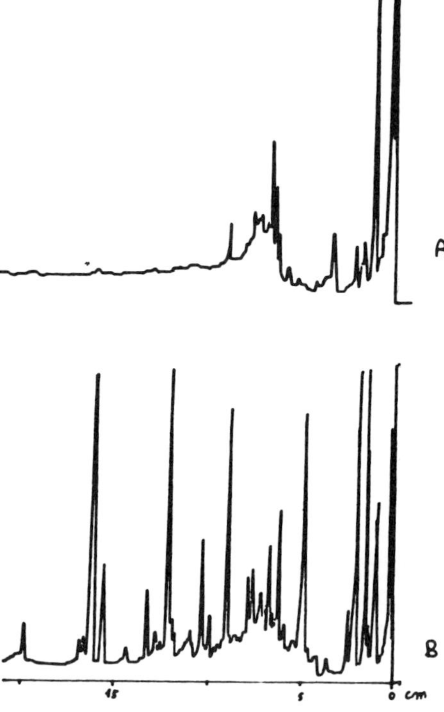

*Figure 4–5.* High performance liquid chromatography. Graphic representation of serum fractions after removal of substances with m.w. > 1500. (A) Normal serum; (B) Uremic serum. Column: Ultrasphere — ODS 4.6 × 150 mm. Stationary phase: RP — 18.5 $\mu$. Precolumn: 4.6 × 35 mm, RP — 18.5 $\mu$. Pressure: 1.20 K psi. Flow rate: 1.0 ml/min. Temperature: ambient. Detector: UV 254 nm. Sensitivity: 0.050 A UFS. Eluent: (A) water, 0.1 M NaCl $O_4$ + 0.07% $H_3PO_4$ (B) $CH_3CN$, 0.1 M NaCl $O_4$ + 0.07% $H_3PO_4$. Program: linear gradient from 0 to 15% B in 40 min. Sample: Preparation: see text. Injection volume: 100 $\mu$l. Paper speed: 0.5 cm/min.

*Problems in Chemical Characterization* It is striking that in chemical studies of MM, a substance with the same chemical composition has rarely been isolated in more than one laboratory. Only two peptides isolated by our group [248] have, at least in terms of amino acid composition, resulted identical to two peptides isolated by other authors [26, 77]: Dzurik's ninth [77] and one of Funck-Brentano's [26], respectively. Reasons for this discrepancy might be that either the fractions from which the substances examined were different, or different substances of the same fractions were examined. Both possibilities seem to be well founded. Preparative and analytical analyses vary so much among different laboratories that fractions thought to be corresponding can contain substances which are, in fact, different. On the other hand, numerous substances are contained in the same fraction. Moreover, given the complexity of these studies, they have been limited to determining the chemical composition only once and in a single patient. Thus, doubts about

92

reproducibility arise, and discrepancies might be attributed not only to the different methods used but also to differences in the subjects examined.


**Serum concentrations and dialysis extraction of middle molecules**

When dialysis efficiency is evaluated, predialysis and postdialysis serum MM concentrations (intradialysis extraction) as well as the predialysis serum MM concentration (interdialysis variation) must be taken into consideration. Dialysis treatment could in theory induce high intradialysis MM extraction and no interdialysis variations. If MM toxicity is assumed, dialysis should be able to reduce not only postdialysis but also predialysis MM concentrations.


**In vitro and in vivo intradialysis middle molecule extraction**

The in vitro dialysis clearance of a substance depends on its mw and chemical structure as well as the physical-chemical characteristics of the dialysis membrane, when dialysis time, blood, and dialysate flow and ultrafiltration rate are unchanged [5, 68, 263]. In vitro polyacrylonitrile is significantly more permeable to vitamin $B_{12}$ than cuprophane [68, 204], and increased cuprophane thickness (from 11 to 18 $\mu$) generally causes a 31–36% reduction in clearance of substances with mw in the MM range (630–1,355) [263].

In vivo chromatographic measurements of MM dialysis clearance have furnished different results. These studies emphasize the error in attributing the same clearance in vivo to dializers studied in vitro [222], and lead to the conclusion that cuprophane and polyacrylonitrile have clearances that are not statistically different when Qb, Qd, dialysis surface area, dialysis time, and ultrafiltration rate are the same [53].

Hemodialysis with (1) different membranes (cuprophane and polyacrylonitrile), (2) different surface areas (from 1.0 to 2.5 m$^2$), (3) different membrane thicknesses (from 13.5 $\mu$ to 35 $\mu$) determines an equal postdialysis reduction (about 40%) of predialysis MM values, when other dialysis parameters are unchanged [22, 53, 219, 222, 264–267].

Deficient in vivo extraction of MM with membranes such as polyacrylonitrile, which in vitro is significantly more permeable to vitamin $B_{12}$ than cuprophane, might depend on the fact that it is electrically charged and can therefore interact with the MM [53], while the uniformity of dialyzers with different dialysis surface areas and membrane thickness might be due to stratification of proteins and leukocytes on the membranes which can nullify the different in vitro dialysis efficiency of the filters [222]. Moreover, the same dialysis extraction with different filters can be explained if the MM have an in vivo mw about half or less than what has been supposed. In this case, the use of more permeable membranes such as polyacrylonitrile or filters with dialysing surfaces larger than 1m$^2$ would not have significant advantages, inasmuch as MM extraction is probably already at its maximum with $1m^2$ cuprophane membranes [53, 219, 222, 225].

*Extraction indexes: actual and apparent*

Another datum stemming from filter permeability studies is that membranes having different thicknesses or chemical structures (with dialysis time and dialysate and blood flow rate being equal) have a higher in vitro clearance for small molecules than for MM, while in vivo, predialysis and postdialysis percent variations of serum urea, serum creatinine, and MM are not statistically different [53, 219]. Two explanations are possible: either the MM are extracted from a compartment which is much smaller than that of the small molecules, or the MM have a much lower intradialysis generation rate than the small molecules. It seems more likely that the MM have a bicompartmental or pluricompartmental kinetics, for example, intra/extracellular with strong resistance at the cell membrane level, rather than a low generation rate. In this case, percent removal of MM from their small distribution volume, despite low membrane efficiency, would take place in the same way as that of the small molecules which have a much larger distribution volume but also a higher facility of passage across membranes of the same filters. The different results obtained in MM extraction measurements using different calculation methods seem to substantiate this hypothesis. If, in fact, MM and urea extraction is evaluated as a percent variation of predialysis and postdialysis plasma concentrations (apparent extraction), statistically significant differences between small and middle molecules are not seen. When, instead, MM and urea extraction are calculated in the dialysate (actual extraction) significant differences are seen. Our studies of three substitutive treatments, short hemodialysis, hemofiltration, and hypertonic hemodiafiltration [265–267] established that actual extractions are different, despite similar 'apparent' extractions of middle and small molecules (table 4–16).

## Interdialysis variations of middle molecules

A great deal of literature demonstrates MM toxicity in vitro (table 4–1), but even now, clinical demonstration of toxicity does not exist. This proof has long been sought in clinical conditions or laboratory data of patients in different hemodialytic treatments that would determine, at least theoretically, an increase or reduction in MM plasma concentrations [6, 47, 62, 70, 197–199, 200–206, 208–211, 217, 229–234, 239]. These studies indicate that the use of elaborate mathematical models to establish how much, in theory, MM plasma concentrations are modified should not be accepted unless corroborated by direct measurements of MM.

The need to measure predialysis MM serum concentrations during a given hemodialysis treatment seems to be substantiated by studies involving MM

94

*Table 4–16.* Actual and apparent extraction index in short dialysis (HD), hemofiltration (HF), and hypertonic hemodiafiltration (HH)

| | Middle Molecules | | Urea | |
| --- | --- | --- | --- | --- |
| | Actual | Apparent | Actual | Apparent |
| HD | 29 ± 4 | 55 ± 5 | 51 ± 3 | 60 ± 8 |
| HF | 37 ± 1 | 68 ± 6 | 49 ± 9 | 53 ± 6 |
| HH | 52 ± 5 | 66 ± 6 | 56 ± 5 | 66 ± 5 |

The reported data were calculated for 4 patients and expressed as average ± SD.

$$\text{Actual Extraction Index} = \frac{\text{Extracted Pool}}{\text{Predialysis Pool}} \times 100$$

$$\text{Apparent Extraction Index} = \frac{\text{Predialysis-Postdialysis Pool}}{\text{Predialysis Pool}} \times 100$$

Extracted Pool = dialysis fluid concentration × dialysis fluid volume

Predialysis Pool = Predialysis Serum Concentration × Total Body Water
Postdialysis Pool = Postdialysis Serum Concentration × Total Body Water
Total Body Water = Dry body weight × 0.6 + (Actual Body Weight − Dry Body Weight)
Dry Weight = Lowest Postdialysis weight without hypotension.

measurements of patients in short dialysis treatment (table 4–11). Patients in short dialysis showed a modest and not constant increase in MM, although a notable increase in MM was expected on the basis of theoretical calculations [175, 198, 266]. Unpredictable variations in MM concentrations have been evidenced by Gotch [222]: the same group of patients underwent dialysis treatment with different dialysis membranes (1.3 versus 2.5 versus 1.3m$^2$) (all other dialytic parameters remained unchanged) for successive periods of 6 months each, without significant variations, at least in the MM group evaluated. It thus is probable that discordant results regarding the clinical effects of MM stem from attributing to different hemodialysis schedules a capacity to modify predialysis MM serum concentrations which, in reality, they did not have.

### Hemofiltration: A substitutive treatment able to reduce predialysis MM serum concentrations

To evaluate MM toxicity, predialysis MM plasma concentrations must not only be significantly modified but these variations must also be maintained for a time period sufficiently long to permit possible clinical or laboratory changes.

A substitutive treatment utilizing highly permeable membranes and convective rather than diffusive force is likely to determine maximum intradialytic and interdialytic variation in the MM pool.

95

Hemofiltration differs from traditional hemodialysis substantially in the large quantities of liquids that are infused and ultrafiltered. It is sustained that a high degree of ultrafiltration promotes a particularly efficient reduction in high molecular weight solutes that are more sensitive to convective force than to diffusion, thus determining a higher MM extraction than in hemodialysis. It is also possible that MM extraction is effected directly from the cell because of the high quantity of infused liquids reducing resistance of MM passage across the cell membrane.

Hemofiltration (HF) should thus bring about a real depletion of MM. Although noteworthy clinical improvement has been reported with hemofiltration and attributed to high MM extraction, there are as yet no long-term studies that quantify the total body pool and extraction index of MM.

## Some personal observations

We evaluated total body pool and actual extraction of the MM in 5 patients in short dialysis and after 3–5 (average 4.5) months and 11–15 (average 13) months of hemofiltration on line.

M.M. concentrations were measured in the serum, dialysate, and hemofiltrate. Dialysate volume varied from 110 to 140 liters; hemofiltrate varied from 33 to 39 liters. All data are reported as averages of two separate samples taken one week apart.

The method used to identify and isolate MM has been previously described. Gel-chromatography was used to measure MM pool concentrations from serum and dialysate. Except for the first peak eluated, the sum of the areas of the peaks was considered as the MM concentration of the sample examined and expressed in $cm^2$. On the basis of MM concentrations in the serum, dialysate, and hemofiltrate, it was possible to calculate the predialytic body and extracted MM pools in hemodialysis and hemofiltration.

High pressure liquid chromatography (HPLC) was used to measure quantitative and qualitative modifications of the MM pattern seen in different substitutive treatments. The HPLC apparatus was connected to a Hewlett Packard 3390A peak recorder able to furnish the elution time and peak area. Peaks eluated from the HPLC of different samples obtained from the serum of the same patient and from different patients were considered corresponding or not on the basis of elution time and peak morphology.

*Predialysis MM body pool in hemodialysis and in hemofiltration*

Hemofiltration can significantly reduce concentrations of the predialysis MM pool found in short dialysis. In table 4–17, we report percent values of the MM pool of each patient after 3–5 months and after 11–15 months of hemofiltration with respect to the MM pool found in short dialysis, set at 100.

Reported in figure 4–6 are the average variations of the predialysis MM

*Table 4–17.* Percent variations of MM pool observed after different time periods (3–5 and 11–15 months) of hemofiltration with respect to the MM pool found in short dialysis (set at 100)

| Patients | Short Dialysis | Hemofiltration | |
|---|---|---|---|
| | | 3–5 ms. | 11–15 ms. |
| C.V. | 100 | 82.3 | 92.5 |
| B.C. | 100 | 54.2 | 63.0 |
| C.B. | 100 | 52.6 | 50.6 |
| M.N. | 100 | 74.9 | 103.0 |
| G.A. | 100 | 48.8 | 63.0 |

Predialysis Pool = see table 4–16.

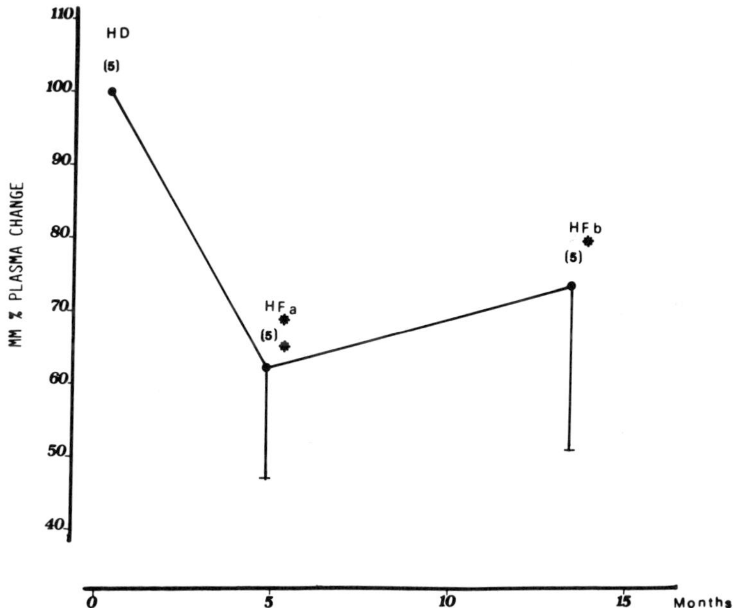


*Figure 4–6.* Average variations in the predialysis MM pool. Predialysis pool: see table 4–16. Hemodialysis = 100%. Hemofiltration 'a' = 63% ± 15 (after 3–5 months). Hemofiltration 'b' = 74% ± 22 (after 11–15 months). Statistical significance was calculated between hemodialysis and hemofiltration 'a' (**), between hemodialysis and hemofiltration 'b' (*), and between hemofiltration 'a' and hemofiltration 'b' (*) with the student's t test for paired data. ** $p < 0.005$. * $p < 0.05$.

pool in hemofiltration with respect to hemodialysis and the degree of significance of the variations brought about by the two substitutive treatments. After 11–15 months of hemofiltration, the MM pool, though significantly lower than the pool in hemodialysis, increases significantly with respect to the MM pool seen after 3–5 months of hemofiltration.

Reported in table 4–18 are the values of the actual MM extraction index in single patients in hemodialysis and after 3–5 months and 11–15 months in hemofiltration. Except for one case, MM extraction is always higher in hemofiltration than in short dialysis.

The average values of the Extraction Index in hemodialysis and hemofiltration are represented graphically in figure 4–7.

*Qualitative and quantitative changes in the MM pattern brought about by the two substitutive treatments* Figures 4–6 and 4–7 show that after 11–15 months of hemofiltration, the body pool increases and the extraction index decreases with respect to values found after 3–5 months. On the basis of these data, it is tempting to speculate that increased generation of some MM or the appearance of new MM not totally removable by hemofiltration might take place.

The results indicated in figure 4–8 seem to substantiate both hypotheses: although the MM concentrations of single patients are highly variable, 6 peaks have average higher serum concentrations in hemofiltration than in hemodialysis, while 7 peaks not present in hemodialysis appear in hemofiltration. The appearance of some for the first time and the increase of others leads to the consideration that hemofiltration not only passivly influences the MM pool through more efficient removal but also determines profound modifications in the metabolism of these solutes.

The hypothesis could be made that MM removal through hemofiltration alters the equilibrium established in hemodialysis through the increased production of different metabolites which are probably representative of catabolic steps different from those that generate the MM found in hemodialysis.

In conclusion, (1) hemofiltration significantly reduces the predialysis MM serum pool found in hemodialysis; (2) hemofiltration has a higher extraction index than hemodialysis; (3) MM depletion induced by hemofiltration, however, involves the accumulation of new substances in the MM weight

*Table 4–18.* Actual MM extraction indexes observed after different time periods (3–5 and 11–15 months) of hemofiltration and in short dialysis

| Patients | Short Dialysis | Hemofiltration | |
|---|---|---|---|
| | | *3–5 ms.* | *11–15 ms.* |
| C.V. | 40.4 | 50 | 47.6 |
| B.C. | 26.5 | / | 41.7 |
| C.B. | 41.9 | 44.7 | 38.2 |
| M.N. | 35.4 | 42.6 | 36.0 |
| G.A. | 24.6 | 52.6 | 51.7 |

Actual Extraction Index = See table 4–16.

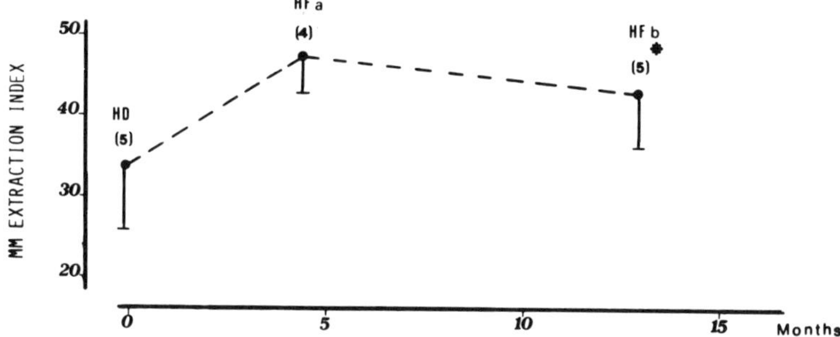

*Figure 4–7.* Average values of the actual extraction index in short dialysis and hemofiltration: Hemodialysis = 34 ± 7. Hemofiltration 'a' = 47 ± 4 (after 3–5 months). Hemofiltration 'b' = 43 ± 6 (after 11–15 months). Statistical significance was calculated between hemodialysis and hemofiltration 'a,' between hemodialysis and hemofiltration 'b,' and between hemofiltration 'a' and hemofiltration 'b' (*) with the Student's t test for paired data. (*) p < 0.05. Actual extraction index: see ABle 4–16.

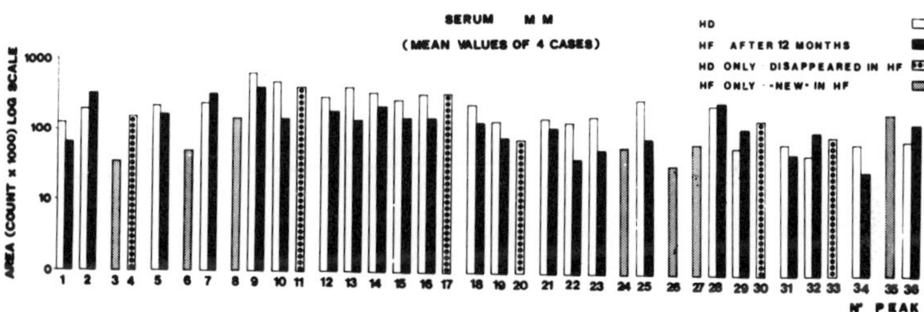

*Figure 4–8.* This figure is a graphic representation of the serum concentrations of 36 MM obtained by HPLC of the MM pool isolated with gel-chromatography from the serum of patients in short dialysis and after 11–15 months in hemofiltration. Seven peaks [▨] (peaks 3, 6, 8, 24, 26, 27, 35) not present in serum in hemodialysis appear ex novo in hemofiltration; six peaks [●●●] (peaks 4, 11, 17, 20, 30, 33) present in serum in hemodialysis are not seen in hemofiltration. Of the remaining 23 peaks [■] [□] , six (peaks 2, 7, 28, 29, 32, 36) have higher serum concentrations in hemofiltration than in hemodialysis, and 17 have higher concentrations in hemodialysis than in hemofiltration.

range not detected in the serum of patients in hemodialysis; (4) the fact that MM can be generated 'during' dialysis treatment raises several questions about the correlation between MM synthesis and biocompatibility of membranes.

## Conclusions

After 15 years of study, the fact that in vivo MM toxicity has yet to be demonstrated has led to doubts about the MM hypothesis itself as well as attempts to find an alternative clinical significance to the MM.

Not all authors agree that the MM are toxic or responsible for the uremic

99

syndrome [214]. Some affirm that these substances are nontoxic catabolites, and that clinical condition depends more on the careful control of calcium, phosphorus, blood pressure, and the hydro-electrolyte balance than on MM [268, 269]. Others hypothesize that in uremic patients, hormonal substances are produced and accumulated in greater quantities to maintain balances upset by reduced renal function (the 'trade-off' hypothesis). High concentrations of these substances would be the expression of metabolic adaptations of the organism to renal failure, and would have the principal function of maintaining homeostasis. Toxic effects would be only secondary manifestations.

Parathormone, or rather, its biologically active fragments, could be one of these substances. Their increase as renal function decreases maintains phosphatemia within normal limits, reducing tubular reabsorption of phosphates in the surviving nephrons. However, the trade-off for the maintenance of phosphate balance is osteodystrophy. Another substance which maintains an otherwise compromised sodium balance in the uremic patient might be the natriuretic factor [94, 95]. The existence of this factor has long been suspected on the basis of clinical and experimental studies [270–272]. It can probably be identified as the atrial natriuretic factor or its active fragments of 26 [273] and 28 amino acids [274, 275] recently isolated.

There is some justification for the slow progress and uncertain results in MM studies. It was hoped that one or a few easily identifiable substances in the MM mw range could substitute urea and creatinine as more reliable indicators of clinical condition in renal failure. With advances in MM studies, however, an enormous number of substances (all of which were theoretically toxic) was found, and consequently, notable problems of separation, isolation, identification, and, above all, standardization arose.

It was expected that predialysis MM concentrations could be easily modified by varying dialysis parameters and filter membranes, and that the etiological relationship between MM and dialysis complications could therefore be easily demonstrated. The difficulty of modifying predialysis MM concentrations became evident together with the fact that dialysis schedules maintain substantially constant MM serum concentrations.

Although MNCV seemed to be an accurate index for establishing MM toxicity and clinical effects of different hemodialysis treatments, the meaning of the MNCV variations reported was almost always difficult to comprehend. In some cases, patient follow-up continued for less than six months: it has been demonstrated that variations in MNCV can take place after prolonged periods (even a year) [2]. In other studies, the variations in MNCV reported were below significant limits (6 m/sec): it has been documented that wide variations occur in the same patient from one day to the next [276]. We should also note that the rare incidence of peripheral neuropathy in patients in peritoneal dialysis was put into question when, after observation of large numbers of dialysed patients, the most serious signs of neuropathy were found in patients in peritoneal dialysis [238, 277–279].

100

It is probable that important contributions to understanding the clinical significance of the MM stem from hemofiltration and hemodiafiltration which are able to significantly reduce MM over extended time periods. This is possible, but not certain, inasmuch as during these substitutive treatments the appearance of new MM, whose clinical significance must still be investigated, has been demonstrated.

The various hemodialysis treatments extract toxic substances chiefly by diffusion and to a lesser degree by convenctive force. Hemofiltration instead extracts MM by convective force. Since the actual MM extraction index is higher for MM in hemofiltration than in hemodialysis, and the predialysis MM concentrations lower in hemofiltration than in hemodialysis, convective force has been demonstrated to be more efficient than diffusion as a means of controlling serum MM concentrations and possible toxicity correlated to them.

These affirmations, on the one hand, contradict the experimental data demonstrating that the mw of the MM is close to the mw of substances extracted by diffusion, and on the other hand, do not explain why each new dialysis treatment almost always determines clinical improvement, independently of how it extracts MM.

While these positive results can be induced both by increased patient care in experimental dialysis and by the active collaboration of patients who strictly follow dietetic and therapeutic indications, they nevertheless tend to be attributed to the extraction of toxic substances, no matter how it occurs. In fact, different substances can be equally toxic yet have different sensitivity to diffusion and convective force. This could explain the beneficial clinical effects of both diffusion and convective force inasmuch as in both cases toxic substances are extracted. It is possible that the extracted MM, more sensitive to diffusion or convective force, create a 'metabolic space' which after a given amount of time (depending on the efficiency of the substitutive treatments) is occupied by other MM only slightly or not at all extractable and just as toxic as the MM extracted. This hypothesis has been confirmed by our results in patients in hemofiltration in whom, after 12–13 months of treatment, a worsening in carbohydrate metabolism has been associated with increased MM concentrations.

On the other hand, it is unrealistic to believe that the complex mechanisms of ultrafiltration, reabsorption, and catabolism of the kidney can be entirely substituted by a filter which only compensates for the ultrafiltrative function. The total elimination of toxic substances and therefore the normalization of both middle and small molecule concentrations is at present unthinkable, as it would also cause depletion of vital substances.

The MM hypothesis has yet to be verified, but a hypothesis, true or false, is intrinsically valuable inasmuch as it stimulates debate and increases knowledge. Researchers certainly recognize that the MM hypothesis has stimulated studies resulting in the manufacturing of new dialysis membranes, the establishment of new dialysis schedules and new substitutive treatments which have profoundly improved the quality of life of patients in substitutive treatment.

## Acknowledgements

The authors would like to thank Nancy Birch Podini for her collaboration in translating and preparing the manuscript.

## References


1. Scribner, B.H. (1965) Discussion. Trans. Amer. Soc. Artif. Int. Organs 11: 29.
2. Jebsen, R.H., Tenckhoff, H. and Honet, J.C. (1967) Natural history of uremic polyneuropathy and effects of dialysis. N. Engl. J. Med. 277: 327–333.
3. Tenckoff, H. and Curtis, F.K. (1970) Experience with maintenance peritoneal dialysis in the home. Trans. Amer. Soc. Artif. Int. Organs 16: 90–95.
4. Tenckoff, H., Shilipetar, G. and Goen, S.T. (1965) One year's experience with home peritoneal dialysis. Trans. Amer. Soc. Artif. Int. Organs 11: 11.
5. Babb, A.L., Popovich, R.P., Graham, T.C. and Scribner, H.B. (1971) The genesis of the square meter-hour hypothesis. Trans. Amer. Soc. Artif. Int. Organs XVII: 81–91.
6. Babb, A.L., Farrel, P.C., Uvelli, D.A. and Scribner, H.B. (1972) Hemodialyser evaluation by examination of solute molecular spectra. Trans. Amer. Soc. Artif. Int. Organs: 98–104.
7. Asaba, H. (1983) Accumulation and excretion of middle molecules. Clin. Nephrol. 19: 116–123.
8. Asaba, H., Bergstrom, J., Furst, P., Oulés, R. and Zimmerman, L. (1976) Accumulation and excretion of middle molecules. Proc. EDTA 13: 481–491.
9. Asaba, H., Bergstrom, J., Furst, P., Johnson, C. and Yahiel, V. (1980) Plasma middle molecules in asymptomatic and 'sick' uremic patients. Artificial Organs 4 (suppl.): 137–142.
10. Chang, T.M.S. and Lister, C. (1980) Middle molecules in hepatic coma and uremia. Artificial Organs 4 (suppl.): 169–172.
11. Chang, T.M.S. and Migchelsen, M. (1973) Characterization of possible toxic metabolites in uremia and hepatic coma based on the clearance spectrum for larger Molecules by the acac microcapsule artificial kidney. Trans. Amer. Soc. Artif. Int. Organs 19: 314–319.
12. Gay, G., Touraine, J.L., Freyria, A.M., Traeger, J. and Navarro, J. (1980) Fractions of middle molecules weight responsible for immunodeficiency in malnourished and burnt patients. Artificial Organs 4 (suppl.): 71–75.
13. Lamperi, S., Buoncristiani, U., Carozzi, S., Cozzani, M., Icardi, A. and Trasforini, D. (1980) Gel-filtration on psoriasic and uremic serum and dialysis fluid. Artificial Organs 4 (suppl.): 156–159.
14. Dzurik, R., Spustovà, V. and Gajdos, M. (1981) In vitro synthesis of middle molecular substances. Proc. 8th Int. Congr. Nephrol.: 600–605.
15. Chapman, G.V., Ward, R.A. and Farrel, P.C. (1980) Separation and quantification of the middle molecules in uremia. Kidney Int. 17: 82–88.
16. Gajdos, M., Spustovà, V., Gerykovà, M. and Dzurik, R. (1981) Erthrocyte transport of middle molecular substances. Proc. EDTA 18: 183–187.
17. Bergstrom, J. and Furst, P. (1976) Uremic middle molecules. Clin. Nephrol. 5: 143–152.
18. Cueille, G., Man, N.K., Sausse, A., Farges, J.P. and Funck-Brentano, J.L. (1981) Further characterization of a neurotoxic uremic middle molecule. Proc. 8th Int. Congr. Nephrol.: 607–617.
19. Furst, P., Zimmerman, L. and Bergstrom, J. (1976) Determination of endogenous middle

molecules in normal and uremic body fluids. Clin. Nephrol. 5: 178–188.

20. Peters, J.H., Gotch, F.A., Keen, M., Berridge, B.J., Jr. and Chao, W.R. (1974) Investigation of the clearance and generation rate of endogenous peptides in normal subjects and uremic patients. Trans. Amer. Soc. Artif. Int. Organs 20: 417–423.

21. Zimmerman, L., Baldesten, A., Bergstrom, J. and Furst, P. (1980) Isotachophoretic separation of middle molecule peptides in uremic body fluids. Clin. Nephrol. 13: 183–188.

22. Dzurik, R., Bozek, P., Reznicek, J. and Obornikova, A. (1973) Blood level of Middle Molecular substances during uraemia and haemodialysis. Proc. EDTA 10: 263–270.

23. Lustemberger, N., Schindhelm, K., Nordmeyer, C., Schuerer, H.J. and Stolte, H. (1980) Renal handling of middle molecules in uremic patients and in the isolated rat kidney. Artificial Organs 4 (suppl.): 110–114.

24. Schiendhelm, K., Schlatter, E., Shurek, H.J. and Stolte, H. (1982) Renal handling of uremic Middle Molecules. Nephron 30: 166–172.

25. Abiko, T., Kumikawa, M., Higuch, H. and Sekino, H. (1978) Identification and synthesis of a heptapeptide in uremic fluid. Biochemical and Biophysical Research Communications 84: 184–194.

26. Funck-Brentano, J.L., Man, N.K., Sausse, A., Zingraff, J., Boudet, J., Becker, A. and Cueille, G.F. (1976) Characterization of a 1100–1300 MW uremic neurotoxin. Trans. Amer. Soc. Artif. Int. Organs 22: 163–166.

27. Fürst, P., Bergström, J., Gordon, A., Johnsson, E. and Zimmerman, L. (1975) Separation of peptides of middle molecular weight from biological fluids of patients with uremia. Kidney Int. 7: S272–S275.

28. Mabuchi, H. and Nakahashi, H. (1981) Analysis of middle molecular peptides in normal and uremic body fluids by high-performance gel-chromatography. J. Chromatogr. 224: 322–326.

29. Mamdani, B.H., Mashouf, Shaykh, M., Evenson, M.A. and Dunea, G. 1979: Chromatographic studies of uremic plasma. Inter. J. Artif. Organs 2: 187–191.

30. Hanicki, Z., Sarnecka-Keller, M., Klein, A. and Slizowska, K. (1974) Middle-sized ninhydrin-positive molecules in uraemic patients treated by repeated haemodialysis. I. Preliminary characteristics. Clin. Chim. Acta 54: 47–54.

31. Cueille, G., Man, N.K., Sausse, A., Farges, J.P. and Funck-Brentano, J.L. (1980) Technical aspects on middle molecules: separation, isolation and identification. Artificial Organs 4 (suppl.): 8–12.

32. Gròf, J. and Menyhàrt, J. (1982) Molecular weight distribution, diffusibility and comparability of middle molecular fractions prepared from normal and uremic sera by different fractionation procedures. Nephron 30: 60–67.

33. Gallice, P., Fournier, N., Crevat, A., Briot, M., Frayssinet, R. and Murisasco, A. (1983) Separation of one uremic middle molecules fraction by high performance liquid chromatography. Kidney Int. 23: 764–766.

34. Navarro, J., Contreras, P., Touraine, J.L., Freyria, A.M., Later, R. and Traeger, J. (1980) Effect of middle molecules on immunological functions. Artificial Organs 4 (suppl.): 76–81.

35. Dzùrik, R., Hupkovà, V., Cernàcek, P., Valovicovà, E. and Niederland, T.R. (1973) The isolation of an inhibitor of glucose utilization from the serum of uraemic subjects. Clin. Chim. Acta 46: 77–83.

36. Leber, H.W., Debus, E., Grulich, U. and Schutterle, G. (1980) Potential role of middle molecular compounds in the development of uremic anemia. Artificial Organs 4 (suppl.): 63–67.

37. Buzio, C., Manari, A., Calderini, C., Montagna, G. and Migone, L. (1980) Serum middle molecules in uremia. Artificial Organs 4 (suppl.): 143–150.

38. Ringoir, S.M.G., van Landchoot, N., and De Smet, R. (1980) Inhibition of phagocytosis by a middle molecular fraction from ultrafiltrate. Clin. Nephrol. 13: 109–112.

39. Champman, G.V. and Farrel, P.C. (1980) Uremic middle molecules: separation and quantification. Artificial Organs 4 (suppl.): 160–165.

40. Brunner, H., Mann, H., Essers, U. and Byrne, T. (1980) Large-scale isolation of middle

and higher molecular weight uremic toxins. Artificial Organs 4 (suppl.): 41–45.

41. Cueille, G., Man, N.K., Sausse, A., Farges, J.P. and Funck-Brentano, J.L. (1980) Characterization of sub-peak b4–2. Middle molecule. Artificial Organs 4 (suppl.): 28–32.

42. Funk-Brentano, J.L., Cueille, G.F. and Man, N.K. (1978) A defense of the middle molecule hypothesis. Kidney Int. 13 (suppl. 8):S31–S35.

43. Smeby, L.H., Jörstad, S., Wideröe, T.E. and Svartass, T.M. (1980) Transport of small, middle, and large molecular weight substances in a dual filtration artificial kidney. Artificial Organs 4 (suppl.): 104–109.

44. Bergström, J., Asaba, H., Fürst, P., Gordon, A., Quadracci, L., and Zimmerman, L. (1976) Middle molecule in uremia. Proc. 6th Int. Congr. Nephrol.: 600–611.

45. Asaba, H., Alverstrand, A., Fürst, P. and Bergström, J. (1983) Clinical implications of uremic middle molecules in regular hemodyalisis patients. Clin. Nephrol. 19: 179–187.

46. Castellani, A., Cristinelli, L., Migozzi, G., Mileti, M., Cannella, G., Mioni, G., Panzetta, G.O. Cecchettin, M., Mombelloni, S. and Maiorca, R. (1975) Short dialysis or personalized dialysis? Opuscula Medico-Technica Lundensia 16: 69–82.

47. Funk-Brentano, J.L., Man N.K., Sausse, A., Cueille, G., Zingraff, J., Drueke, T., Jungers, P. and Billion, J.P. (1975) Neuropathy and middle molecule toxins. Kidney Int. 7: S352–S356.

48. Gotch, F.A. (1980) A quantitative evaluation of small and middle molecule toxicity in therapy of uremia. Dialysis & Transplantation 9: 183–194.

49. Lutz, W. (1980) A uremic peptide containing polyamine: formation and possible role in uremic hypertriglyceridemia. Physiol. Chem. & Physics 12: 451–456.

50. Bergström, J. (1981) Uremic toxins and patient rehabilitation in uremia-pathobiology of patients treated for 10 years or more. In C. Giordano and E.A. Friedman (eds.). Milano: Wichting, pp. 198–199.

51. Man, N.K., Cueille, G., Zingraff, J., Boudet, J., Sausse, A. and Funck-Brentano, J.L. (1980) Uremic neurotoxin in the middle molecular weight range. Artificial Organs 4: 116–120.

52. Man, N.K., Cueille, G., Zingraff, J., Drueke, T., Jungers, P., Sausse, A., Boudet, J. and Funk-Brentano, J.L. (1978) Evaluation of plasma neurotoxin concentration in uraemic polyneuropathic patients. Proc. EDTA 15: 164–169.

53. Asaba, H., Fürst, P., Oulès, R., Yahiel, V., Zimmerman, L. and Bergström, J. (1979) The effect of hemodialysis on endogenous middle molecules in uremic patients. Clin. Nephrol. 11: 257–266.

54. Abiko, T., Kumikawa, M. and Sekino, H. (1979) Inhibition effect of rosette formation between human lymphocytes and sheep erythrocytes by specific heptapeptide isolated from uremic fluid and its analogs. Biochemical and Biophysical Research Communication 84: 945–952.

55. Rola-Plesz Zynski, M., Bolduc, D., Forand, S., Plante, G.E. and St. Pierre, S. (1983) Cellular immune function in uremia: altered cytotoxic and suppressor cell responses to an immunomodulating heptapeptide. Clinical Immunology and Immunopathology 28: 177–184.

56. Abiko, T., Kumikawa, M., Ishiraki, M., Takahashi, H. and Sekino, H. (1978) Identification and synthesis of a tripeptide in ecum fluid of an uremic patient. Biochemical and Biophysical Research Communication 83: 357–364.

57. Abiko, T., Onodera, I. and Sekino, H. (1980) Characterization of an acidic tripeptide in neurotoxic dialysate. Chem. Pharma. Bull. 28: 1629.

58. Abiko, T., Onodera, T. and Sekino, H. (1979) Isolation, structure and biological activity of the trp-containing pentapeptide from uremic fluid. Biochemical and Biophysical Research Communication 89: 813–821.

59. Hanicki, Z., Cichocki, T., Sarnecka-Keller, M., Klein, A. and Komorowska, Z. (1976) Influence of middle sized molecule agregates from dialysate of uremia patients on lymphocyte transformation in vitro. Nephron 17: 73–80.

60. Cichocki, T., Hanicki, Z., Klein, A., Komorowska, Z., Sarnecka-Keller, M. and Sulowicz,

104

W. (1980) Influence of middle-molecular-weight solutes from dialysate on the migration rate of leukocytes. Kidney Int. 17: 231–236.

61. Touraine, J.L., Navarro, J., Corre, C. and Traeger, J. (1975) Inhibitory effect of medium sized molecules from patients with renal failure on lymphocyte stimulation by phytohemag-glutinin. Biomedicine 23: 180–184.

62. Hurst, K.S., Saldanha, L.F., Steinberg, S.M., Galen, M.A., Lowrie, E.G., Gagnea, S.A., Lazzarus, J.M., Strom, T.B., Carpenter, C.B. and Merril, J.P. (1975) The effects of varying dialysis regimens on lymphocytes stimulation. Trans. Am. Soc. Artif. Int. Organs 21: 329, 333.

63. Navarro, J., Gerlier, D., Touraine, J.L., Later, R., Contreras, P., Dore, J.F. and Traeger, J. (1979) A potent inhibitor of cell proliferation in middle molecules isolated from the urine of uremic patients. Biomedicine 31: 261–264.

64. Traeger, J., Navarro, J., Contreras, P., Touraine, J.L. and Later, R., Freyria, A.M. (1981) Immunological activity of middle molecules. Proc. 8th Int. Congr. Nephrol.: 625–629.

65. Ota, K., Sanaka, T., Agishi, T. and Nakajima, O. (1980) Influence of uremic middle molecules on blood cells. Artificial Organs 4: 113–115.

66. Delaporte, C., Gros, F., Jonsson, C. and Bergstrom, J. (1980) In vitro cytotoxic properties of plasma fractions from uremic patients. Artificial Organs 4 (suppl.): 68–70.

67. Bergstrom, J. (1975) Uraemic toxicity. Proc. EDTA 12: 579–585.

68. Man, N.K., Terlain, B., Paris, J., Werner, G., Sausse, A. and Funck-Brentano, J.L. (1983) An approach to middle molecules identification in artificial kidney dialysate, with reference to neuropathy prevention. Trans. Amer. Soc. Artif. Int. Organs 19: 320–324.

69. Funck-Brentano, J.L., Man, N.K., Sausse, A., Cueille, G., Zingraff, J., Drueke, T., Jungers, P. and Billion, J.P. (1974) Polynevrite uremique et moyennes molecules. Rein et Foie, maladies de la nutrition 16B: 317–326.

70. Man, N.K., Cueille, G., Zingraff, J., Drueke, T., Jungers, P., Sausse, A., Billon, J.P. and Funck-Brentano, J.L. (1974) Investigations on clinico-chemical correlations in uraemic polyneuritis. Proc. EDTA 11: 214–221.

71. Cloix, J.F., Cueille, G. and Funck-Brentano, J.L. (1976) Inhibition of bovine renal adenylate cyclase by urinary products. Biomedicine 25: 215–218.

72. Le Moel, G., Strecker, G., Cueille, G., Boudet, J., Man, N.K., Galli, A. and Agneray, J. (1980) Uremic middle molecules: analytical study of middle molecular weight fractions subpeak b4–2. Artificial Organs 4 (suppl.): 17–21.

73. Boudet, J., Cueille, G., Benoist, J.M., Man, N.K. and Funck-Brentano, J.L. (1980) In vitro frog sural nerve test: a monitor for detecting neurotoxin solutes. Artificial Organs 4 (suppl.): 94–97.

74. Odeberg, H., Olsson, I. and Thysell, H. (1973) The effect of uremic serum on granulocyte iodination capacity. Trans. Amer. Soc. Artif. Int. Organs 19: 484–485.

75. Dzurik, R., Adam, J. and Reznicek, J. (1972) The ineffectiveness of haemodialysis in removing peptides inhibiting glucose utilization. Proc. EDTA 9: 142–145.

76. Tison, P., Cernacek, P., Silvanova, E. and Dzurik, R. (1981) Uremic toxins and blood platelet carbohydrate metabolism. Nephron 28: 192–195.

77. Dzurik, R., Adam, J. and Grega, B. (1972) Inhibition of glucose utilization in rat diaphragm by peptides of uraemic serum isolated by high voltage electrophoresis. Internat. Urol. and Nephrol. 4: 297–301.

78. Dzurik, R., Hupkova, V., Holoman, J. and Valovicova, E. (1971) Abnormal carbohydrate metabolism in uraemia. Internat. Urol. and Nephrol. 3: 409–413.

79. Gajdos, M. and Dzurik, R. (1973) Erythrocyte glycolysis in uraemia: dynamic balance caused by the opposite action of various factors. Internat. Urol. and Nephrol. 5: 331–336.

80. Lindsay, R.M., Dennis, B.N., Bergstrom, J.C., Jonsson, C. and Furst, P. (1980) Platelet function as an assay for uremic toxins. Artificial Organs 4 (suppl.): 82–89.

81. Gallice, P., Fournier, N., Crevat, A., Saingra, S. Frayssinet, R., Murisasco, A. and Sicardi, F. (1980) In vitro inhibition of platelet aggregation by uremic middle molecules. Biomedicine 33: 185–188.

82. Rinaudo, J.B., Bernard, P., Crest, M., Moret, J.M., Murisasco, A., Saingra, S., Frayssinet, R., Crevat, A., Gallice, P., Fournier, N. and Sicardi, F. (1980) Some aspects of middle molecules toxicity. Artificial Organs 4 (suppl.): 90–93.

83. Rinaudo, J.B., Gallice, P., Crevat, A., Saingra, S. and Murisasco, A. (1979) Action of middle molecules from chronic renal insufficiency treated by haemodialysis on mitochondrial respiration. Biomedicine 30: 215–218.

84. Bernard, P., Crest, M., Rinaudo, J.B., Gallice, P., Fournier, N., Crevat, A., Murisasco, A., Saingra, S. and Frayssinet, R. (1982) A study of the cardiotoxicity of uremic middle molecules on embryonic chick hearts. Nephron 31: 135–140.

85. Mabuchi, H. and Nakahashi, H. (1983) Isolation and partial characterization of platelet aggregation inhibitors in the blood of dialyzed patients. Nephron 35: 112–115.

86. Leber, H.W., Baumgarten, C., Goubeaud, G., Matthias, R. and Schutterle, G. (1975) Globin synthesis in uraemia. Proc. EDTA 12: 355–361.

87. Leber, H.W., Spiegelhalter, R., Ulm, A., Gobeaud, G. and Rawer, P. (1980) Influence of middle molecules on the anemia of uremic patients. Artificial Organs 2: 378–381.

88. Goubeaud, G., Leber, H.W., Schott, H.H. and Schutterle, G. (1977) Middle molecules and haemoglobin synthesis. Proc. EDTA 11: 371–376.

89. Gutman, R.A. and Huang, A.T. (1980) Inhibitor of marrow thymidine incorporation from sera of patients with uremia. Kidney Int. 18: 715–724.

90. Rege, A.B., Moriyama, Y. and Fisher, J.W. (1974) Characterization of a serum inhibitor of erythropoiesis. Federation Proceeding 33: 597.

91. Moriyama, Y., Rege, A. and Fisher, J.W. (1975) Studies on an inhibitor of erythropoiesis. II. Inhibitory effects of serum from uremic rabbits on heme synthesis in rabbit bone marrow cultures (38483). Proc. Soc. Exp. Biol. Med. 148: 94–97.

92. Brunner, H., Mann, H., Essers, U., Schultheis, R., Byrne, T. and Heintz, R. (1978) Preparative isolation of middle molecular weight fractions from the hemofiltrate of patients with chronic uremia. Artificial Organs 2: 375–377.

93. Brunner, H., Mann, H., Essers, U., Schultheis, R., Byrne, T. and Heintz, R. (1978) Zur methodik der praparativen gelchromatographischem isolierungvon sogenannten Mittelmolekulen aus hamofiltrate. Donausymposium fur Nephrologie 3: 135–144.

94. Bourgoignie, J.J., Klahr, S. and Bricker, N.S. (1971) Inhibition of transepithelial sodium transport in the frog skin by a low molecular weight fraction of uremic serum. J. Clin. Invest. 50: 303–311.

95. Bourgoignie, J.J., Kaplan, M., Eun, C., Favre, H., Hwang, K.H., Blumenfeld, Y. and Bricker, N.S. (1975) On the characterization of natriuretic factor. Clinical Research 23: 429A.

96. Bourgoignie, J.J., Hwang, K.H., Espinel, C., Kalhr, S. and Bricker, N.S. (1972) A natriuretic factor in the serum of patients with chronic uremia. J. Clin. Invest. 51: 1514–1527.

97. Kinniburgh, D.W. and Boyd, N.D. (1981) Isolation of peptides from uremic plasma that inhibit phenytoin binding to normal plasma proteins. Clin. Pharmacol. Ther. 30: 276–280.

98. Menyhart J. and Grof, J. (1977) Composition, toxicity and diffusibility of middle molecular weight substances (MMS) prepared from sera of healthy and uremic individuals. Journal of Molecul. Med. 2: 371–380.

99. Grof, J. and Menyhart, J. (1977) Non diffusible toxic polypeptides in uraemic sera: a new group of uraemic toxins. Acta Chirurg. Academ. Scientiarum Humgaricae 18: 283–287.

100. Dall'Aglio, P., Savi, M., Silvestri, M.G., Buzio, C. and Migone, L. (1975) Leukocytes migration inhibition of uremic serum and its fractions. Proc. 6th Int. Congr. Nephrol.: 372.

101. Ehrlich, K., Holland, F., Turnham, T. and Klein, E. (1981) Osmotic concentration of polypeptides from hemofiltrate of uremic patients. Clin. Nephrol. 14: 31–35.

102. Pogglitsch, Von H., Petek, W., Waller, J. and Stubchen-Kirchner, H. (1977) Hamodynamisch wirksame nieder und mittel-molekulare metabolite in hamofiltrat niereninsuffizienter patienten. Wiener Klinische Wochenschrift 89: 812–819.

103. Lutz, W., Markiewicz, K. and Klyszejko, S. (1974) Investigations on the activity of lactic

dehydrogenase and its inhibitors in the serum of uremic patients during hemodialysis. Acta Med. Pol. 15: 97–104.

104. Lutz, W. (1975) Studies on formation of complexes of insulin with basis peptides isolated from the plasma of uremic patients. Acta Med. Pol. 16: 159–170.

105. Lutz, W. (1976) The influence of strongly basic uremic peptide on liberation of lipoproteinlipase activity from human adipose cells. Acta Med. Pol. 17: 55–70.

106. Milutinovic, S., Breyer, D., Jankovic, N., Molnar, V., Stefovic, A. and Rocic, B. (1983) Inhibitor of insulin binding to erythrocytes in plasma of uremic patients. Nephron 34: 99–103.

107. Braguer, D., Chauvet-Monges, A.M., Sari, J.C., Crevat, A., Durand, C., Murisasco, A., Elsen, R. (1983) Inhibition in vitro of the polymerization of tubulin by uremic middle molecules: Corrective effect of isaxonine. Clin. Nephrol. 20: 149–154.

108. Drutz, D.J. (1979) Altered cell-mediated immunity and its relationship to infection susceptibility in patients with uremia. Dialysis & Transplantation 8: 320–368.

109. Dammin, G.J., Couch, N.P. and Murray, Y.E. (1956) Prolonged survival of skin homografts in uremic patients. Ann. N.Y. Acad. Sci. 64: 967–976.

110. Morrison, A.B. Maness, K. and Tawes, R. (1963) Skin homograft survival in chronic renal insufficiency. Arch. Path. 75: 139–143.

111. Smiddy, F.G., Burwell, R.G. and Parsons, F.M. (1961) Influence of uraemia on the survival of skin homografts. Nature 190: 732–734.

112. Boulton-Jones, J.M., Cameron, J.S. and Vick, R. (1972) Immune response in uremia. Kidney Int. 2: 179.

113. Kirkpatrick, C.H., Wilson, W.E.G. and Talmage, D.W. (1964) Immunologic studies in human organ transplantation. I. Observation and characterization of suppressed cutaneous reactivity in uremia. J. Exp. Med. 119: 727–742.

114. Touraine, J.L., Touraine, F., Revillard, J.P., Brochier, J., Traeger, J. (1975) T-Lymphocytes and serum inhibitors of cell-mediated immunity in renal insufficiency. Nephron 14: 195–208.

115. Willson, W.E.C., Kirkpatrick, C.H. and Talmage, D.W. (1964) Immunologic studies in human organ transplantation. III. The relationship of delayed cutaneous hypersensitivity to the onset of attempted kidney, allograft rejection. J. Clin. Invest. 43: 1881–1891.

116. Jensson, O. (1958) Observations on the leukocyte blood picture in acute uraemia. Brit. J. Haemat. 4: 422–427.

117. Riis, P. and Stougaard, J. (1975) The peripheral blood leukocytes in acute anuria. Dan. Med. Bull. 6: 90–94.

118. Touraine, J.L., Navarro, J., Corre, C. and Traeger, J. (1975) Effects of middle molecules from uremic patients in vitro lymphocyte proliferation and rosette formation. Proc. 6th Int. Congr. Nephrol. Abstracts 411.

119. Gombos, E.A., Jeffersson, D.M., Ganesh Bhat, J. (1974) Adequate dialysis and immune response. Kidney Int. 6: 5A.

120. Kasakura, S. and Loewenstein, K. (1967) The effect of uremic blood on mixed leukocyte reactions and on cultures of leukocytes with phytohemagglutinin. Transplantation 5: 283–289.

121. Silk, M.R. (1967) The effect of uremic plasma on lymphocyte transformation. Invest. Urol. 5: 195–199.

122. Moynihan, P.C., Jackson, J.K. (1966) Lymphocyte transformation in acute uraemia. Nature 212: 206–216.

123. Contreras, P., Later, R., Navarro, J., Touraine, J.L., Freyria, A.M. and Traeger, J. (1982) Molecules in the middle molecular weight range. Nephron 32: 193–201.

124. Hutchins, R.H., Hegstrom, R.M. and Scribner, B.H. (1966) Glucose intollerance in patients on long-term intermittens dialysis Ann. Intern. Med. 65: 275–285.

125. Yamada, T. and Nakagawa, S. (1976) Analysis of uremic ultrafiltrate: a possible coincidence of highly toxic small molecular fraction with guanidine derivatives. Trans. Amer. Soc. Artif. Int. Organs. 22: 155–161.

126. Bozzini, C.E., Devoto, F.C.H. and Tomjo, J.M. (1966) Decreased responsiveness of hematopoietic tissue to erythropoietin in acutely uremic rats. J. Lab. & Clin. Med. 68: 411–417.

127. Fisher, J.W., Hatch, F.E., Roh, B.L., Allen, R.C. and Kelley, B.J. (1968) Erythropoietin inhibitor in kidney extracts and plasma from anemic uremic human subjects. Blood 31: 440–452.

128. Markson, J.L. and Rennie, J.B. (1956) The anemia of chronic renal insufficiency: the effect of serum from azotemic patients of the maturation of normoblasts in suspension cultures. Scot. Med. J. 1: 320–322.

129. Valovicova, E., Spustova, V., Dzuric, R. and Cernacek, P. (1974) The utilization of glucose in the brain slices during uraemia. Internat. Urol. and Nephrol. 6: 239–242.

130. Leber, H.W., Sinning, P. and Schutterle, G. (1974) Porphobilinogen and porphyrin synthesis in reticulocytes from uraemic patients. Proc. EDTA 11: 383–390.

131. Leber, H.W., Spiegelhalter, R. and Schutterle, G. (1978) New aspect concerning uraemic haemolysis: increased susceptibility of erythrocytes to peroxidation. Proc. EDTA 15: 437–440.

132. Bergstrom, J., Furst, P. and Zimmermann, L. (1979) Uremic middle molecules exist and are biologically active. Clin. Nephrol. 11: 229–238.

133. Lote, C.J., Gent, J.P. Walstencroft, J.H. and Srelke, M. (1976) An inhibitory tripeptide for cat spinal cord. Nature 264: 188–189.

134. Savazzi, G.M., Buzio, C. and Migone, L. (1982) Lights and shadows on the pathogenesis of uremic polyneuropathy. Clin. Nephrol. 18: 219–229.

135. Coben, B.D. (1962) Abnormal carbohydrate metabolism in uraemia. Ann. Intern. Med. 57: 204–213.

136. Hampers, C.L., Lowrie, E.G., Soeldner, J.S. and Merril, J.P. (1970) The effect of uremia upon glucose metabolism. Arch. Intern. Med. 126: 870–874.

137. Westervelt, B.F., Jr. and Schreiner, G.E. (1962) The carbohydrate intollerance of uremic patients. Ann. Intern. Med. 57: 226–276.

138. Cerletty, J.M., Engbring, H.H. (1967) Azotemia and glucose intolerance. Ann. Intern. Med. 66: 1097–1108.

139. Chamberlain, M.J. and Stimmler, L. (1967) The renal handling of insulin. J. Clin. Invest. 46: 911–919.

140. Hampers, C.L., Soeldner, J.S., Doak, P.B. and Merril, J.P. (1966) Effect of chronic renal failure and hemodialysis on carbohydrate metabolism. J. Clin. Invest. 45: 1719–1731.

141. Horton, E.S., Johnson, C. and Lebovitz, H.E. (1968) Carbohydrate metabolism in uremia. Ann. Intern. Med. 68: 63–74.

142. Perkoff, G.T., Thomas, C.L., Newton, J.D., Sellman, J.C., Tyler, F.H. (1958) Mechanism of impaired glucose tollerance in uremia and experimental hyperazotemia. Diabetes 7: 375–383.

143. Dzurik, R. and Valovicovà, E. (1970) Glucose utilization in muscle during uremia: in vitro study. Clin. Chim. Acta 30: 137–142.

144. Dzurik, R. and Krajci-Lazary, B. (1967) The effect of uremic serum on carbohydrate metabolism in rat diaphragm. Separatum Experientia 23: 798–801.

145. Gambhir, K.K., Archer, H.A., Nerurkar, S.G., Cruz, I.A. and Sanders, M. (1981) Erythrocyte insulin receptors in chronic renal failure. Nephron 28: 4–10.

146. Emerson, P., Wilkinson, J.H. and Withycombe, W.A. (1964) Effect of oxalate on the activity of lactate dehydrogenase isoenzymes. Nature 202: 1337–1338.

147. Fujimoto, Y. and Wilkinson, J.H. (1970) Effect of the urea-urease system and the carbonate ion on the activities of lactate dehydrogenase isoenzymes. Biochim. Biophys. Acta. 206: 38–45.

148. Wilkinson, J.H., Fujimoto, Y., Senesky, D., Ludwig, G.D. (1970) Nature of the inhibitors of lactate dehydrogenase in uremic dialysates. J. Lab. Clin. Med. 75: 109–119.

149. Ringoir, S., Wieme, R.J. (1972) Serum LDH in haemodialysis. Clin. Chim. Acta 42: 315–320.

108

150. Balestri, P.L., Rindi, P., Biagini, M. and Giovannetti, S. (1972) Effects of uraemic serum, urea, creatinine and methylguanidine on glucose metabolism. Clin. Sci. 42: 395–404.

151. Dzurik, R., Adam, J., Valivicova, E., Reznicek, J. and Zvara, V. (1971) The effect of haemodialysis on blood peptide levels. Proc. EDTA 8: 167–173.

152. Lindsay, R.M., Friesen, M., Koens, F., Linton, A.L., Oreopoulos, D. and Veber, G. (1976) Platelet function in patients on long term peritoneal dialysis. Clin. Nephrol. 6: 335–339.

153. Saltzman, E.W. and Neri, L.L. (1966) Adhesiveness of blood platelets in uremia. Thromb. Diath. Haemorrh. 15: 84–92.

154. Evans, E.P., Branch, R.A. Bloom, A.K. (1972) A clinical and experimental study of platelet function in chronic renal failure. J. Clin. Path 25: 745–753.

155. Castaldi, P.A., Rozenberg, M.C. and Stewart, J.H. (1966) The bleeding disorder of uraemia. Lancet 2: 66–69.

156. Horowitz, H.I., Cohen, B.D., Marinez, P. and Papayoancu, M.F. (1967) Defective ADP-induced platelet factor 3 activation in uremic. Blood 30: 331–334.

157. Horowitz, G.I., Stein, J.M., Cohen, B.D. and White, J.G. (1970) Futher studies on the platelets inhibitory effect of guanidino succinic acid and its role in uremic bleeding. Amer. J. Med. 49: 336–345.

158. Rabiner, S.F. and Hrodek, O. (1968) Platelet factor 3 in normal subjects and patients with renal failure. J. Clin. Invest. 47: 901–912.

159. Schöndorf, T.H. and Hey, D. (1974) Platelet function tests in uremic and under acetylsalicylic acid administration. Haemostasis 3: 129–131.

160. Stewart, Y.H. and Castaldi, P.A. (1967) Uraemic bleeding: a reversible platelet defect corrected by dialysis. Q. J. Med. 36: 409.

161. Lindsay, R.M., Friesen, M., Aronstam, A., Andrus, F., Clark, W.F. and Linton, A.L. (1978) Improvement of platelet function by increased frequency of hemodialysis. Clin. Nephrol. 10: 67–70.

162. Nenci, G.G., Berrettini, M., Agnelli, G., Parise, P., Buoncristiani, U. and Ballatori, U. (1979) Effect of peritoneal dialysis haemodialysis and kidney transplantation on blood platelet function. Nephron 23: 287–292.

163. Glare, R.P., Morgan, J.M., Morgan, R.E. (1967) Uncoupling of oxidative phosphorylation by ultrafiltration of uremic serum. Proc. Soc. Exp. Biol. Med.: 125–172.

164. Martinelli, R., Rodriguez, L.E.A., Machado, A.E.C. and Rocha, H. (1976) The effect of acute uremia on liver mitochondrial activity. Nephron 17: 155–160.

165. Yamada, T., Yoshida, A., Koshikawa, S. (1969) Alteration of oxidative phosphorylation in uremia. Jap. Circulat. J. 33: 59–63.

166. Farrel, P.C., Grib, N.L., Fry, D.L.L., Popovich, R.P., Broviac, J.W. and Babb, A.L. (1972) A comparison of in vitro and in vivo solute-protein binding interactions in normal and uremic subjects Trans. Amer. Soc. Artif. Int. Organs 18: 268–276.

167. Depner, T.A. and Gulyassy, P.F. (1980) Plasma protein binding in uremia: extraction and characterization of an inhibitor. Kidney Int. 18: 86–94.

168. Gulyassy, P.F. and Depner, T.A. (1979) Abnormal drug binding in uraemia. Dialysis & Transplantation 8: 19–23.

169. Reidenberg, M.M. (1977) The binding of drugs to plasma proteins and the interpretation of measurements of plasma concentrations of drugs in patients with poor renal functions. Am. J. Med. 62: 465–470.

170. Andreasen, F. (1974) The effect of dialysis on the protein binding of patients with acute renal failure. Acta Pharmacol. Toxicol. 34: 234–294.

171. Porter, R., Layzer, R. (1975) Plasma albumin concentration and diphenylhydantoin binding in man. Arch. Neurol. 32: 298–303.

172. Shoeman, D. and Azarnoff, D. (1972) The alterations of plasma proteins in uremia as reflected in their ability to bind digotoxin and diphenylhydantoin. Pharmacology 7: 169–177.

173. Schoots, A.C., Mikkers, E.P., Cramers, C., De Smet, R.U. and Ringoir, S. (1984) Uremic

toxins and the elusive Middle Molecules. Nephron. 38: 1–8.

174. Schumacher, K., Schneider, W., Alzer, G. and Oerkermann, H. (1972) The influence of urea on protein synthesis of stimulated lymphocytes. Klin. Wochenschrift 50: 86–91.

175. Navarro, J., Contreras, P., Touraine, J.L., Freyria, A.M., Later, R. and Traeher, J. (1982) Are middle molecules responsible for toxic phenomena in chronic renal failure? Nephron 32: 301–307.

176. Emerson, P. and Wilkinson, J.H. (1965) Urea and oxalate inhibition of the serum lactate dehydrogenase. J. Clin. Path. 18: 803–807.

177. Emerson, P., Withycombe, W.A. and Wilkinson, J.H. (1965) Inhibition of lactate dehydrogenase by sera of uraemic patients. Lancet 2: 571–572.

178. Rabin, E.Z., Algom, D., Freedman, M.H., Guenthier, L., Dardick, I. and Tattrie, B. (1981) Ribonuclease activity in renal failure. Nephron 27: 254–259.

179. Ku, G., Hird, U.M., Varghese, Z., Almed, K.Y., Fiter, M., Ng, C.M. and Moorhead, J.F. (1974) Inhibition of DNA synthesis by guandine compounds in uraemia. Proc. EDTA 11: 427–432.

180. Lonergan, E.T., Semar, M., Lange, K. (1970) Transketolase activity in uraemia. Arch. Intern. Med. 126: 851–854.

181. Record, B.N., Princhard, J.W., Gallagher, B.B., Seligson, D. (1969) Phenolic acids in experimental uremia. I. Potential role of phenolic acids in the neurological manifestations of uremia. Arch. Neurol. 21: 387–394.

182. Wardle, E.N. and Williams, R. (1980) Polymorph leukocyte function in uraemia and jaundice. Acta Haematol. 64: 157–167.

183. Jörstad, S., Smeby, L.C., Wideröe, E. and Berg, K.J. (1980) Toxicity of middle molecules: clinical evaluation using a selective filtration artificial kidney. Artif. Organs 4 (suppl.): 98–103.

184. Jörstad, S., Smeby, L.C., Wideröe, E. and Berg, K.J. (1980) Removal of uremic toxins and regeneration of haemofiltrate by a selective dual haemofiltration artificial kidney (SEDUFARK) system Clin. Nephrol. 13: 85–92.

185. Balestri, P.L., Biagini, M., Rindi, P. and Giovannetti, S. (1970) Uremic toxins. Arch. Intern. Med. 126: 843–845.

186. Molinas, F.C. (1973) Inhibition by phenol and phenolic acids of platelet release reaction. Thromb. Diath. Haemorrh. 30: 334–338.

187. Davis, J.W., Field, M.C., Jr., Phillips, P.E. and Graham, B.A. (1972) Effect of exogenous urea, creatinine and guanidinosuccinic acid on human platelet aggregation in vitro. Blood 39: 388–397.

188. Horowitz, H.I. (1970) Uremic toxins and platelet function. Arch. Intern. Med. 126: 623–628.

189. Carrol, H.Y. (1985) Energy production and utilization by human platelets in the presence of some guanidines and phenols (uremic toxins) that inhibit aggregation. Thromb. Diath. Haemorrh. 43: 63–71.

190. Rabiner, S.F. and Molinas, F. (1970) The role of phenol and phenolic acids on the thrombocytopathy and defective platelet aggregation of patient with renal failure. Am. J. Med. 49: 346–351.

191. Lascelles, P.P. and Taylor, W.H. (1966) The effect upon tissue respiration in vitro of metabolites which accumulate in uraemic coma. Clin. Sci. 31: 403–413.

192. Mills, D.C.B. and Smith, J. (1972) The control of platelet responsive by agents that influence cyclic AMP metabolism. Ann. NY Acad. Sci. 201: 391–399.

193. Hicks, J.M., Young, D.S. and Wootton, I.D.P. (1964) The effect of uraemic blood constituents on certain cerebral enzymes. Clin. Chim. Acta 9: 228–231.

194. Pressman, B.L. (1968) Ionophorous antibiotics as models in biological transport. Federation Proceeding 27: 1283–1288.

195. Kersting, F. and Brass, H. (1977) The effects of uraemic compounds on oxygen consumption and mechanical activity of isolated guinea pig hearts. Proc. EDTA 11: 472–479.

196. Giovannetti, S., Cioni, L., Balestri, B.L. and Biagini, M. (1968) Evidence that guanidines and some related compounds cause haemolysis in chronic uraemia. Clin. Sci. 34: 141–148.

110

197. Milutinovic, J., Halar, E.M., Harker, L.A., Babb, A.L. and Scribner, B.H. (1971) Further experience with hemodialysis at 100 ml/min dialysate flow rate. Proc. Dialysis Transplant Forum 1: 48–52.

198. Graham, Christopher T., Cambi, V., Harker, L.A., Hurst, P.E., Babb, A.L. and Scribner, B.H. (1971) A study of hemodialysis with lower ed dialysate flow rate. Trans. Amer. Soc. Artif. Int. Organs 17: 92–95.

199. Cambi, V., Dall'Aglio, P., Savazzi, G., Arisi, L., Rossi, E. and Migone, L. (1972) Clinical assessment of hemodialysis patients with reduced small molecules removal. Proc. EDTA 9: 67–73.

200. Rattazzi, T., Wathen, R., Comty, C., Raij, L., Leonard, A. and Shapiro F. (1974) The comparison of low flow (QD 200) to regular flow (QD 500) dialysis. Trans. Amer. Soc. Artif. Int. Organs 20: 402–408.

201. Rosenzweig, J., Babb, A.L., Vizzo, J.E., Scribner, B.H. and Ginn, H.E. (1971) Large surface area hemodialysis. Proc. Dialysis Transplant Forum 1: 56–59.

202. Funck-Brentano, J.L., Man, N.K. and Sausse, A. (1975) Effect of more porous dialysis membranes on neuropathic toxins. Kidney Int. 7: S52–S57.

203. Funck-Brentano, J.L., Sausse, A., Man, N.K., Granger, A., Zingraff, J., Jungers, P. and Rondon-Nucete, A. (1972) Une nouvelle méthode d'hemodialyse associant une membrane à haute perméabilité pour les Moyennes Molécules et un bain de dialyse en circuit fermé. Proc. EDTA 9: 55–65.

204. Man, N.K., Granger, S., Rondon-Nucete, M., Zingraff, J., Jungers, J., Sausse, S. and Funck-Brentano, J.L. (1973) One year follow-up of short dialysis with a membrane highly permeable to middle molecules. Proc. EDTA 10: 236–246.

205. Scribner, B.H., Babb, A.L., Strand, M.C. and Milutinovic, J. (1973) Current status of the middle molecules hypothesis. 6th Annual Contractor' Conference. Artif. Kidney Prog.: 60–61.

206. Ginn, H.E., Bugel, H.J., James, L. and Hopkins, P. (1971) Clinical experience with small surface area dialyzers. Proc. Dialysis Transplant Forum 53: 53–55.

207. Teehan, B.P., Smith, L.H., Gilgore, S. and Sigler, M.H. (1974) Adverse effects of large surface area dialysis on motor nerve conduction velocity. Proc. Dialysis Transplant Forum 4: 166–170.

208. Mirahmadi, Kai, J.K., Miller, J.H., Gorman, S.T. and Rosen, S.M. (1974) Clinical evaluation of patients dialysed with double Gambro 4 hours, three times per week. Proc. EDTA 11: 121–126.

209. Cambi, V., Savazzi, G., Arisi, L., Buzio, C., Dall'Aglio, P., Rossi, E. and Migone, L. (1973) Dialysis schedules and peripheral neuropathy. Proc. EDTA 10: 271–280.

210. Lowrie, G., Steinberg, S., Galen, A., Gagneux, A.S., Lazarus, J.M., Gottlieb, M.N. and Merrill, J.P. (1976) Factors in the dialysis regimen which contribute to alterations in the abnormalities of uremia. Kidney Int. 10: 409–422.

211. Teschan, P.E., Ginn, H.E., Bourne, J.R. and Ward, J.W. (1976) Neuro-behavioral responses to 'middle molecule' dialysis and transplantation. Trans. Amer. Soc. Artif. Int. Organs 22: 190–194.

212. Ben Ari, I., Oren, A. and Berlyne, G.M. (1976) Short duration-high area regular dialysis using two UF2 coil in series. Nephron 16: 74–80.

213. Kjellstrand, C.M., Petersen, R.J., Evans, R.L., Shideman, J.R., Von Hartitzsch, B., Buselmeier, T.J. (1973) Considerations of the middle molecule hypothesis II: neuropathy in nehprectomized patients. Trans. Amer. Soc. Artif. Int. Organs. 19: 325–335.

214. Kjellstrand, C.M., Evans, R.L., Petersen, R.J., Shideman, J.R., Hartitzsch, B., Buselmeier, T.J. (1975) The unphysiology of dialysis: a major cause of dialysis side effects? Kidney Int. 7: S30–S34.

215. Kjellstrand, C.M. and Evans, R.L. (1975) Considerations of new dialysis schedules: theoretical evaluation and review of literature. Opuscola Medico-Technica Lundensia 16: 26–37.

216. Babb, A.L., Strand, M.J., Uvelli, D.A., Milutinovic, J., Scribner, B.H. (1975) Quantitative description of dialysis treatment: a dialysis index. Kidney Int. 7: S23–S29.

111

217. Milutinovic, J., Strand, M., Casaretto, A., Follette, W., Babb, A.L., Scribner, B.H. (1974) Clinical impact of residual glomerular filtration rate on dialysis time. A preliminary report. Trans. Amer. Soc. Artif. Int. Organs 20: 410–416.

218. Valek, A., Dzurik, R., Spustova, V., Valkova, D. (1980) Concentration of plasma middle molecular weight substances and clinical condition of patients undergoing short-time regular dialysis teatment. Artificial Organs 4 (suppl.): 173–176.

219. Ringoir, S. and Desmet, R. (1978) Serum chromatography pattern in different dialysis strategies. Int. J. Artif. Organs 1: 218–223.

220. Bergstrom, J., Furst, P., Asaba, H. and Gordon, A. (1975) Middle molecules in uremia. Opuscola Medico-Tecnica Lundensia 16: 50–56.

221. Gotch, A.F. and Sargent, J.A. (1980) Modeling of middle molecules in clinical studies. Artificial Organs 4 (suppl.): 133–136.

222. Gotch, A.F., Sargent, J.A. and Peters, J.H. (1975) Studies on the molecular etiology of uremia. Kidney Int. 7: S276–S279.

223. Schiendhelm, K., Lustenberger, N., Nordmeier, C., Farrell, P. and Stolte, H. (1982) Middle molecules in patients with predialysis chronic renal failure: a comparative clearance study. Clin. Nephrol. 17: 200–205.

224. Gotch, A.F., Sargent, J.A., Keen, M., Lam, M., Prowit, M., Grady, M. (1976) Clinical results of intermittent dialysis therapy guided by ongoing kinetic analysis of urea metabolism. Trans. Amer. Soc. Artif. Int. Organs 22: 175–179.

225. Chapman, G.V. and Farrell, P.C. (1981) Uremic middle molecules Int. J. Artif. Organs 4: 52–54.

226. Zimmerman, L., Jornvall, H., Bergstrom, P., Furst, P., Sjovall, Y. (1980) Characterization of middle molecules compounds. Artificial Organs 4 (suppl.): 33–36.

227. Zimmerman, L., Furst, P. Bergstrom, P., Jornvall, H. (1980) A new glycine containing compound with a blocked amino-group from uremic body fluids. Clin. Nephrol. 14: 107–111.

228. Menyhart, J. and Grof, J. (1981) Many hitherto unknown peptides are principal constituents of uremic middle molecules. Clin. Chem.: 1712–1716.

229. Graefe, U., Steinhausen, D., Knoll, O., Alterhoff, G. and Loew, H. (1979) Dissociation between in clinical and biochemical aspect of uremia and mathematical modeling.Opuscola Medico-technica Lundensia 22: 1–6.

230. Shaldon, S., Florence, P., Fontanier, P., Polito, C. and Mion, C. (1975) Comparison of two strategies for short dialysis using 1 m$^2$ and 2 m$^2$ surface area dialysers. Proc. EDTA 12: 596–603.

231. Teehan, B.P., Gacek, E.M., Heymach, G., Brown, J., Smith, L.J., Sigler, M.H., Gilgore, G.S. and Schleifer, C.R. (1977) A clinical appraisal of the dialysis index. Trans. Amer. Soc. Art. Int. Organs 23: 548–554.

232. Milutinovic, J., Babb, L.A., Eschbach, W.J., Follette, C.W., Graefe, U., Strand, M.J., Scribner, B.H. (1978) Uremic neuropathy. Evidence of middle molecule toxicity. Artificial Organs 2: 45–54.

233. Teschan, P.E., Ginn, H.E., Bourne, J.R., Ward, J.W., Schaffer, J.D. (1983) A prospective study of reduced dialysis. Trans. Amer. Soc. Artif. Int. Organs 6: 108.

234. Raja, R.M., Kramer, M.S., Rosenbaum, J.L. (1978) Long-term short hemodialysis. Implications to dialysis index. Trans. Amer. Soc. Artif. Int. Organs 24: 367–374.

235. Cambi, V., Savazzi, G., Arisi, L., Bignardi, L., Bruschi, G., Rossi, E., Migone, L. (1974) Short dialysis schedules. Finally ready to become a routine. Proc. EDTA 11: 112–120.

236. Chapman, G.V., Mahoni, J.F. and Farrell, P.C. (1980) A crossover study of short time dialysis. Clin. Nephrol. 13: 78–84.

237. Cambi, V., Savazzi, G., Arisi, L., Bignardi, L., Buzio, C., Pandolfo, E., Rossi, E. and Migone, L. (1974) Emodialisi a tempi brevi (10, 5–12 ore settimanali). Minerva Nefrologica 21: 275–281.

238. Cambi, V., Arisi, L., Bignardi, L., Garini, G., Rossi, E., Savazzi, G. and Migone, L. (1975) Short dialysis after three years. Progress report. Opuscula Medico Technica Lundensia 16: 40–46.

239. Maiorca, R., Castellani, A., Migozzi, G., Panzetta, G.O. and Usberti M. (1974) Short time personalised dialysis: good results in spite of high levels or small and middle molecules. Proc. EDTA 11: 146–152.

240. Barber, S., Appleton, D.R., Kerr, D.N.S. (1975) Adequate dialysis. Nephron 14: 209–227.

241. Adjei, S., Ashcroft, R., Clarkson, B.A., Elliott, R.W., Kerr, D.N.S. and Robson, A.M. (1964) Effect of ultrafiltration on efficiency of dialysis with twin coil kidney. Proc. EDTA 1: 303–307.

242. Nolph, K.D., Stoltz, M.L., Carter, C.B., Fox, M. and Maher, J.F. (1970) Factor affecting the composition of ultrafiltrate from hemodialysis coils. Trans. Amer. Soc. Artif. Int. Organs 16: 495–497.

243. Hilderson, J., Ringoir, S., Waeleghem, J.P., Egmond, J., Hael, J.P. and Schelstraete, K. (1975) Short dialysis with a polyacrylonitrilmembrane (RP6) without the use of a closed recirculating dialyzate delivery system. Clin. Nephrol. 4: 18–22.

244. Buzio, C., Montagna, G., Calderini, C., Manari, A. and Migone, L. (1980) Methodology for identification of serum middle molecules. Artificial Organs 4 (suppl.): 23–27.

245. Buzio, C., Manari, A., Montagna, G., Arisi, L., Calderini, C. Savazzi, G., Migone, L. (1980) Le Medie Molecole in uremia. Minerva Nefrologica 27: 483–494.

246. Buzio, C., Del Monte, G., Manari, A., Montagna, G. and Migone, L. (1979) Middle molecules in uremia. Isolation techniques, chemical determination, biological tests, effects of dialysis. Opuscola Medico-Technica Lundensia 22: 17–34.

247. Migone, L, Dall'Aglio P. and Buzio, C. (1975) Middle molecules in uremic serum, urine and dialysis fluid. Clin. Nephrol. 3: 82–93.

248. Buzio, C., Manari, A., Montagna, G., Calderini, C. and Migone, L. (1981) Uremic middle molecules. Uremia Pathobiology of patients treated for 10 years or more. In C., Giordano and E.A. Friedman (eds.). Milano: Wichting, pp. 200–207.

249. Leber, H.W., Gobeaud, G. and Spiegelhalter, R. (1979) Middle molecules in renal failure. Ann. Clin. Biochem. 16: 389–395.

250. Furst, P., Bergstrom, J. and Gordon, A. (1974) Separation of middle molecular solutes in biological fluids. Rein et Foie, Maladies de la Nutrition 16B: 278–285.

251. Furst, P., Asaba M., Gordon, A., Zimmerman, L. and Bergstrom, J. (1974) Middle molecules in uraemia. Proc. EDTA 11: 417–426.

252. Mabuchi, H. and Nakahashi, H. (1983) Medium-sized peptide in the blood of patients with uremia. Nephron 33: 232–237.

253. Mabuchi, H. and Nakahashi, H. (1982) Profiling of urinary mediumsized peptides in normal and uremic urine by high-performance liquid chromatography. J. Chromat. 233: 107–113.

254. Oulés, R., Emond, C., Claret, G., Brauger, B., Mion, H. and Mion, C. Middle Molecule accumulation in uraemia: an 'extra uremic factor?' Artificial Organs 4 (suppl.) 177–183.

255. Dall'Aglio, P., Buzio, C., Cambi, V., Arisi, L. and Migone, L. (1972) La retention de moyennes molecules dans le sérum urémique. Proc. EDTA 9: 409–415.

256. Saito, A., Kanazawa, I., Chung, T.G. and Maeda, K. (1980) Analytical study for separation of middle molecules. Artificial Organs 4 (suppl.): 13–16.

257. Shoots, A.C., Mikkers, E.P., Claessens, H.A., De Smet, R.U., Landschoot, N. and Ringoir, S. (1982) Characterization of uremic middle molecular fractions by gas-chromatography, mass-spectrometry, isotachophoresis and liquid-chromatography. Clin. Chem. 28: 45–49.

258. Bergstrom, J., Furst, P. and Zimmermann, L. (1981) Separation and identification of uremic middle molecules. Introduction. Proc. 8th Int. Congr. Nephrol.: 595–599.

259. Manari, A., Buzio, C., Calderini, C., David, S., Montagna, G., Quaretti, P., Gròf, J. and Migone, L. (1982) Modificazioni del profilo sierico delle Medie Molecole (MM) in pazienti a diversa anzianità dialitica. Minerva Nefrologica 29: 93–100.

260. Manari, A., Buzio, C., Calderini, C., Montagna, G. and Migone, L. (1981) Limiti ed errori nella tecnica di separazione delle medie molecole (MM) sieriche. Un contributo al miglioramento della metodica. [Milano: Wichting (Ed.) Nefrologia, Dialisi, Trapiano, pp. 365–366.]

261. Gròf, J and Menyhàrt J. (1981) Isotachophoretic analysis of 500–5,000 Dalton molecular

mass solutes in biological fluid samples of human origin. In F.M. Everaerts Amsterdam: Analytical Isotachophoretic, pp. (ed.). 99–107.

262. Le Moel, G., Strecker, G., Troupel, S., Dolegeal, M., Jacobs, C., Galli, A. and Agneray, J. (1980) Carbohydrate content of middle molecular weight substances (MMWS) in uraemic patients. Artificial Organs 4 (suppl.): 37–40.

263. Hartitzsch, B., Hoenich, N.A., Peterson, R.J., Buselmeier, T.J., Kerr, D.N.S. and Kjellstrand, C.M. (1973) Middle molecule clearance in current dialysers. Proc. EDTA 10: 522–527.

264. Peters, J.H. and Gotch, F.A. (1975) Artificial kidneys: Biochemical evaluations. Proc. 8th Ann. Contract. Conf., DHEW Publication (NIH): 44–45.

265. Arisi, L., Buzio, C., Cambi, V., Calderini, M.C., David, S., Manari, A., Montagna, G., Zanelli, P. and Migone, L. (1981) Estrazione di medie molecole in differenti trattamenti emodepurativi. Milano Wichting (Ed.) Nefrologia, Dialisi e Trapianti, pp. 367–368.

266. Cambi, V., Buzio, C., Arisi, L., Calderini, M.C., David, S., Bono, F., Manari, A., Zanelli, P. (1981) Vascular stability and middle molecules removal in hypertonic hemodiafiltration. Proc. EDTA 18: 681–688.

267. Manari, A., Calderini, M.C., Buzio, C., Montagna, G., Arisi, L., David, S., Zanelli, P. and Cambi, V. (1981) Capacità estrattiva delle medie molecole endogene di diverse modalità di depurazione extracorporea: emodialisi, emofiltrazione, emodiafiltrazione ipertonica, emoperfusione. Risultati preliminari. Atti del Convegno di Nefrologia e Dialisi, Torre Pelice: 33–35.

268. Bricker, N.S. (1972) On the pathogenesis of the uremic state. N. Engl. J. Med. 20: 1093–1099.

269. Bricker, N.S. and Fine, L.G. (1978) The trade-off hypothesis: current status. Kidney Int. 13: 55–58.

270. De Wardener, H.E., Mills, I.H., Clapham, W.F. and Hayster, C.J. (1961) Studies on the efferent mechanism of the sodium diuresis which follows the administration of intravenous saline in the dog. Clin. Sci. 21: 249–258.

271. Mills, J.H., De Wardener, H.E., Hayter, C.J. and Clapham, W.F. (1961) Studies on the afferent mechanism of the sodium chloride diuresis which follows intravenous saline in the dog. Clin. Sci. 21: 259–264.

272. Cort, J.H., Pliska, V. and Dousa, T. (1968) The chemical nature and tissue source of natriuretic hormone. Lancet 1: 230–234.

273. Atlas, S.A., Kleinert, H.D., Camargo, M.J., Januszewicz, A., Scalley, J.E., Laragh, J.H., Maack, T., Schilling, J.W., Lewicki, J.A. and Jotuson, L.K. (1984) Purification, sequencing, and synthesis of natriuretic and vasocative rat atrial peptide. Nature 309: 717–719.

274. Kangawa, K. and Matsuo, H. (1984) Purification and complete aminoacid sequence of $\alpha$-human atrial natriuretic polypeptide ($\alpha$hANP). Biochem., Biophys. Res. Commun. 118: 131–139.

275. Flynn, T.G., deBold, M.L. and deBold, A.J. (1983) The aminoacid sequence of an atrial peptide with potent diuretic and natriuretic properties. Biochem. Biophys. Res. Commun. 117: 859–865.

276. Kominami, N., Tyler, R., Hampers, C.L. and Merril, J.P. (1971) Variation in motor nerve conduction velocity in normal and uremic patients. Arch. Intern. Med. 128: 235–242.

277. Oreopoulos, B.G., Gordon, R.D., Blair, H., Meema, E. and Deveber, G.A. (1975) Evolution of uremic neuropathy and renal osteodystrophy in patients undergoing chronic paritoneal dialysis. Abstract Am. Soc. Artif. Internal Organs 4: 47.

278. Thomas, P.K., Hollinrake, K., Lascelles, R.G., O'Sullivan, D.J., Baillod, R.A., Modrhead, J.F. and MacKenzie, J.C. (1971) The polyneuropathy of chronic renal failure. Brain 94: 761–780.

114

# 5. Features of uremic peripheral polyneuropathy in the light of experience with the short hemodialysis schedule (shs)

Giorgio M. Savazzi

Of all the complex functional and structural changes in various organs and systems brought on by uremia, those involving the peripheral nervous system (PNS) have certainly been most widely investigated. Nevertheless, as long as subjective and objective symptomatology were the only data on which neurological impairment could be assessed in the uremic patient, interest in the PNS was no greater than in the other systems affected by this disorder. However, an intent look in the PNS flourished when regular dialysis treatment (RDT) became available and it then became known that the degree of peripheral neuropathy could be finely recorded electromyographically (EMG) and re-checked in the same patient at suitable intervals, giving the nephrologist the possibility — or, at times, the illusion — of tracing back from the neurological impairment to the degree of uremic toxication. Changes of EMG indices were considered early indicators from which to predict more serious uremic symptomatology, and this meant that substitutive treatment of the renal function could be started in proper time, or suggestions could be made for checking and improving the efficiency of dialytic treatment. This chapter's aim is to describe the main aspects of the natural history and evolution of peripheral polyneuropathy during long-term hemodialysis treatment. A semeiologic, histoenzymological, and ultrastructural profile is built up, in the light of the data refering to the patients who in 1971, in Parma, were moved from the traditional dialysis treatment of the sixties to that encouraging experience known as the short hemodialysis schedule (SHS) [1, 2]. Comments are made on facts, traps, illusions, and errors implicit in the EMG indices used at the time, and we take a look at the degree of neuropathy of patients who for many years have been and are today living with this type of dialysis technique.

**Natural history of peripheral nerve function in uremia: NCV changes, signs, and symptoms in patients on short hemodialysis schedule (SHS)**

The most significant EMG indices that in uremia, as in other polyneuro-pathies with a different etiology, may show early alterations before

*Vincenzo Cambi (editor) Professor of Nephrology*
© *1987 Martinus Nijhoff Publishing, Boston. ISBN 0-89838-858-9. Printed in The United States.*

symptoms, are set out in table 5–1. Maximum motor nerve conduction velocity (Max MNCV), more simply known as motor NCV, has been accepted as a sensitive indicator of neuropathy in the uremic patient, and has been widely verified in conservative and chiefly in dialysis treatment [3, 4]. While some Max MNCV indications were up to expectations, many others were conflicting and distracting! Figure 5–1 summarizes a large number of Max MNCV records obtained on a vast case list of patients checked throughout conservative treatment, then during SHS from 1971–1980. Despite its limitations, reviewed in detail below, when Max MNCV is checked in a large population, its time course gives an idea of the functional decay of the nervous system in uremia; the PNS is damaged more in relation to the severity of terminal uremia than to its duration. In fact, only in the terminal phases of conservative treatment some patients present a very rapid drop of Max MNCV (1–2 months) which is never recuperated, whereas in most patients this improves in 2–6 months after starting dialysis. The clinical history of this minority of patients brings to light frequent causes of catabolism (undernutrition, urinary or gastrointestinal protein loss, infections and fever, marked acidosis, and tendency to hyperpotassiemia); collection of the symptoms show that most of them presented distal paresis, total lack of the Achilleus jerks, dysesthesias, and paresthesias. Even after starting

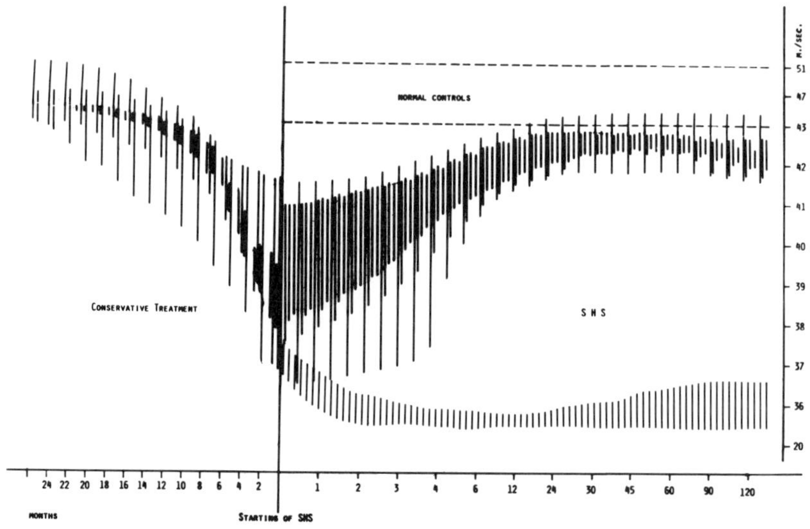



*Figure 5–1.* Changes of posterior tibial nerve maximum motor nerve conduction velocity in 47 patients, checked throughout 25 months before starting dialysis and than throughout 10 years of short hemodialysis schedule. There is a rapid drop of nerve conduction velocity in the latest periods of conservative treatment which improves in most of patients after starting dialysis. Subnormal values are rapidly recovered after the start of SHS. Patients that in conservative treatment reach the most severe symptomatic degree of polyneuropathy and the slowest NCV values are at risk to no more improve this EMG index. (See further details in the text.)

116

*Table 5–1.* Some Electrophysiological indices pathologically modified by uremia

— Changes in shape, duration, and amplitude of motor unit action potentials
— Changes in recruitment of motor unit action potentials
— Appearance of fibrillation potentials
— Slowed maximum and minimum motor nerve conduction velocity
— Changes in shape, duration, and applitude of evoked orthodromic sensory action potentials
— Slowed maximum and minimum sensory nerve conduction velocity
— Changes in evoked (visual, auditory, somatosensory) potentials

hemodialysis a check of symptoms indicates that they take longer to eliminate, and objectively loss of distal jerks persists; however, although Max MNCV values and EMG indices in general remain forever extremely pathological, with time patients recover their motor function. This discrepancy between EMG findings and symptomatology should not lead one to believe that the functional improvement means cure of the PNS. In these cases, in fact, the most frequent histological finding is not at all the restitutio ad integrum of the nerve fibers but the appearance of collateral sprouts from surviving axons (see later) which restore function to a small proportion of muscle fibers, so that with time partial functional recovery is seen. In the overall population the changes of Max MNCV during conservative treatment (figures 5–1) can be related to the progression of polyneuropathic symptoms from their earliest stages to their most disabling manifestations (table 5–2).

Figure 5–1 also shows the course of Max MNCV after the start of SHS: subnormal values were rapidly recovered within 2–6 months. From the cronological pattern of onset, progression, and severity of the symptoms set out in table 5–2, a typical course can be laid out for polyneuropathy in uremia: the onset of symptoms is mainly sensorial taking the form of

*Table 5–2.* Progression of polyneuropathy in 47 patients in conservative treatment (signs and symptoms 6 months, 3 months, and before starting SHS.

|  | 6 Months | 3 Months | Before Starting SHS |
|---|---|---|---|
| Impaired vibratory sensation | 12 | 21 | 39 |
| Paresthesia-disesthesia | 2 | 7 | 21 |
| Restless legs syndrome | 0 | 1 | 9 |
| Burning foot syndrome | 0 | 2 | 11 |
| Reduction of kee jerks | 2 | 5 | 8 |
| Loss of knee jerks | 0 | 4 | 5 |
| Reduction of ankle jerks | 14 | 29 | 20 |
| Loss of ankle jerks | 6 | 18 | 27 |
| Muscular hypotrophies | 2 | 7 | 21 |
| Paresis | 0 | 0 | 5 |
| Cumulative Upper limbs signs and symptoms | 0 | 0 | 6 |

*Table 5–3.* Changes of recruitment in abductor hallucis muscle and of posterior tibial nerve max MNCV from conservative treatment to SHS: 47 consecutive patients

| Patient | Conservative treatment | | After 6 Months of SHS | | After 12 Months of SHS | |
|---|---|---|---|---|---|---|
| | Recruitment | PTN Max MNCV | Recruitment | PTN Max MNCV | Recruitment | PTN Max MNCV |
| G.C. | MI | 38 | MI | 41 | MI | 40 |
| B.C. | NI | 37 | MI | 40 | MI | 44 |
| C.C. | NI | 41 | NI | 44 | NI | 43 |
| A.B. | MI | 35 | MI | 42 | MI | 43 |
| S.G. | FI | 39 | FI | 44 | FI | 44 |
| M.Q. | NI | 33 | NI | 39 | MI | 41 |
| N.C. | NI | 32 | NI | 40 | MI | 40 |
| O.C. | MI | 34 | FI | 36 | FI | 38 |
| M.T. | NI | 27 | NI | 26 | NI | 30 |
| A.A. | NI | 22 | NI | 26 | NI | 25 |
| F.F. | FI | 38 | MI | 40 | MI | 40 |
| R.G. | NI | 36 | MI | 37 | MI | 37 |
| M.C. | MI | 41 | MI | 44 | MI | 46 |
| B.I. | MI | 42 | FI | 45 | FI | 44 |
| A.B. | MI | 30 | MI | 38 | MI | 41 |
| D.G. | MI | 39 | MI | 39 | FI | 43 |
| G.L. | NI | 35 | NI | 40 | NI | 39 |
| R.F. | FI | 44 | MI | 46 | MI | 45 |
| D.A. | NI | 36 | NI | 35 | NI | 35 |
| R.B. | NI | 38 | FI | 42 | FI | 44 |
| B.M. | MI | 38 | NI | 37 | NI | 38 |
| P.I. | NI | 35 | MI | 35 | MI | 39 |
| D.A. | NI | 41 | NI | 39 | NI | 39 |
| V.C. | MI | 40 | MI | 39 | MI | 42 |
| G.C. | MI | 36 | MI | 38 | MI | 39 |
| G.P. | MI | 37 | MI | 41 | MI | 40 |
| B.G. | NI | 36 | MI | 38 | MI | 38 |
| R.P. | NI | 39 | NI | 38 | NI | 38 |

| | | | | | |
|---|---|---|---|---|---|
| F.S. | NI | 27 | MI | 26 | MI | 26 |
| A.Q. | NI | 39 | MI | 39 | FI | 46 |
| S.G. | MI | 31 | NI | 39 | NI | 30 |
| M.E. | MI | 29 | MI | 40 | MI | 45 |
| N.C. | FI | 44 | FI | 47 | FI | 48 |
| O.C. | MI | 41 | MI | 44 | MI | 43 |
| M.T. | NI | 36 | MI | 40 | MI | 42 |
| A.E. | NI | 39 | NI | 39 | NI | 38 |
| I.B. | NI | 39 | MI | 44 | MI | 44 |
| L.F. | MI | 40 | FI | 44 | FI | 48 |
| M.G. | MI | 37 | MI | 39 | MI | 41 |
| G.M. | NI | 42 | MI | 42 | MI | 41 |
| C.V. | NI | 40 | MI | 42 | MI | 41 |
| C.G. | NI | 36 | MI | 35 | MI | 38 |
| R.P. | NI | 39 | MI | 39 | MI | 40 |
| A.E. | NI | 25 | NI | 30 | NI | 29 |
| G.S. | MI | 34 | MI | 35 | MI | 34 |
| N.C. | NI | 39 | MI | 42 | MI | 43 |
| O.B. | NI | 40 | MI | 43 | MI | 43 |

|  |  |  |
|---|---|---|
| NI = 26 | NI = 13 | NI = 11 |
| MI = 17 | MI = 28 | MI = 28 |
| FI = 4 | FI = 6 | FI = 8 |

The rating scale for the degree of neuropathy in each single patient is indicated in table 5–4. This table indicates a progressive improvement but not total recovery of peripheral nerve function passing from conservative treatment to SHS.

dysesthesia and paresthesia, insidiously involving first the lower limbs; the restless legs syndrome comes under this heading, believed to be due to axon damage and to demyelination of the sheath of the finest dendritic branches, but involvement of the autonomic nervous system cannot be excluded, as then comes the 'burning foot' syndrome, a painful burning paresthesia; vibratory sensation in the feet is reduced early.

Neuromuscular impairment starts as easy fatiguability and limited capacity for effort; at this stage, while jerks weaken, starting with the Achilles tendon reflexes and then progressing up to the patellar one, a careful examination of the muscle mass, especially distal muscle, reveals initial slight hypotrophies. By the time the first distal paresis occurs, the Achilles jerk has long been lost; the small distal muscles of the feet are the first to be compromised, giving rise to the 'dropped foot' that causes these patients problems with tripping. But even at this stage major symptoms in the arms may still be undetectable. Obviously the sequence and severity of symptoms, as uremia advances, vary widely in individual patients. However, a search for and analysis of the most common symptoms found in this caselist of 47 patients in conservative treatment just before beginning SHS (table 5–3) leads to two conclusions: sensory nerves are affected before the motor ones and legs before and much more severely than the arms. Thus the characteristics distinguishing poly-neuropathy in our patients are not qualitatively different from those of subjects receiving other types of dialysis schedules.


**Uremic neuropathy as a criterion of adequate dialysis**

In the sixties dialytic treatment was still in its experimental, pionering stage and was based on virtually empirical criteria regarding its efficacy in removing uremic solutes. There was a widely felt need for an index of the efficiency of dialysis, but we had to wait until the seventies for the topic to be tackled in terms of kinetics of typical solutes, such as middle molecules or kinetic modelling of urea nitrogen [5–6].

In consideration of the polyneuropathy arising in uremia, noted parti-cularly in dialyzed patients, and drawing on the now routine EMG technique, as early as 1964 it had been noted that some EMG indices were modified by uremia [7]. This would, however, have remained just one of the many factors making up the multifaceted clinical picture of the uremic syndrome had it not been for the fact that about the same time, slowing of NCV was reported as an early sign of worsening of neuropathy, related to inadequate dialysis treatment [8].

This led to numerous studies of the relations between degree of neuropathy, as assessed by NCV, and indices of nitrogen retention [9, 10]. An inverse linear relationship between motor and/or sensory Max NCV and serum creatinine levels was obtained by Blagg and associates [10] confirmed by Van Der Most Van Spijk and associates [11] and Jennekens and associates

120

[12] in the uremic patient under conservative treatment. This knowledge certainly formed an important part of the overall clinical and blood biochemistry picture on which to base the decision when to start a patient on chronic dialysis treatment. This same relationship was held to be valid in dialysis patients by Cadilhac and associates. [13], and it was soon generally agreed that slowly of Max NCV in patients in dialysis treatment was a sign of worsening of their polyneuropathy due to inadequate dialysis. Later, however, the reliability of this single EMG index as a guide to the adequacy of dialysis was criticized by several authors [14]. Nephrological needs were, in fact, frequently left unfulfilled by the acritical use of Max NCV in dialyzed patients [15] without taking due account of the many technical variables that could affect its value and limit its sensitivity, especially when used as the sole means of obtaining a prompt and presumably precise definition of the severity of neuropathy in the dialyzed patient.

Max NCV thus proved unsuitable for monitoring the adequacy of dialytic treatment, especially when employed with the overambitious aim of distinguishing the best among several dialytic techniques.

Unequivocal conclusions concerning the role and limits of Max NCV as a guide to adequacy of dialysis treatment were provided by Savazzi and associates [16] who investigated the relationship between glomerular filtration rate (GFR) and degree of polyneuropathy in conservative and hemodialyzed patients. The relationship between GFR and the degree of neuropathy confirmed in conservative treatment was not found in dialysis patients: this lack of relation between the so-called 'dialysis index,' and the degree of neuropathy did not confirm the utility of Max NCV and other simple but reliable EMG indices of neuropathy in tailoring adequate or personalized dialysis schedules. Despite the limited sensitivity of Max NCV, there is no denying that when it is repeated over long periods in the same patient, in exactly reproduced conditions of technical execution, it has some practical significance. It offers an acceptable means of checking for significant improvement or worsening in the degree of neuropathy.

This criterion, applied to the dialytic experience gained in Parma, suggested that when the passage from traditional dialysis to SHS caused no worsening in the long run, indicating that the peripheral nervous system had stabilized under the new regimen, we were justified in shifting terminal uremic patients directly to SHS. The validity of this decision has been confirmed by the results to date, not only regarding improvement of peripheral neuropathy but also the patients' clinical and rehabilitational status and general subjective well-being [2].


**Methods**

Since 1970 we have been using maximum motor nerve conduction velocity (Max MNCV) for periodic checks on patients treated by experimental dialysis

121

schedules and/or SHS. In 1973 we added standard electromyographic (EMG) examination. Of the various EMG parameters considered, we lay emphasis on the presence or absence of fibrillation, and on recruitment of motor units since these lend themselves to mathematical expression (table 5–4). In our dialysis unit, Max MNCV was elicited and recorded using a Hewlett Packard 1510 A dual-channel electromyograph with a variable persistence storage scope and camera; the examination was always done by the same physician in our laboratory. The orthodromic single stimulation was a square wave pulse width, variable from 200–500 msec delivered through a pair of electrodes placed to ensure a distal position of the cathode. Supramaximal stimuli were used for recording, and we measured the latent period from the shock artefact to the point where the recorded action potential first begins to leave the baseline.

In positioning the needle within the muscle, care was taken to ensure that the initial deflections of the muscle action potentials (MAP) were such as to permit measurement of the intervals of the corresponding points, and only equal morphologies of the MAP were considered. Particular care was taken when recording the EMG, to the temperature of the limb, since this has great influence on conduction velocity [17]. Recordings were made at a room temperature of 26–28°C, and the surface temperature of the limb was measured using a thermocouple. Bipolar needle pick-up electrodes were selected as routine. Average maximum conduction velocity of our normal controls is 47 ± 4 m/sec for the posterior tibial nerve and 49 ± 5 mt/sec for the peroneal nerve (knee to ankle). Max MNCV values always refer to measurements made before dialysis. Despite the reliability limits of nerve conduction data — as later underlined — the course of this parameter, when checked periodically in the same patient over long periods of time, and the technical accuracy ensured by the examination being made with particular care by the same physician using the same equipment, do improve its reliability and increase the significance of its findings, to the extent that it provides a long-term record of the severity of neuropathy in patients on dialysis.


**Clinical significance and limits of Max MNCV**

Of the many EMG indices that show alterations in uremia, Max MNCV has aroused general interest since the sixties on account of its practical appeal: it is easy, speedy, and simple, and gives numerical results which can therefore be compared with subsequent and past readings for the same patient. In addition, numerical terms do not allow subjective interpretations by the investigator, whereas this can happen for other EMG aspects of equal or finer significance of neuropathy but mainly morphological in expression. Of paramount importance is a convincing linear correlation between Max MNCV and serum creatinine levels during conservative treatment (figure

122

*Table 5–4.* Degree of neuropathy (DN) obtained by Max MNCV, then by coupling Max MNCV with the recruitment of MU and then adding the finding of fibrillation potentials in 40 patients in SHS

| Patients | PTN-Max MNCV (m/sec) | DN (PTN-Max MNCV) | Recruit-ment | DN (PTN-Max MNCV) + Recruitment | Fabrillation Potentials | DN (PTN-Max MNCV) + Recruitment + Fibrillation |
|---|---|---|---|---|---|---|
| M.C. | 51 | 0 | MI | 3 | P | 4 |
| I.B. | 30 | 2 | NI | 4 | P | 5 |
| A.B. | 46 | 0 | NI | 2 | A | 2 |
| D.G. | 47 | 0 | MI | 1 | A | 1 |
| L.G. | 46 | 0 | MI | 1 | A | 1 |
| R.F. | 40 | 1 | NI | 3 | P | 4 |
| A.D. | 39 | 1 | NI | 3 | P | 4 |
| R.B. | 37 | 2 | NI | 4 | A | 4 |
| G.F. | 49 | 0 | MI | 1 | A | 1 |
| B.M. | 50 | 0 | MI | 1 | A | 1 |
| P.I. | 41 | 1 | MI | 2 | A | 2 |
| L.B. | 42 | 1 | NI | 2 | A | 2 |
| P.B. | 39 | 1 | MI | 2 | A | 2 |
| G.G. | 41 | 1 | NI | 2 | A | 2 |
| T.T. | 47 | 2 | NI | 4 | A | 4 |
| G.R. | 42 | 1 | FI | 1 | A | 1 |
| A.G. | 41 | 1 | MI | 2 | A | 2 |
| L.F. | 42 | 1 | NI | 3 | P | 4 |
| M.G. | 48 | 0 | NI | 2 | P | 3 |
| L.M. | 40 | 1 | MI | 2 | A | 2 |
| V.C. | 42 | 1 | FI | 1 | A | 1 |
| G.C. | 42 | 1 | NI | 3 | A | 3 |
| G.P. | 38 | 2 | NI | 4 | P | 5 |
| G.B. | 36 | 2 | MI | 3 | A | 3 |
| P.R. | 39 | 1 | NI | 3 | P | 4 |

*Table 5–4.* Continued.

| Patients | PTN-Max MNCV (m/sec) | DN (PTN-Max MNCV) | Recruit-ment | DN (PTN-Max MNCV) + Recruitment | Fabrillation Potentials | DN (PTN-Max MNCV) + Recruitment + Fibrillation |
|---|---|---|---|---|---|---|
| F.S. | 38 | 2 | MI | 3 | P | 4 |
| B.M. | 44 | 0 | MI | 1 | A | 1 |
| G.C. | 43 | 0 | MI | 1 | A | 1 |
| C.B. | 33 | 2 | NI | 4 | A | 4 |
| G.L. | 46 | 0 | MI | 1 | A | 1 |
| C.P. | 39 | 1 | MI | 2 | A | 2 |
| A.B. | 53 | 0 | MI | 1 | A | 1 |
| S.G. | 49 | 0 | MI | 1 | A | 1 |
| M.Q. | 42 | 1 | NI | 3 | P | 4 |
| N.C. | 41 | 1 | FI | 1 | P | 2 |
| O.C. | 42 | 1 | NI | 3 | A | 3 |
| T.M. | 42 | 1 | MI | 2 | P | 3 |
| A.A. | 47 | 0 | NI | 2 | A | 2 |
| F.F. | 38 | 2 | MI | 3 | A | 3 |
| R.G. | 42 | 1 | MI | 2 | A | 2 |

The table indicates progressive DN in 50 patients in long-term SHS, coupling the recruitment of MU in abductor hallucis muscle to posterior tibial nerve Max MNCV (PTN-Max MNCV) (column 5) and then adding to this the presence of fibrillation potentials (column 7) to compare to the DN indicated by PTN-Max MNCV alone (column 3). The rating scale for the DN in each patient is as follows:

PTN-Max MNCV: $\geq$43 m/sec. (normal)  DN = 0  
         from 39 to 43 m/sec.DN = 1  
         $\leq$38 m/sec.  DN = 2  
Recruitment: (FI) Interference  DN = 0  
      (MI) Mixed Interference  DN = 1  
      (NI) No Interference  DN = 2  
Fibrillation Potentials: Absent  DN = 0  
         Present  DN = 1

5–2) The observation that as uremia progresses Max MNCV gradually decreases is long-standing and inconfutable; unfortunately the opposite, i.e., that substitutive treatment with resolution of subjective symptomatology leads to restoration of normal NCV, is not likewise true because NCV values become normal in only very few patients (table 5–3). Nevertheless in the seventies Max MNCV did have a real clinical significance as frequently severe neuropathies were encountered either as a result of conservative treatment prolonged to the very extreme degrees of uremia because of the limited availability of substitutive treatment in those years, or because of the substantial improvements of the neuropathy resulting from the start of hemodialysis. In practice it soon became evident that whereas the switch from conservative treatment to hemodialysis resulted in significant improvement in nerve conduction indices in the 2–6 months after the start of dialysis, no further significant improvement or change was seen in patients whose clinical conditions were stable, even when the duration of dialysis was progressively reduced to 4 hours 3 times a week or 3 hours each other day (figure 5–3) compatibly with what later became known as 'adequate dialysis' treatment. The relative sensitivity and clinical significance of Max MNCV arises from many different reasons: first the formula (velocity = space/time) used in calculating NCV is subject to imprecision in practical esecution, contrary to what the physical expression might suggest. Even following a very careful and

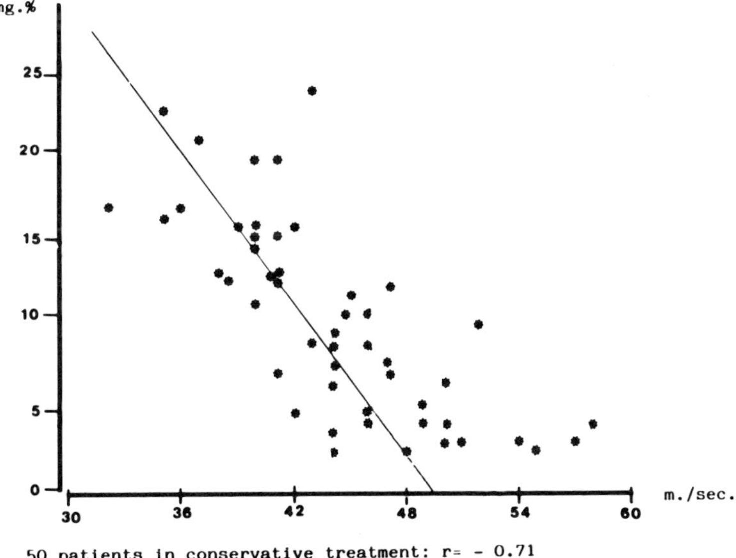



*Figure 5–2.* The interdependence between major degrees of renal failure and the polyneuropathy is confirmed by a significant inverse relationship between PTN-Max MNCV and creatininemia. In our laboratory the normal mean control values of PTN Max MNCV are 47±4 m/sec.; especially values inferior to 40 m/sec. have been found increasingly associated with a more evident neurological damage.

125

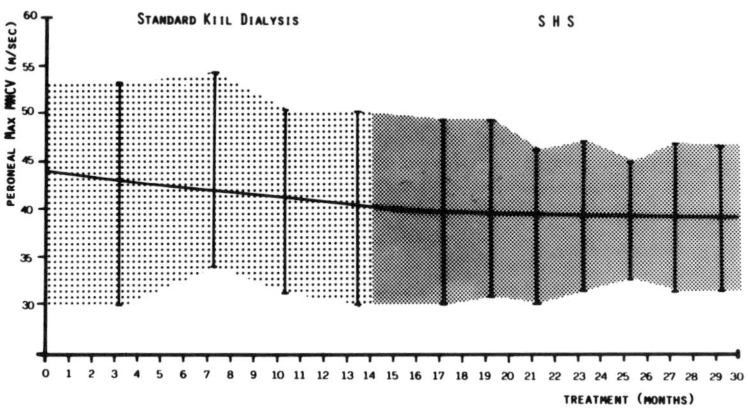


*Figure 5–3.* A longitudinal control of peroneal Max MNCV in 13 patients, before in standard Kiil dialysis and later in SHS; neither deterioration of MNCV nor clinical neuropathy appeared during 30 months.

rigorous method, findings in the same subject at different times usually vary by 8% [18] and uremic patients have been found to present wider than normal variability [19]. To make things worse, the temperature in the vicinity of the nerve consistently affects the conduction [17]. Serum potassium and calcium levels, and chiefly any sudden variation affect NCV. Thus these physical variants by themselves are enough to modify results and lead to mistakes in their clinical interpretation if a hypothermic limb is not warmed or if there are sudden electrolyte changes with therapy or dialysis. Second the peripheral nerve segment to which conduction refers is made up of several hundred fibers that vary greatly in thickness and myelination, thresholds of excitability and hence conduction. Because the conduction velocity increases with nerve fibers' size, electrical charges which pass through these faster fibers are responsible for the start of an oscilloscopic deflection where Max MNCV is calculated that represents the evoked compound muscle potential; therefore, Max MNCV assesses the function of the most heavily myelinated and largest diameter fibers and is therefore properly called Maximum MNCV. The same considerations exist for Max Sensory MCV, i.e., nerve conduction obtained on a sensory nerve. For technical reasons linked to the EMG amplification system, the limited depolarization of even only a few nerve fibers triggers the oscilloscopic deflection of the evoked potential on whose start the latency time is calculated. Therefore, if only a few fibers less severely damaged by uremia are able to bring about a nearly normal conduction, the resulting Max MNCV is not representative of the anatomopathological conditions of the nerve as a whole [20].

Finally, in uremia axonal degeneration and segmental demielination are uneven not only in different fibers but also in different tracts of the same fiber [21] and appear first and more severely in the distal segments of an increasing numer of axons; but the way NCV is calculated (in the formula

126

V=S/T, the time is the difference between proximal and distal latency time) excludes any indication concerning the axon terminals that are the principal site of earlier and greater pathological involvement. Hence the importance of a criterion taking account of these limitations and providing a basis in a uremic patient for relating a certain NCV value to an objective degree of polyneuropathy. A normal Max MNCV does not exclude the presence even of appreciable neuropathy, usually still subsymptomatic. Borderline values generally indicate definite neuropathy and coexist with changes in more sensitive EMG indices; clearly pathological values indicate severe neuropathy and usually coexist with symptoms and precise histological damage to the axon populations. The limits of NCV as a sensitive measure of the degree of neuropathy are more evident when compared with other EMG indices routinely checked by the neurologist seeking to diagnose and establish the severity of neuromuscular impairment in single patients. Max motor and sensory NCV are indicators of whether large-diameter, fast-conducting nerve fibers are intact or not; spontaneous activity at rest usually signifies muscle fibers' denervation or may be a signal of intrinsic muscle fibers' cell distress. Investigation of the motor unit action potential (MUP) parameters during weak voluntary contraction gives a picture of the anatomofunctional situation of the motor unit (MU) — see further details later — and the modality and capacity for recruitment of MU during maximal muscular voluntary effort indicates, when anomalies are present, the existence of denervation or muscle lesions. Undeniably it is impossible to unify in an expression simple as a number given by NCV the many details provided by the multiple electro-physiological parameters listed above. This is why routine EMG has never acquired much favor for nephrological purpose. Any significant change in electrophysiological indices, including NCV, can be traced to real structural changes in the nerve or muscle or both, obviously related to real changes in the degree of uremia.

This tightknit relationship easily explains the disappointment of those who in the seventies expected omens of the clinical future or portents of better treatment in different dialysis schedules and methods, differing in technical content but with basically the same effects in eliminating uremia, from significant changes in the electrophysiologic indices of neuropathy. In the context of experience with SHS, it was noted that once subnormal NCV values were obtained, usually within 2–3 months of starting regular dialysis treatment, a corresponding rapid resolution was noted in the subjective symptoms of neuropathy, after which no further significant changes took place. This led to other EMG parameters being employed with Max MNCV to draw up a composite picture of the neuropathy, reflecting more closely the real state of the peripheral nerve, and casting light on aspects that were not sufficiently clarified by nerve conduction data alone. Since EMG aspects differing so widely in the severity of the neuropathy they represented could be converted to numerical expressions, and on account of the well-proved clinical worth of EMG experience as a whole, we focused on the presence or absence of spontaneous electrical activity (fibrillation) and on motor unit (MU) recruitment during maximal voluntary contraction. Table 5–4 epitomizes three EMG indices, the Max MNCV on the posterior tibial nerve, the recruitment of MU during maximum voluntary contraction in abductor hallucis muscle, and fibrillation if present in 50 patients treated by SHS (4 hours 3 times a week). The recruitment of MU can be considered a straightforward EMG index, sufficiently reproducible and therefore reliable, that has been successfully coupled with Max MNCV to gain a better idea of the degree of neuropathy closer to each patient's or caselist's real neurological impairment, than that given by NCV alone. This shows that the coupling of simple EMG indices, well-tried in everyday neurological practice which are known to be modified by precise physiopathological events, can give reliable indications to the practicing nephrologist (table 5–4). These clinical indications are sometimes more elucidatory than sophisticated electrophysiological indices taken singly.

If, therefore, with the experience of the eighties almost behind us, we take a fresh look at the EMG investigations of neuropathy in SHS patients made in the seventies, the obvious conclusion is that the degree of neuropathy was certainly not finely assessed, but the overall findings were useful for clinical purposes, especially as a means of checking that no significant worsening was occurring with time. In the meantime, from the severity of neuropathy observed in most terminal uremic patients moved through SHS to regular dialysis treatment we can see such worthwhile improvements in EMG parameters and symptoms in relatively short times, that there can be no doubt about the efficacy of SHS, even for specific treatment of neuropatic complications.


**The motor unit in normal conditions and its regressive changes and repair in SHS**

A schematic knowledge of the normal motor unit [22] (MU) is basic for understanding some EMG, histopathological and ultrastructural changes that are clinically important for assessing uremic polyneuropathy. The MU is an anatomofunctional structure, consisting of a lower motor neuron and all the muscle fibers on which its terminal arborizations synapse (figure 5–4). Within a muscle region all the fibers linked to this neuron are laid out in a roughly spherical three-dimensional array. Since these muscle fiber cells overlap and intermingle with muscle fibers belonging to other MU, the muscle fibers from a single MU are hardly ever contiguous. The motor unit potential (MUP) is thus the outcome of electrical phenomena resulting from asynchronous depolarization of the muscle fiber cells when activated by depolarization of its specific motor neuron. The MUP is normally visualized as a biphasic or triphasic oscilloscopic deflection due to concurrent complex electrical phenomena in the context of a conducting volume (the whole muscle and the

128

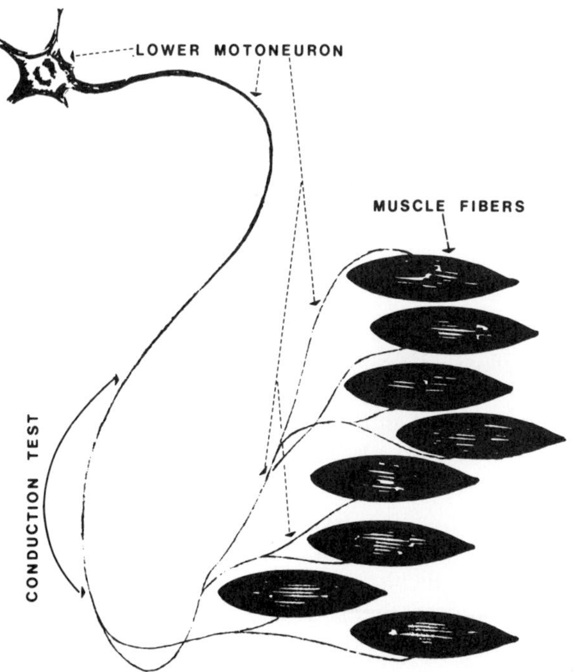


*Figure 5–4.* The motor unit (MU) is an anatomofunctional structure made up of one second-order motor neuron and all the muscle fibers supplied by it. The MU can be studied under electrophysiological, histological, histochemical and ultrastructural profile and allows a panoramic knowledge in regard to normality and to regressive or ameliorative changes.

tissues lying above the electrode lead) and is therefore the electronic image of functional activation of MU. While the duration of MUP correlates in general with the spatial arrangement of the muscle fibers, the size reflects the number, size, and spatial array of muscle fibers within the MU; finally, morphology depends on more complex components including the harmonious nonsynchronous firing of the activated muscle fibers within the same MU. Values outside the band of normal for shape and duration of the MUP indicate functional or structural alterations of the MU that can be ascribed either to the nerve section or to the muscle section or both.

**Integrated activation of the motor unit: the recruitment of MU**

The physiological purpose of the MU is to achieve tension, and the integrated contraction of many MU aims at the execution of effort and movement. A healthy muscle, when completely relaxed, does not produce any electrical activity; weak voluntary contraction causes some MU to fire; and the shape, amplitude, and duration of its MUP are easily distinguished. Voluntary contraction force can be obtained and progressively increased by the interaction of two phenomena: an increase in the frequency-discharge of one MU and the involvement of a larger number of MU. This interaction is called recruitment. When the contraction force is progressively increased a larger number of MU are called into action, and maximum voluntary effort will lead to an oscilloscope tracing with crowding and superposition of potentials to the point where the characteristics of a single MUP can no longer be distinguished among its fellows. This EMG pattern, known as 'interference,' indicated that all possible MU have been recruited in the normal way.

When the nerve fiber is consistently damaged and nerve conduction does not progress to the muscle section of the MU, that MUP is lost on oscilloscope tracing and the interference pattern is no longer seen even if the patient makes his/her maximal voluntary contraction. A moderate loss of MUP results in a mixed interference pattern and severe loss in minimal recruitment (no interference). The recruitment of MU, too, is subject to limitations in sensitivity. Its detection can be inaccurate because of poor technique or poor cooperation by the patient in producing a maximal effort. The tracings are subjectively evaluated by the physician carrying out the examination and it is difficult to distinguish small differences from one tracing to another and compare them. This is why only three different pattern gradings can be easily identified: interference, mixed or subinterference, and minimal or no interference (figure 5–5).

Compared to the clinical indications that NCV gives by itself recruitment alone does not seem to offer substantial advantages for a better definition of the degree of neuropathy. However, one can find cases where NCV is still within the normal range, while recruitment of MU is already altered in a muscle innervated by the nerve on which NCV was still normal, thus indicating a damage previously undetected by NCV. This discrepancy becomes clearer if one remembers the different physiopathologies that modify the two indices, NCV linked to the changes in the nerve fibers that together compose the nerve as a whole, and recruitment of a single MU, dependent on a single axon among the many that compose the nerve.


**Regressive MU changes and reparative phenomena in uremia: data concerning SHS**

Because the histological picture of damage to nerve fibers in uremia begins and shows the most severe axonmyeline changes in the peripheral end-branches of the longest nerves, the most abnormal EMG patterns can be expected from these peripheral districts; in any case, the most marked histological and functional alterations involve the MU distally and are electromyographically shown by changes in the MUP. A first approach to the size and type of the damage to the MU in uremia is provided by EMG tracings that show regressive changes in MU recruitment during maximum muscular

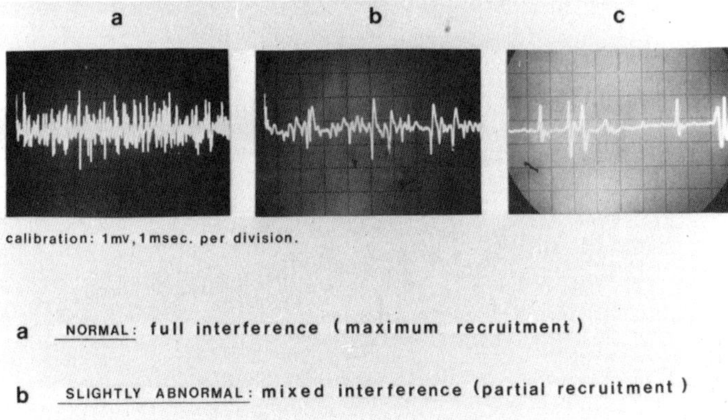


*Figure 5–5*. Different E.M.G. patterus of recruitment obtained by maximum muscular contraction.

voluntary contraction (figure 5–5) with reduction of the mean amplitude of the potentials and a loss of MUP. This loss causes the mixed interference pattern indicative of moderate loss of MU, functional if not yet anatomical, hence indicating moderate neuropathy. More severe EMG recruitment alterations in which few MUP are detectable (no interference pattern) are indicative of at least functional dysfunction of a large number of MU, hence severe neuropathy. The pathogenesis of these EMG alterations lies in the degree of damage to the axon. If the damage is irreversible the MU is forever impaired and its MUP is lost while the muscle fibers belonging to this MU either become atrophic and lost to the contractile function or join other MU through sprouting (see later). If damage to the nerve fibers is within the limits of possible repair, muscle fibers will be restored to function and MUP will reappear in the EMG effort tracings as indication of improved recruitment. That in more severe uremic neuropathy the loss of MUP in the voluntary contraction tracings means real loss of neuromuscular structures is confirmed by peripheral biopsy of the sural nerve where the number of myelinated and unmyelinated fibres is markedly reduced in patients on either conservative or substitutive treatment. But the improvement of MU recruitment with repopulation of the EMG tracings after the start of substitutive therapy indicate that the loss of MUP in uremia does not always and necessarily imply anatomical loss. Table 5–4 illustrates the improvement of recruitment of MU in the abductor hallucis muscle during maximum voluntary contraction, in patients previously on conservative treatment after 6 and 12 months' short dialysis schedule (4 hours thrice weekly). These examples illustrate that in muscle two opposing events arise during uremic polyneuropathy, likely any other form of chronic neuropathy: regressive events leading to the detachment of muscle fibers from their primary motor neuron, and repair events leading to restoration of function. Not only in theory, this unstable balance is related to the level of uremic toxication in the nerve parenchyma and to modifications reflecting the effectiveness of treatment; two extremes might be exemplified by the ingravescent neurological symptoms in terminal uremia and the symptomatological and functional recovery set in motion by a successful transplant. Partial denervation found to different degrees but nearly always present in the uremic patient and documented morphologically by a loss of axon and electromyographically by loss of MUP indicates that functional recovery after these patients have begun substitutive treatment cannot only be ascribed to repair to nerve fibers but sometimes chiefly to sprouting of surviving axons. Sprouting is the term employed when distal branchings of a less severely damaged motor neuron manage to 'hook up' some muscle fibers from the pathological pool of the denerved ones and restore their function. More than repair of fibers, sprouting is the explanation of the functional improvement in paresic uremic patients in whom, once substitutive therapy is started, motor performance can be restored to some extent despite large-scale, definitive loss of motor neurons, a loss indicated by the persistence of no interference in EMG voluntary contraction patterns. On the whole, the final balance between regression and repair of the MU in uremia is almost always negative because in terminal conservative treatment there is always a definitive loss of axons; EMG confirms that this negative balance persists even after prolonged dialysis, SHS included, when repopulation of the tracings under effort fails to occur or is only partial (table 5–3). Morphologically, such EMG loss of MUP finds its counterpart in the nerve, where fascicular biopsy shows irrecuperable loss of axons, and in the muscle which presents aspects of partial denervation in the form of sparse atrophic muscle fibers and small-group atrophy also indicative of denervation. A further proof of the loss of MU in uremia is obtained by a fascinating EMG technique that can be performed in the small distal muscles of the limbs and that provides a count of the functioning MU in each muscle examined [23]. The extensor digitorum brevis muscle, for example, works properly from 199

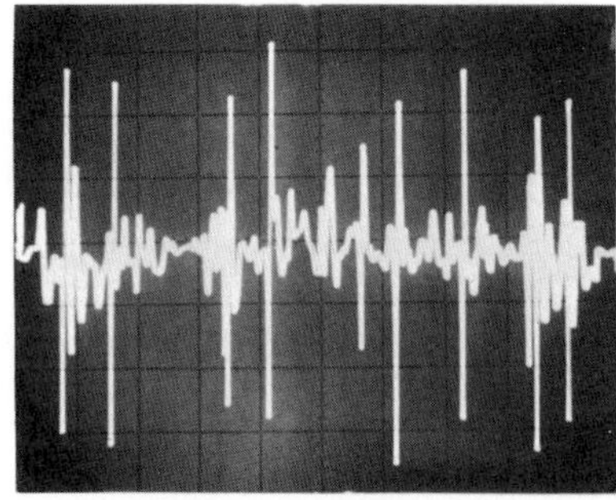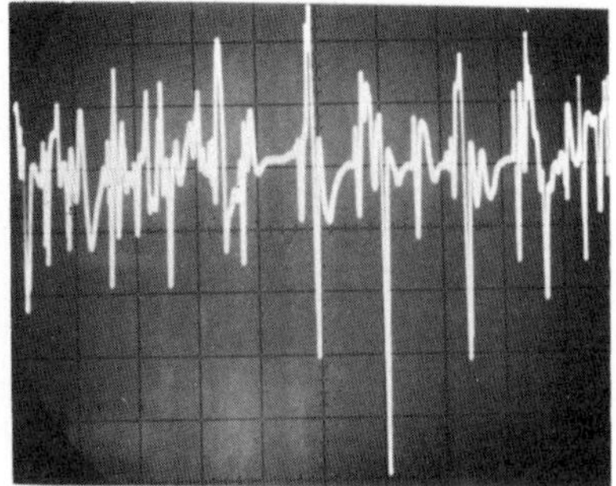

*Figure 5–6.* A Mixed interference pattern (loss of motor unit potentials) and evidence of sprouting (high voltage potentials) during maximum voluntary contraction, in abductor hallucis muscle of 2 patients submitted to SHS from 59 months (right tracing) and 72 months (left tracing). Calibration: 1 mV, 20 msec. per division.

132

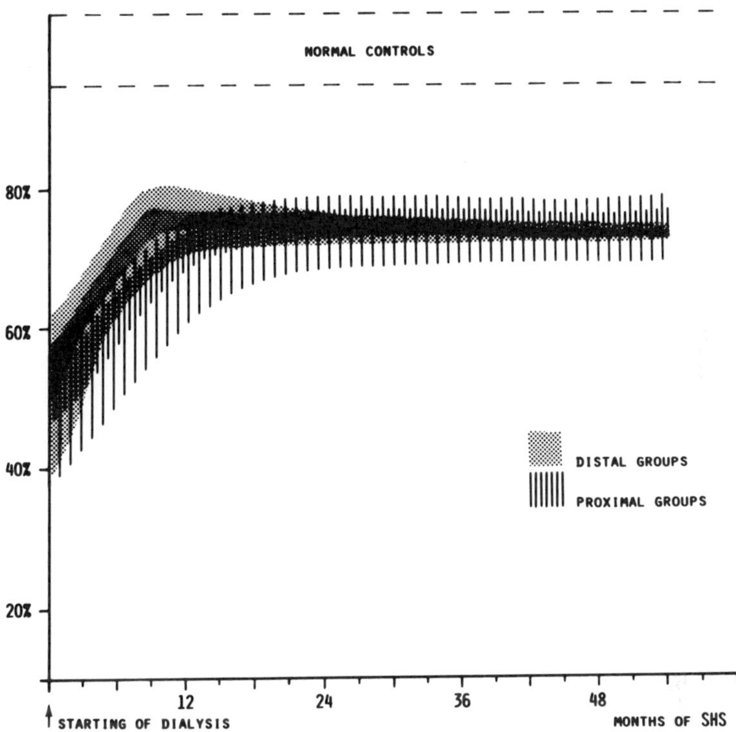


*Figure 5–7.* Analogy of behavior between muscular performance and nerve conduction velocity (see figure 5–1) after starting dialysis.

∓ 60 MU [23], each one lifting an average of 1,6g. (24). The use of this technique, although the results are not universally considered reliable, when applied on uremic patients and those on SHS confirms the loss of MU [25] at least functional, while EMG findings of MUP of higher amplitude in the same patients indicate the existence of sprouting (figure 5–6). From the functional viewpoint, sprouting tends to increase the contractile force of the 'extended' MU beyond its original capacity in relation to the increase of muscle fibers, but such units are less efficient than expected ]26], and that such compensation is partial in relation to functional needs is demonstrated by ergometric investigations in the upper and lower limbs of uremic subjects. In this respect the performance of our patients on SHS (figure 5–7) is comparable to other populations of dialysed patients described in the literature [27].

**The degree of damage to nerve fibers in uremia: data from patients in SHS**

The subjective symptoms and the reduction of reflexes, the paresis, are all initially reported in the feet and find a histological explanation by the fact

133

that, at different levels along the uremic peripheral nerve, there is a loss of nerve fibers per bundle, progressing from the proximal to distal nerve segments. A drop in the number of fibers amounting to 4% at mid-calf but reaching 50% at the ankle has in fact been reported from a study of uremic patients [28]. A systematic approach to assessing uremic peripheral nerve damage calls for fascicular biopsy (figure 5–8) of the sural nerve at the ankle; a 1–2 cm long cylinder should be sampled, containing 4–6 nerve bundles, for an optical study, for teasing, for the fiber density, and for ultramicroscopic study of the histological preparation.

Since in uremia the loss of nerve fibers is never massive, optical microscope preparations do not provide an accurate evaluation of the degree of damage, and only in the most severe cases can the loss of axon be easily perceived from the increased proportion of collagen structures. In contrast the density of fibers per square mm of tissue provides a reliable assessment of the loss of axons, and the distribution curve of fiber diameters indicates whether the loss involves mainly small, medium, or large fibers. Both in conservative treatment and in patients in dialysis treatment (figure 5–9 refers to data from patients in SHS), the loss usually involves all fiber populations with a preference for the larger ones, so that the distribution curve of the nerve axons shows a tendency to reduction or loss of the second peak, attributable to myelinated axons between 8 and 10–12 $\mu$ in diameter. By teasing (figure 5–10), a single axon can be separated from the other and stained in osmic acid; this more detailed qualitative study of the myelin fiber, and of the sheath

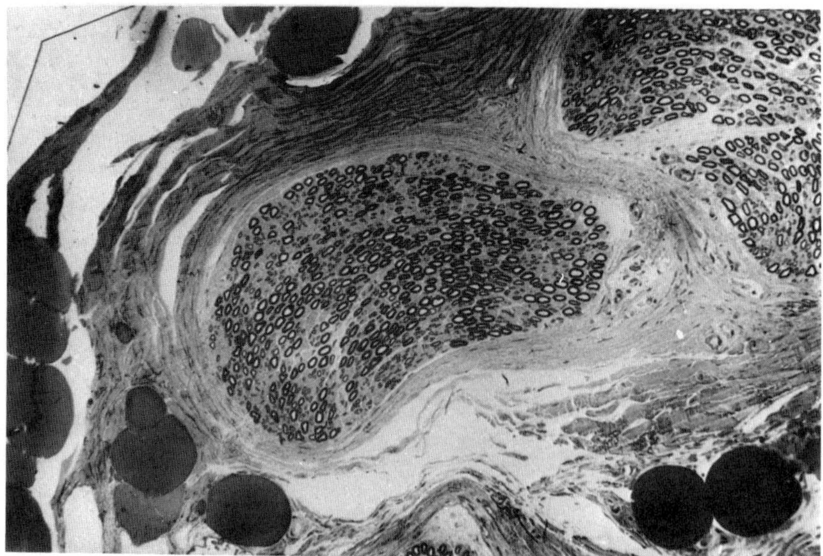

*Figure 5–8.* Epoxy-resin embedded semithin section: thiomine and acridine stain × 100. Transverse section of right sural nerve of a 39-year-old patient in SHS for 15 months, showing slight loss of larger-diameter axons with replacement of collagen structures.

134

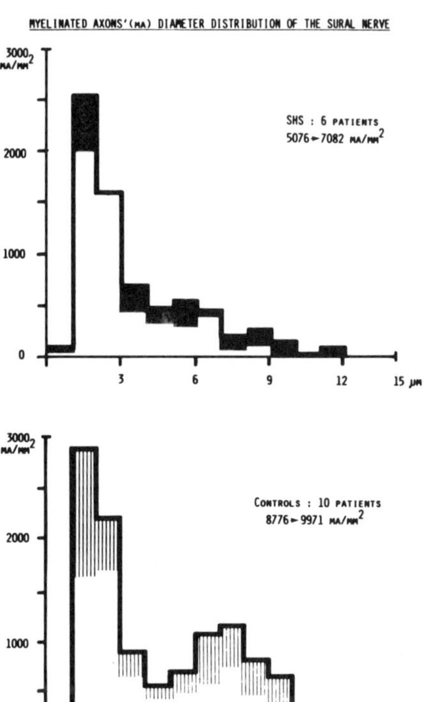


*Figure 5–9.* Density of myelinated fibers per square mm of tissue in 6 patients in SHS (min. 36, max. 62 months). As opposed to the controls see how the distribution curve shows a reduction of the second peak, indicating preferential loss of the larger axons between 8–12 $\mu$ in diameter; in effect, the loss involves all fiber populations. The very small diameter axons are in fact remyelinated axons belonging to the small axons group, because in the remyelinated tracts the sheath is thinner than in the intact axon.

in particular, indicates that the most common damage in uremics is non-homogeneous with demyelinated axons running alongside others that are intact or only slightly altered. In the same fiber, apparently normal myelinated segments may alternate with demyelinated segments. Such regressive events of segmental demyelination may be encountered together with areas of remyelination. This is revealed by shorter irregular intervals between Ranvier's nodes (figure 5–10); in the remyelinated tracts the sheath is generally thinner than in intact axons. Nerve conduction begins with graded electrical discharges at the axon hilloch and when the generator potential is sufficient to exceed the threshold for nerve excitability, the action potential is produced by skipping from one node of Ranvier to the next so normal nerve conduction velocity essentially depends on the length of intact myelinated segments of the axons being normal. Demyelination begins with retraction of the Schwann cell processes from the node of Ranvier, which increases the

135

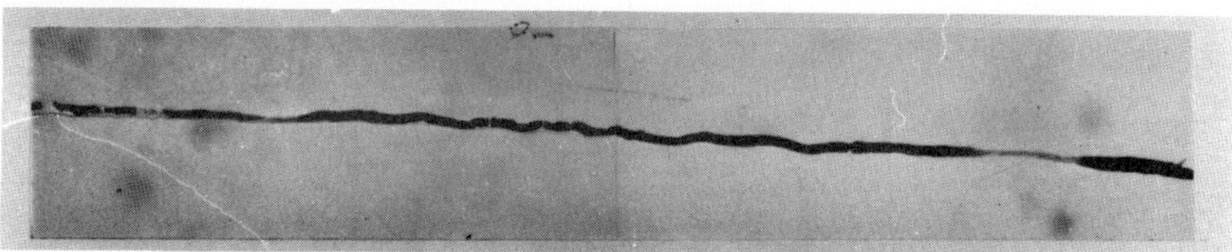

*Figure 5–10.* Patient G.C., 32 years old, SHS for 13 months. Teased fiber exhibiting paranodal segments or large portions of internodal demyelination coexisting with shorter areas of re-myelination. In this patient quantitative studies of the frequency distribution of myelinated fiber size failed to show the normal bimodal pattern because of a prevalent loss of 9–12 $\mu$ myelinated axons. Symptomatology characterized by right foot drop was resolved in 3 months of SHS. Peroneal Max MNCV at the moment of the sural nerve biopsy was 39 m/sec.

axon plasma-membrane area. This results in difficulty in propagation of the action potential. Then, when the lesion progresses and the internodal stretches of the axon are stripped of myelin, propagation of the potential is no longer possible. These histological changes represent the morphological basis of the progressive slowing and subsequent nonevocable nerve conduction velocity. Remyelination is a repair process seen also in conservative treatment but especially after substitutive treatment has begun. Even though reparative remyelination can restore nerve conduction, the shorter length of repaired myelin jackets keeps the NCV slower than in the predisease state, so that function returns and symptoms disappear, but conduction velocity remains forever slower than normal. In addition to remyelination of the nerve fibers, distal degeneration of axons may be followed by sprouting. These two repair methods provide the morphological explanation of the functional improvement, including resolution of pareses, observed after the beginning of dialysis or after renal transplantation [29, 30]. Ultrastructural examination (figure 5–11) defines myelin, and above all, axon damage. The former is represented by aspects of demyelination, sliding of myelin sheaths away from the axons, and sometimes complete extrusion of the axons. Remyelination may sometimes by exuberant with whorls of myelin lamellae without axonal content, making up the so-called 'onion bulbs.' Axonal damage appears as an increase in the ratio of neurofilaments to neurotubules due to abundance of neurofilaments [30] and to a relative scarcity of neurotubules, dilatation and vesiculation of the smooth endoplasmic reticulum profine, and clustered degenerating mitocondria. Reshuffling of nerve structure involves amyelinic fibers as well: some of these fibers are replaced by connective stroma within the nerve bundle forming 'collagen pockets.' Therefore this morphological finding unequivocally indicates loss of axon structures, as indicated in figure 5–9.

## Muscular distress in uremia: data concerning SHS

Long-term chronic hemodialyzed patients rarely show symptoms of muscular damage, and reduced strength, easy fatiguability, and hypotrophies are

136

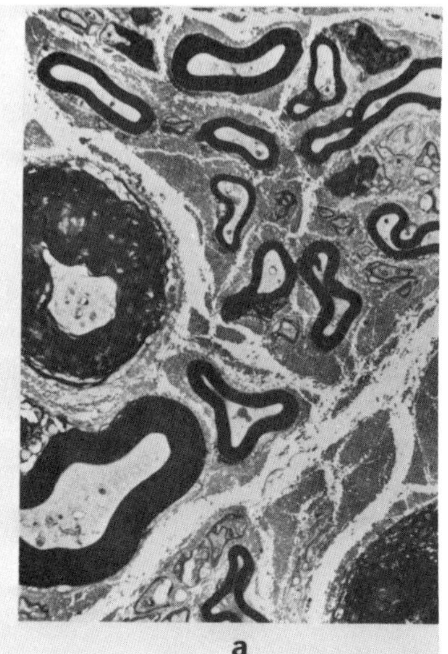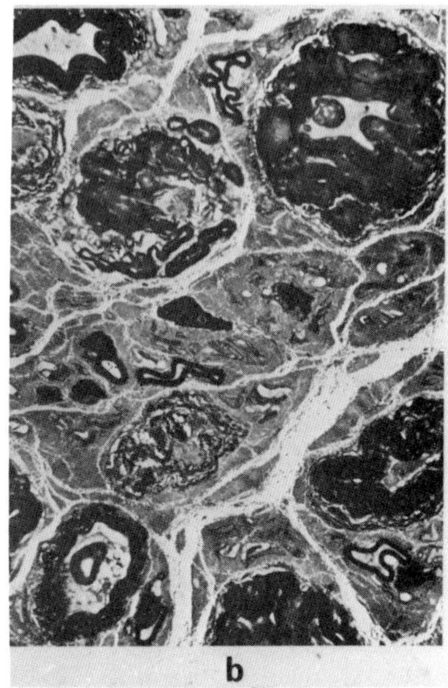

*Figure 5–11.* (a) Reshuffling and loss of larger myelinated fibers coexisting with remyelinated fibers and consistent loss of amyelinic fibers, a picture of endoneural fibrosis. (b) Widespread aspects of demyelination and increased proportion of endoneural collagen.

frequently underestimated. This muscular distress is in the majority of cases so subtle that it is not even clearly perceived by the patient him/herself. However, the incidence of symptoms involving the musculature largely depends on how much care is put into searching for them by careful semeiology, and is demonstrated by EMG examination and appropriate morphological investigation. This disability is functionally identified by ergometric measurement which clearly show subnormal strength in the terminal phases of conservative uremia, by an improvement but not a restoration of normal values some months after the start of dialysis, and then a slight but gradual decline during long-term dialysis treatment (figure 5–7). It is well known that a muscular distress can be 'neurogenic' or 'myogenic.' In this light the existence of neuropathy in the case of uremia might suggest that muscle damage is always and totally secondary. However, recent knowledge gained in neuromuscular disorders convincingly shows that some neurogenic atrophies closely mimic the clinical picture of some types of primary muscle damage and vice versa. Therefore, it is often risky if not impossible to definitely assess the degree and make a precise qualitative diagnosis of myopathy on clinical and EMG grounds alone, without employing modern morphological investigation methods like histoenzymology and untra-structure. These diagnostic problems exist also in patients in conservative treatment or in SHS where in most cases, the EMG findings unequivocally suggest that the muscle impairment is secondary to concomitant neuropathy (slowed Max motor and Max sensory NCV, lost MUP under voluntary

137

control, MUP parameters indicative of neuropathy); nevertheless in sporadic but significant cases there are smaller, highly polyphasic MUP of decreased amplitude and duration, a high-pitched sound at the londspeaker, and sudden recruitment of MU in relation to the strength of contraction, thus justifying doubts about muscular primary impairment. These EMG patterns arise in cases with diffusely distributed neuropathic changes, as in uremia, initially involving the distal nerve branches of the MU (axonal twig dysfunction), with a reduction in the number of active muscle fibers able to generate force, so that these MU must fire faster to achieve the desired summated tension. Thus during voluntary contraction a pattern of excessively reduced complex morphology, excessively discharging MUP evolves, suggesting a wrong diagnosis of myogenic damage or any case giving diagnostic doubts. The disarray, rearrangement, and loss of contractile structures found on histoenzymological and ultrastructural examination of the uremic muscle provide an immediate explanation for the reduced functional performance and add qualitative data to further our understanding of muscular disability in uremia.

**The normal muscle's histochemical profile**

In humans, modern histochemical methods permit the distinction between two main muscle fiber types, I and [31, 32] II, differing in terms of quantitative enzyme content (table 5–5). Type I fibers, rich in cytochrome oxidase, succinate dehydrogenase, and nicotinamide-adenine-dinucleotide diaphorase (NADH), have an array of enzymatic systems chiefly promoting a preferential oxidative metabolism. Type II fibers are rich in mitochondrial glycerophosphate dehydrogenase, phosphorylases, and lactic acid dehydrogenase, and perform a preferentially anaerobic metabolism through the glycolytic pathway. These enzymatic and functional differences between the muscle types are closely linked to their type of innervation. Retrograde

*Table 5–5.* Main fiber types in human muscle

|  | Type I Fibers | Type II Fibers |
| --- | --- | --- |
| *Function* | resistant | fatiguable |
| (twitch) | slow | fast |
| *Structure* | | |
| Fiber size | small | large |
| Mitochondria | rich | poor |
| Z Line | thick | thin |
| *Metabolism* | oxidative | glycolytic |
| *Histochemical reaction* | | |
| Myosin ATPase pH 9.4 | light | dark |
| Myosin ATPase pH 4.6 | dark | light |
| NADH | dark | light |

chromotolysis and retrograde transport studies have established the existence of different types of anterior horn motor neurons; large alpha and medium motor neurons are rich in phosphorylase and poor in succinic dehydrogenase and are therefore mainly glycolytic in metabolism. These motor neurons supply type II muscle fibers, discharge at a higher threshold, require higher discharge rates before reaching stable firing, develop fast-twitch high tension, but are less capable of substained discharge. There is also a larger number of muscle fibers per MU, making for swift, strong force. On the whole such MU are anaerobically dependent. In contrast, smaller motor neurons low in phosphorylase and high in succinic dehydrogenase activity, reflecting a preferentially oxidative metabolism, supply type I muscle fibers; these are recruited on milder effort, are capable of slow but prolonged and relatively rhythmic discharge, and the number of muscle fibers per MU is small. Thus type I MU orchestrate precision and fineness of movements, while type II MU allow swift, strong force. Muscle fibers within a MU shown uniform histochemical, biochemical, and physiological properties but are distributed throughout the muscle, intermingling with fibers belonging to other MU. Thus the final histochemical aspect of a muscle section on biopsy is a mosaic, chequerboard pattern of muscle fibers of different enzymatic types.

**The uremic muscle's histochemical profile**

Nearly all uremic patients present atrophy of type II fibers; adjunctive atrophy of type I fibers, less marked at first, becomes important in cases with severe symptomatology, evident muscle impairment, and long-term dialysis treatment [33, 34]. Hemodialyzed patients have a higher atrophy factor for type II fibers than conservatively treated patients [34]. The expression of extreme atrophy, consisting of angulated fibers and small-group atrophy, is indicator of neurogenic muscle damage and is a constant finding in hystoenzymological preparations from uremic patients in conservative or dialytic treatment [34].

Table 5–6 summarizes the histological and histochemical aspects of muscles from a population treated on SHS for 64–123 months. Atrophy of type II and adjunctive atrophy of type I fibers are confirmed in these patients. Preincubation of ATPase preparations at low pH values is a means of showing up type II fiber subtypes A, B, and C. The latter cannot really be considered a separate subtype, as they are more like undifferentiated forms or precursors of the A and B subtypes and in normal conditions are rarely found in human muscle. These type II C fibers have been found increased in uremic muscle, where they might be taken as marker of denervation–reinnervation [30].

Preferential or earlier atrophy of type II muscle fibers (figure 5–12) a very important reason for muscle disability, has been seen in animals after denervation and in patients with diseases involving the upper and lower motor neurons. This finding could be taken as secondary to the underlying

*Table 5–6.* Histological, histochemical, and ultrastructural aspects of the muscle from patients in SHS.

| Sex (Months of SHS) | Mean Diameter (u) of Muscle Fiber Type | | Hypertrophy Factor | | Atrophy Factor | | MUP Amplitude (uV) | Type grouping | |
|---|---|---|---|---|---|---|---|---|---|
| | I | II | I | II | I | II | | I | II |
| F (57) | 45 | 24 | 0 | 0 | 432 | 870 | 5500 | +++ | 0 |
| M (47) | 44 | 42 | 0 | 220 | 366 | 682 | 6700 | ++ | 0 |
| M (76) | 47 | 24 | 0 | 0 | 450 | 980 | 4500 | + | + |
| F (131) | 54 | 52 | 0 | 0 | 109 | 217 | 6800 | + | 0 |
| M (90) | 57 | 62 | 290 | 150 | 50 | 250 | 5000 | + | 0 |
| F (112) | 56 | 35 | 50 | 0 | 125 | 1080 | 6500 | + | + |
| M (52) | 50 | 38 | 62 | 10 | 72 | 685 | 4500 | + | + |
| F (37) | 56 | 37 | 0 | 0 | 131 | 986 | 9800 | ++ | ++ |
| M (49) | 60 | 62 | 57 | 60 | 22 | 24 | 2500 | 0 | 0 |
| F (54) | 45 | 29 | 0 | 0 | 470 | 820 | 8500 | ++ | + |
| Normal values          F | 61 | 65 | 0–300 | 0–500 | 0–150 | 0–150 | 2500–4000 | 0 | 0 |
| M | 53 | 49 | 0–400 | 0–150 | 0–100 | 0–200 | | | |

Morphological and Histoenzymatic data refer to gastrocnemius muscle biopsy. EMG data have been obtained from abductor hallucis muscle by standard needle electrode.
The first column indicates the sex (M, F) of the patient and the duration in months of SHS.
The next three columns are divided into two parts and refer to type I and type II muscle fibers.
See the absence of compensatory hypertrophy and the widespread atrophy of type II fibers.

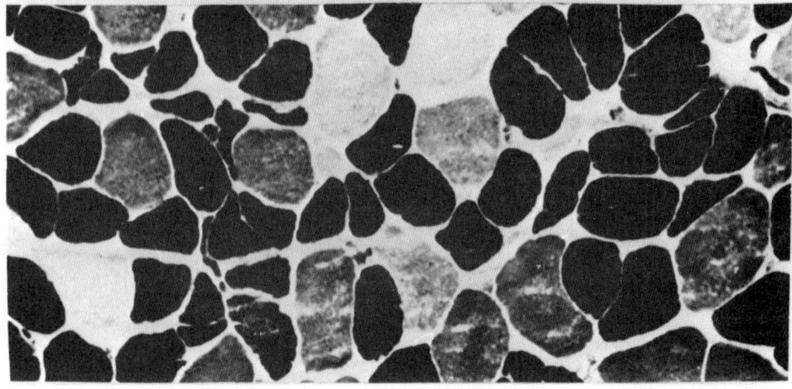

*Figure 5–12.* Preferential atrophy of type II muscle fibers in the uremic patient. Patient RP, 36 years old, in SHS for 2 months. ATPase pH 4.35 reaction: widespread atrophy of fibers type II that look darker.

neuronal damage [35] but it can also occur associated with inanition, chronic steroid intoxication, or malignancies [36], and has been found in disuse secondary to bedrest or joint affections [35]. More uncertain are the causes of fiber type I atrophy, which is less dependent on neuronal trophic impulses and probably more susceptible to direct toxic muscle noxae [27]. Because immobilization influences the size of type I fibers, less physical activity and reduced muscle tone might be important in explaining type I atrophy in the uremic patient. In addition, there is no denying, a priori, the possibility of a direct toxic effect on the muscle of uremia and/or chronic hypoxia (see the ultrastructural findings below) in analogy with primary toxic myopathies. In light microscopy preparations another important finding concerning type I muscle fibers is the possible presence of subsarcolemmal rims, which turn out under electron microscopy to be mitochondrial accumulations [34]. Even though the correlations between these morphological findings and metabolic alterations remain uncertain, some damage must be suspected to the energy metabolism, abundantly represented in the mitochondrial apparatus of type I fibers. In uremic patients, especially those who have undergone long-term SHS, the appearance of targetoid fibers merits attention (figure 5–13). Best seen with the oxidative enzyme reaction, these consist of muscle fibers with a central unstained zone, fading into a relatively normal peripheral region. Such fibers, usually associated with denervating diseases, are condidered a characteristic manifestation of the subsequent reinnervation of the denervated myofiber and are generally encountered in chronic peripheral neuropathies with a slowly progressive course. The presence of these targetoid fibers [34], indicative of denervation and reinnervation in progress, is in line particularly in SHS patients with the finding of type grouping [30], muscle areas where the normal mosaic chequerboards of different histochemical fiber types has been replaced with clusters of one fiber type next to clusters of

141

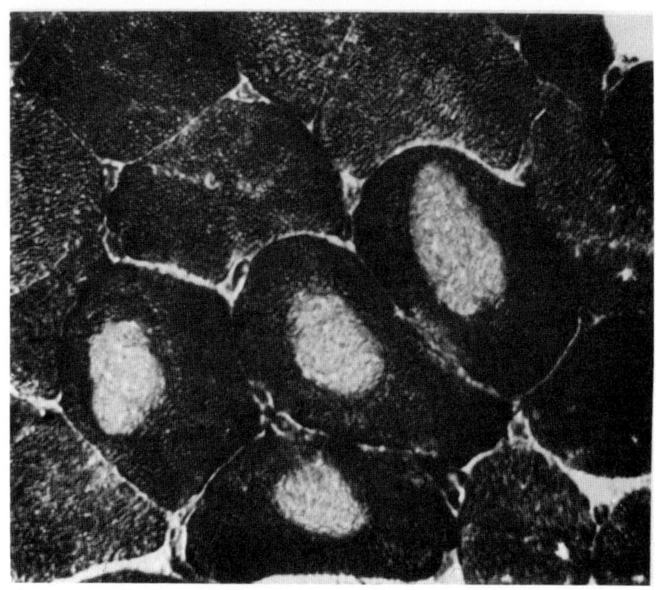

*Figure 5–13.* A group of four targetoid fibers (histoenzymatic NADH-TR preparation) with a central unstained zone fading into the stained periphery of a targetoid fiber in the gastrocnemius muscle of patient GC, 51 years old, treated by SHS for 13 months. This patient began hemodialysis treatment with marked motor symptoms consisting in dropping right foot, diffuse hypotrophy of the distal muscles of the lower limbs. The paresis regressed after 2 months of SHS. The EMG effort tracings after 12 months of dialysis were characterized by no interference and sporadic high amplitude MUP (7,500–11,500 $\mu$V).

another type [35]. Because type grouping is associated with collateral sprouting, consisting, as already seen, of new nerve sprouts growing out from surviving nerve axons to supply denervated muscle fibers, this finding reflect reinnervation. Under the EMG profile, sprouting increases the amplitude of MUP on account of the increase of muscle fibers within the same MU and the new abnormal contiguous relations between muscle fibers belonging to the same MU. The EMG equivalent of ample areas of type grouping are MUP of high voltage, usually over 10,000 $\mu$V, markedly polyphasic in form, and of prolonged duration indicating a large amount and complex modality of depolarization of large muscle areas, but the uremic patient presents sporadic MUP usually between 4,000 and rareky exceeding 10.000 $\mu$V, only very slightly prolonged if not normal, or even sometimes reduced in duration and simple in form, inserted in EMG tracings characterized by reduction in the mean amplitude and with loss of MUP (figure 5–6). Such potentials are the reflection of well-synchronized depolarization in smaller muscle areas, and indicate sluggish reinnervation, with consequent partial, poorly efficient functional recovery. Except for rare reports [37], most uremic patients, including those in dialysis treatment, do not present hypertrophy of muscle

142

fibers [30, 38, 39] that are not involved in the priority finding of atrophy, hypertrophy aimed at naturally compensating the functional loss of the atrophic fibers. In patients on SHS we have also not found evidence of compensatory hypertrophy. Although in dialyzed patients this might be interpreted as a result of disuse, this hypothesis does not fit all patients, and a possible explanation is that the pathogenic factor(s) responsible for the widespread atrophic damage also prevent any compensatory hypertrophy. In conclusion, preferential atrophy of type II fibers, however aspecific it may be, the increase in type II C fibers, the angulated fibers found dotted in the muscle, and the small-group atrophy, the presence of targetoid fibers, and the limited areas of type grouping all suggest the presence of denervation and a sluggish limited compensatory reinnervation. It largely places uremic muscle disability under the heading of myopathy secondary to innervation damage, so the neuropathy appears amply responsible for the muscle damage. Nevertheless, uremic muscle presents quantitatively less marked but qualitatively important changes, such as fiber size changes, central nuclei, and rare phagocytic fibers [37]; all these aspects are more common in primary forms of muscle disability, and are in any event not dependent on innervation. This is why disability due to direct muscle fiber damage in uremia can justifiably be postulated as deriving either from direct uremic toxicity or — particularly in patients with a long history of dialysis — from ischaemic damage, as suggested by the fact that the arterial tree is impaired in a large percentage of patients, judging from the vascular calcifications, well-documented by x-ray of soft tissues, and from the occlusions to small vessels in muscle tissue, shown by ultrastructural examination of muscle preparations [34].


## Ultrastructural findings in muscle from patients on SHS

The submicroscopic alterations found first in the muscle involve the myofibrillar sarcoplasm, i.e., the contractile matrix of skeletal myofibers. As degeneration proceeds, lysis of the myofilaments extends to increasingly large areas of the fiber, and the myofibril becomes smaller until complete breakdown. The lost contractile matrix is replaced by amorphous, finely granular sarcoplasmic material consisting of particulate glycogen, lipofuscin granules, lipid droplets, and mitochondria (figure 5–14). As a result of these changes, the Z discs of adjacent myofibrils are no longer arranged in register, and some Z discs show streaming while the Z disc material extends into I bands. A curious finding is rare intermyofibrillar crossovers, suggesting a limited attempt of inefficient morphofunctional compensation. Therefore, disarray and loss of the contractile structure explain, in terms of strict morphological profile, the main muscular symptoms of dialyzed patients: early reduction of muscle strength, easy fatiguability, and, finally, muscle atrophy [34]. In patients in SHS findings indicative of reinnervation, in the

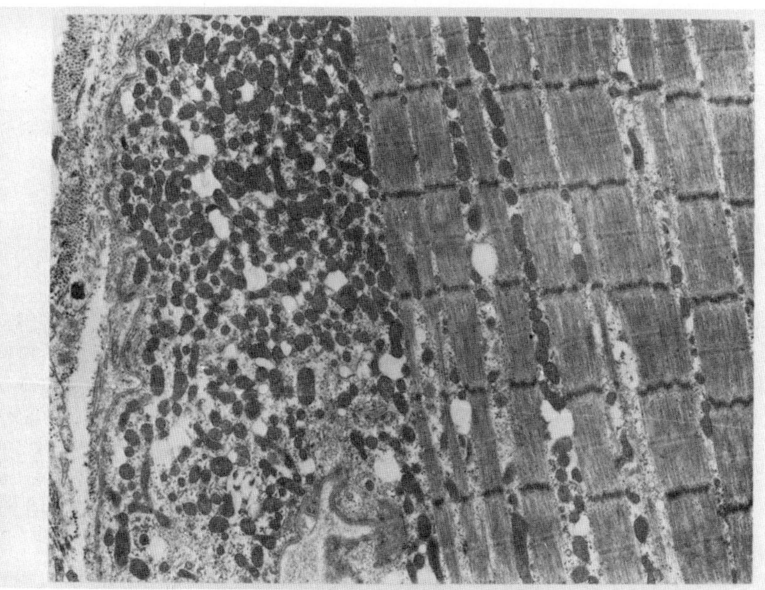

*Figure 5–14.* Areas of lost contractile matrix and substitution with amorphous sarcoplasmic material, streaming of Z discs, hypertrophy, and hyperplasia of the mitochondrial apparatus remain in the gastrocnemius muscle biopsy of patient PP, 29 years old, 31 months after starting SHS.

form of targetoid or target fibers, are frequently encountered, but such fibers are inefficient in terms of mechanical performance. Parallel to the gradual extension of the alterations to the myofibrillar sarcoplasm, modifications start to appear in the extrafibrillar sarcoplasm, slowly becoming more marked. The mitochondria increase and account [40] for true hypertrophy becoming oval, lengthening transversely to lie perpendicular to the main axis of the myofibrils; this 90° reorientation depends on ex vacuo phenomena, because loss of whole myofibrils removes the mechanical support for the mitocondria. The number of crystae increases extending the respiratory surface for each mitochondrion; at this stage, hyperplasia is the main finding in the mitochondrial apparatus (figure 5–14). All these changes in the extrafibrillar sarcoplasm probably indicate an attempt to expand metabolic respiratory capacity to meet the growing needs of a contractile muscle apparatus where the progressive loss of contractile structures indicates that even mitochondrial hypertrophy and hyperplasia are not enough to keep up with the constantly increasing metabolic requirements of the remaining myofibers [34]. Direct uremic toxicity to the muscle fiber cell, in the context of clinically demonstrable toxicity to the parenchymas cannot be excluded, but alterations to the microcirculation can be taken clearly as the histopathological basis of the ischaemic damage to muscle in uremia. The endomysial capillaries in both conservatively treated and dialyzed patients show a thickened, reduplicated

144

amorphous-looking basal lamina, but in long-term dialyzed patients in particular, these capillaries present deposits of electro-dense material resulting from salt precipitation, with the formation of intraluminal occlusions (calcospherites) [34]. These submicroscopic findings of uremic intramuscular microangiopathy with reduction of the capillary lumen are probably the hystopathological basis of deficiences in muscle microcirculation and of reduced tissue oxygenation, possibly linked with alterations to the mitocondrial respiratory chain, which could represent the direct damage to the muscle fiber. Thus ultrastructural investigation of uremic skeletal muscle gives a picture compatible with alterations secondary to neurogenic damage; these include initially focal but gradually growing alterations to the myofibrillary sarcoplasm, the early 'sawtoothed' profile of the sarcolemma, the deep infolding of the nucleolemma of the nuclear membranes suggesting nuclear segmentation. The mitochondrial changes, however, have greater probative value in direct damage of the primary type.


**Conclusions**

Considering only patients aged under 50 years, so as to exclude those with possible age-related modifications of EMG parameters, 47 patients have been checked by periodic EMG controls for a full 14 years, and just another under 100 patients have been followed closely since they started SHS in the years after. SHS has unequivocally demonstrated to provide a guarantee over time of stable neuromuscular performance, compatible with everyday life and with a range of work requiring different muscle output.

In addition, the start of SHS has proved a means of eliminating in a short time, usually not more than 2 or 3 months, the most debilitating subjective and objective symptoms of uremic polyneuropathy, such as disesthesia and paresis. Despite these satisfactory functional results there is, however, no denying that the EMG, histological, histoenzymatic, and untrastructural findings indicate unequivocally a compromise of the nerve and muscle parenchyma.

It is nevertheless important to stress that any comparison, however limited, of electrophisiological and morphological findings in the SHS population as opposed to populations treated by other forms of dialysis, shows that the former are under PNS profile, often better off than the latter, in any case never worse. This experience emerging from SHS patients allows us to realize that the degree of neuromuscular damage in the hemodialyzed patient does not appear to depend strategically on the type of dialysis available, in the range of today's adequate dialysis treatment, but on two sources of neuromuscular damage. The first component, main reason of damage to the PNS, is the devastating toxication to the nervous parenchyma of the final stages of conservative treatment, when glomerular filtration rates are extremely reduced and acidosis and electrolyte disorders are rampant, with catabolism arising from protein-caloric malnutrition, intercurrent infections and protein losses: briefly the complications of terminal uremia.

This stage of terminal uremia is marked by anatomical, hence definitive loss, of neurons confirmed at nerve biopsy level by optical microscopy, teasing and ultrastructural investigation for myelinated fibers, and by the finding of collagen pockets as an example of substitution of amyelinic fibers with collagen structures at the ultrastructure. In line with these parenchymal regressive events of the MU are the EMG effort tracing that show a constant loss of MUP, indicating that the damage of the MU is not merely functional and that there is no hope of recovery with time.

The muscle shows widespread signs of distress largely secondary in type and cannot achieve satisfactory functional and structural recovery probably because during chronic dialysis treatment, it does not matter which schedule is, an attenuated intoxication, resurgent in the intervals between dialysis, persists as a direct and/or mediate damage to nerve and muscle. This second component is difficult to quantify because we still lack a so sensitive and reliable electrophysiological, or it does not matter other index, from which to establish, over time, the actual degree of neuropathy in the same patient or in dialyzed populations treated by different approaches.

In the history of the substitutive treatment of uremia, Max sensory NCV was perhaps the only pointer, when dealing with the severe degrees of uremic neuropathy of the sixties, probably adequate for the nephrological requirements of those years.

Max motor NCV provided a useful reference index for excluding only worsening of the PNS in patients treated by SHS: in our experience, here indicated, the significativity of this index dipends on the long-term control in a wide omogeneous population, but Max motor MCN was an illusion in helping establish adequate dialytic strategies for short-term controls and limited groups of patients.

Derisory clinical advantages over traditional EMG indices are today provided by somatosensory, visual, and auditory potentials, and therefore a sensitive quantification of the uremic neuropathy still remains an unresolved puzzle for the clinical purposes of the nephrologist.

But the passing of the years has cut the problem down to a less stressing size since wider availability of substitutive treatment of the renal function, and expecially its proper starting, has reduced the neuronal damage of terminal uremia.

This explains why uremic neuropathy today is less of an objective clinical problem, and seems to be slowly fading toward oblivion.


**Acknowledgments**

For invaluable discussion with and suggestions from Dr. E. Govoni (Institute of Electronmicroscopy, University of Bologna) who supplied ultrastructural preparations, and Dr. A. Marbini (Institute of Neurology, University of

146

Parma) who supplied light and histenzymologic preparations, I would like to extend my gratitude.


## References


1. Cambi, V., Arisi, L., Bignardi, L., Bruschi, G., Rossi, E., Savazzi, G. and Migone, L. (1974) Short dialysis schedule. Finally ready to become a routine? Proc. Europ. Dial. Transpl. Ass. XI: 112.
2. Cambi, V., Garini, G., Savazzi, G., Arisi, L., David, S., Zanelli, P., Bono, F. and Gardini, F. (1983) Short dialysis. Proc. Europ. Dial. Transpl. Ass. XX: 111–121.
3. Funck-Brentano, J.L., Chaumont, P., Mery, J.P., Vantalon, J. and Zingraff-Kok, J. (1964) Intérêt de la mesure de la vitesse de conduction nerveuse dans la surveillance des malades urémiques, soumis à des hémodialyses répétées. Proc. Europ. Dial. Transpl. Ass. I: 23–29.
4. Heron, J.R., Konotey-Ahuluf, I.D., Shaloom, S. and Thomas, P.K. (1965) Nerve conduction in chronic renal failure treated by dialysis. Proc. Europ. Dial. Transpl. Ass. II: 138–143.
5. Babb, A.L., Strand, M.J., Uvelli, D.A., Milutinovic, J., Scribner, B.H. (1975) Quantitative description of dialysis treatment: a dialysis index. Kidney Int. (Suppl. 2): S23–S29.
6. Gotch, F.A., Sargent, J.A., Keen, M.L. and Lee, M. (1974) Individualized quantified dialysis therapy in uremia. Proc. Clin. Dial. Transplant Forum 4: 27–35.
7. Preswick, G., and Jeremy, D. (1964) Subclinical polyneuropathy in renal insufficiency. Lancet 2: 731–732.
8. Jebsen, R.H., Tenckoff, H. and Honet, J.C. (1967) Natural history of uremic polyneuropathy and effects of dialysis. N. Engl. J. Med. 277: 327–333.
9. Williams, I.R., Davison, A.M., Mawdsley, C. and Robson, J.S. (1973) Neuropathy in chronic renal failure. In *New Developments in EMG Clinical Neurophysiology*, Vol. 2, J.E. Desmedt (ed.). Basel: Karger, pp. 390–399.
10. Blagg, C.R., Kemble, F. and Taverner, D. (1968) Nerve conduction velocity in relationship to severity of renal disease. Nephron 9: 290–299.
11. Van Der Most Van Spijk, D., Hoogland, R.A. and Dijkstra. (1973) Conduction velocities compared and related to degrees of renal insufficiency. In *New Developments in EMG Clinical Neurophysiology*, Vol. 2, J.E. Desmedt (ed.). Basel: Karger, pp. 381–389.
12. Jennekens, F.G.I., Dorhout Mees, E.J. and Van Der Most Van Spijk, D. (1971) Clinical aspects of uraemic polyneuropathy. Nephron 8: 414–426.
13. Cadilhac, J., Dapres, G., Fabre, J.L. and Mion, C. (1973) Follow-up study of motor conduction velocity in uraemic patients treated by hemodialysis. in *New Developments in EMG Clinical Neurophysiology*, Vol. 2, J.E. Desmedt (ed.). Basel: Karger, pp. 372–380.
14. Savazzi, G.M., Arisi, L., Bignardi, L., Rossi, E., Cambi, V. and Allegri, L. (1976) La velocità di conduzione nervosa motoria massima nella polineuropatia di pazienti uremici sottoposti a trattamento di differente tecnica e durata: valore e limiti. Rivista di Neurologia 46: 25–35.
15. Savazzi, G.M. (1981) Editorial: nerve conduction times in uraemia. Internat. J. Artificial Organs 4: 211–212.
16. Savazzi, G.M., Cambi, V. and Migone, L. (1980) The influence of glomerular filtration rate on uremic polyneuropathy. Clinical Nephrol. 13: 64–72.
17. Johnson, E.W. and Olsen, K.J. (1960) Clinical value of motor nerve conduction velocity determination. J.A.M.A. 172: 2030.
18. Pinelli, P., Lanzi, G., Savoldi, F. and Zebri, F. (1961) Questioni attuali sulla misura di velocità di conduzione delle fibre nervose motorie nell'uomo. Riv. Pat. Nerv. Ment. 82: 377–394.
19. Kominami, N., Tyler, H.R., Hampers, C.L. and Merrill, J.P. (1971) Variations in motor nerve condution velocity in normal and uremic patients. Arch. Int. Med. 128: 235–239.
20. Buchtal, F. (1973) Sensory and motor conduction in polyneuropathies. In *New Developments*

*in EMG Clinical Neurophysiology*, Vol. 2, J.E. Desmedt (ed.). Basel: Karger, p. 259.

21. Savazzi, G.M., Marbini, A., Gemignani, F., Cavatorta, A., Govoni, E., Bragaglia, M.M. (1985) The peripheral nervous system in dialyzed uremic patients: regressive motor unit changes. In *Advances in Nephrology and Dialysis*, Contr. Nephrol. Vol 45. Basel: Karger, pp. 42–59.

22. Engel, W.K. and Warmolts, J.R. (1973) The motor unit. In *New Developments in EMG Clinical Neurophysiology*, Vol. 1. Basel: Karger, pp. 141–177.

23. Mc Comas, A.J., Fawcett, P.R.W., Campbell, M.J. and Sica, R.E.P. (1971) Electrophysiological estimation of the number of motor units within a human muscle. J. Neurol. Neurosurg. Psychiat. 34: 121–131.

24. Mc Comas, A.J., Sica, R.E.P., Campbell, M.J., Upton, A.R.M. (1971) Functional compensation in partially denervated muscles. J. Neurol. Neurosurg. Psychiat. 34: 453–460.

25. Savazzi, G.M., Allegri, L., Arisi, L., Bignardi, L., Garini, G., Rossi, E., Cambi, V. and Migone, L. (1975) La polineuropatia uremica: parte II. Le modificazioni uremiche della unità motoria. In *Attualità Nefrologiche e Dialitiche*, Vol. 7. Roma: Pensiero Scientifico Editore, pp. 306–319.

26. Leuman, J.A.R. (1959) Quantitative Electromyographic changes associated with muscular weakness. J. Neurol. Neurosurg. Psych. 22: 306–310.

27. Bundschu, H.D. (1974) Uremic myopathy. In *Renal Insufficiency*. Stuttgart: Georg Thieme Publishers, pp. 280–286.

28. Thomas P.K., Hollinrake, K., Lascelles, R.G., O'Sullivan, D.J., Baillod, R.A., Moorhead, J.F. and MacKenzie, J.C. (1971), The polyneuropathy of chronic renal failure. Brain 94: 761–780.

29. Said, G., Boudier, L., Serva, J., Zingraff, J. and Drucke, T. (1983) Different patterns of uremic polyneuropathy: clinicopathologic study. Neurology 33: 567–574.

30. Savazzi, G.M., Cambi, V., Migone, L., Marbini, A., Govoni, E. and Bragaglia, M.M., Juvarra, G. and Dall'Aglio, P.P. (1980) The influence of uraemic neuropathy on muscle: EMG, histoenzymatic and ultrastructural correlations. Proc. Europ. Dial. Transpl. Ass. 17: 312–317.

31. Brooke, M.H. and Engel, W.K. (1968) The hystographic analysis of human muscle biopsy with regard to fiber types. Neurology 19: 221–233.

32. Karpaty, G. and Engel, W.K. (1968) Correlative histochemical study of scheletal muscle after suprasegmental denervation, peripheral nerve section and scheletal fixation. Neurology 18: 681–692.

33. Bundschu, H.D. (1978) Myopathy in clinical and experimental uremia. Riv. Neurobiol. 24: 26–36.

34. Savazzi, G.M., Govoni, E., Bragaglia, M.M., Cambi, V. and Migone, L. (1982) Ultrastructural findings of uraemic muscular damage: functional implications. Proc. Europ. Dial. Transpl. Ass. 19: 258–264.

35. Dubowitz, V. and Brooke, N.H. (1973) *Muscle Biopsy: A Modern Approach*. London: Saunders Company, — pp. 79–82.

36. Warmolts, J.R., Re, P.K., Lewis, R.J. and Engel, W.K. (1975) Type II muscle fiber atrophy (II atrophy): an early systemic effect of cancer. Neurology 25: 374.

37. Ahonen, R.E. (1980) Light microscopic study of striated muscle in uremia. Acta Neuropathol. 49: 51–55.

38. Bundschu, H.D. and Schlote, W. (1974) Elektronen mikroskopische untersuchungen der skelettmuskulatur bei terminaler Niereninsuffizienz. J. Neurol. Sci. 23: 243–254.

39. Bautista, J., Gil-Necija, E., Castilla, J., Chinchon, I. and Rafel E. (1983) Dialysis myopathy. Acta Neuropathol. 61: 71–75.

40. Shah, A.J., Sahgal, V., Quintamilla, A.P., Subramani, V., Singh, H. and Hughes, R. (1983) Muscle in chronic uremia. A histochemical and morphometric study of human quadriceps muscle biopsies. Clin. Neuropathol. 2: 83–89.

# 6. Nutritional status and nitrogen metabolism in patients treated with short dialysis

Luca Arisi

## Nitrogen metabolism and nutritional status of the pre-dialysis patient

Wasting and malnutrition are common features in predialysis patients [1–3]. Aside from the accumulation of nitrogenous waste products, many abnormalities are recognized. Both serum proteins, especially those with rapid turnover [4–6], and intracellular proteins [6–7] are frequently depressed. Free amino acid patterns in serum [4, 8–10], muscle [11–12], red blood cells [13], and white cells [14] are frequently deranged, together with their interorgan fluxes and organ-specific metabolism. This has been verified in skeletal muscle [15], in the liver and the splanchnic bed [16], the brain [17], and the failing kidney itself [18–19].

Quantitative and qualitative alterations in the utilization of various amino acids infused in vein have been observed [20]. Reduced intestinal absorption [21] and interference [22] among amino acids have also been demonstrated. Moreover, postprandial amino acid metabolism has been found to be abnormal, evidencing altered interorgan fluxes and hepatic escape, chiefly of nonessential amino acids [23].

Even though abnormalities in aminoacid metabolism are also evidenced in well-nourished patients with chronic renal failure, it is worth noting that many of them are shared by protein-calorie malnourished patients with normal renal function. The two clinical conditions are distinguished by the following biocemical conditions: in malnutrition, serum glycine is characteristically increased, cystine is decreased together with the urea cycle aminoacids [24–25], whereas in uremia, glycine is normal, cystine is increased [26], arginine is normal, and citrulline is increased due to argininosuccinate lyase inhibition [27, 28]. Other defects in aminoacid metabolism considered specific to uremia include impaired hydroxilation of phenylalanine [29, 30], accelerated valine catabolism [31], and altered protein-binding of tryptophan [32, 33]. If and how much the biochemical abnormalities of chronic renal failure provoke protein-calorie malnutrition or are in turn affected by it has not yet been clarified.

Other factors contribute to malnutrition in uremic patients: first of all, restricted dietary intake complicated by anorexia and vomiting due to uremic

*Vincenzo Cambi (editor) Professor of Nephrology*
© *1987 Martinus Nijhoff Publishing, Boston. ISBN 0-89838-858-9. Printed in The United States.*

intoxication, stress and drugs [34–36], as well as prescribed fasting for diagnostic procedures [37]. Moreover, in uremia, fasting is accompanied by a greater catabolic response [6], even though protein degradation is not affected [38].

Other causes of nutritional impairment include abnormal aminoacid uptake and release by the diseased kidney [18, 34–41], intercurrent illnesses [42, 43] due to the immune deficit [44, 45], and several abnormal hormonal activities directly or indirectly involved in nitrogen metabolism. Tissue resistance to insulin action is well documented [46]. Hyperglucagonemia is also present [47], although its role in glucose intolerance is minimal [48]. Nevertheless, hepatic gluconeogenesis has been found either increased [49] and not suppressed by dialysis [50] or normal [51]. Elevated growth hormone [52] and decreased testosterone [53] levels are also present. Hyperparathyroidism may also be responsible for the catabolic trend [54, 55]. Thyroid hormone levels are frequently deranged: circulating thriiodothyronine levels are decreased [56, 57]: this could be of particular importance in view of the observed inverse correlation of the nitrogen sparing capacity to the T3 level [58]. Other metabolic derangements, such as acidosis [59, 60], potassium deficiency [61], and retained toxins [62] (see chapter 4) may be responsible for nitrogen catabolism.

Although dietary restrictions and their consequences play a principal role in the development of wasting, protein restriction in patients in advanced renal failure still appears mandatory: in fact, protein liberalization exacerbates uremic symptoms [8, 63] and accelerates the progression of renal damage [64–66].


**Dialysis therapy**

Subjects suffering from protein-calorie malnutrition who have normal renal function recover completely after a few months' refeeding [25]. In dialyzed patients, however, many of the signs of altered metabolism [14, 67–73] and malnutrition persist despite the qualitative and quantitative improvement in dietetic intake usually accompanying the beginning of dialysis treatment. In fact, nutritional conditions at that time seem particularly decisive inasmuch as dialysis does not generally improve the nutritional state [70–75], and malnutrition directly influences dialysis morbidity and mortality [74].

In our dialysis population, we demonstrated that standard short dialysis treatment (4 hours thrice weekly) generally blocks this tendency to lose weight with the exception of patients suffering from nephrosclerosis who only experience a moderate slowing down of weight loss with the beginning of dialysis therapy (table 6–1) [75].

We also observed that the major weight loss occurs in previously overweight patients, and that it involves chiefly fat. This is the same phenomenon seen in obese subjects during marked energy restriction [76].

150

*Table 6–1.* Body weight loss and relative body weight loss per year from diagnosis of the disease until stabilization in dialysis (A) and from stabilization to the present time (B).

| | A | | B | |
| | Real | Relative | Real | Relative |
|---|---|---|---|---|
| GN  male | −3.9 ± 6.5 | −6 ± 8 | +0.2 ± 1.7 | 0 ± 2 |
|     female | −1.6 ± 3.0 | −4 ± 6 | +0.4 ± 2.1 | 0 ± 4 |
| PN  male | −2.0 ± 5.3 | −3 ± 7 | +0.2 ± 1.3 | 0± 2 |
|     female | −1.2 ± 3.1 | −3 ± 4 | −0.2 ± 1.6 | −1 ± 3 |
| NS  male | −4.8 ± 9.5 | −5 ± 13 | −1.6 ± 2.2 | −2 ± 3 |

GN = Glomerulonephritis
PN = Pyelonephritis
NS = Nephrosclerosis

*Table 6–2.* Cross-sectional nutritional evaluation of our dialysis population

| | | |
|---|---|---|
| Hct | 30 ± 6 | |
| Duration of treatmt. (years) | 4.9 ± 2.9 years | |
| Average age (years) | 52 ± 13 | |
| Total Proteins g/dl | 6.9 ± 0.4 | |
| Albumin g/dl | 3.9 ± 0.3 | |
| Pseudocholinesterase | 3045 ± 637 | |
| | *Male* | *Female* |
| Relative Body Weight | 89 ± 11 | 96 ± 16 |
| % Fat | 15 ± 5 | 28 ± 5 |
| % Standard triceps skin fold | −38 ± 29 | −21 ± 25 |
| Muscle Circ. | 239 ± 2.0 | 231 ± 2.1 |
| % Standard muscle circ. | 95 ± 8 | 96 ± 9 |

The average values of some nutritional indices of our population are shown in table 6–2. With a few exceptions, they are substantially in line with values presented by other authors [70, 72, 73, 77].

Kopple [78] and our group [79] have reported somewhat similar observations on patients treated for over 10 years: Kopple and associates compared anthropometric indexes of populations with different dialysis ages (0–5, 6–9, 10 years) and observed a marked reduction, chiefly of fat, in patients with a longer dialysis age; after 5 years, however, this stabilized.

Our group, instead, studied weight range over the years in two populations: one with a dialysis age of at least 10, the other of at least 5. Similar to Kopple's series, our first group showed significant but moderate weight loss for 5 years, followed by stabilization. In the second group, instead, average weight remained stable.

In comparing our cases it became evident that the turning point from net weight loss to stability in the patient group with a longer dialysis age coincided with the years in which short dialysis (4 hours thrice weekly) was established in our unit as an alternative [80, 81] to more prolonged treatments. Thus short dialysis seems to involve a tendency to lower catabolism. Analogous improvement was seen in the hematocrit, total serum protein, and serum albumin [79, 82].

In evaluating nutritional status, including nitrogen metabolism, anthropometric, and liver secretory protein measurements, though widely used (and useful from the epidemiological point of view), are at times difficult to interpret in the individual patient; moreover, they are not sufficiently sensitive to evaluate the short-term effects of variations in dietetic or dialytic treatment. In this case, Baker and associates [83] maintain that the validity of anthropometric and humoral measurements is usually no greater than overall clinical judgment. For these reasons, a number multi-parametric studies has been undertaken in order to identify the most sensitive indices of nutritional status and nitrogen metabolism.

For example, Guarneri and colleagues [72] compared food intake, anthropometric indexes, serum proteins as well as measurements of skeletal muscle content of alkali-soluble proteins (noncollagen proteins) of DNA, RNA, and fat in two dialysis populations. Food intake of one group was decidedly poor, and, in fact, anthropometric indexes for fat and muscular mass were significantly more compromised; other serum and muscle indexes were no different from those of the other group. Noteworthy, however, is that the RNA:DNA muscular ratio, which expresses the protein synthesizing capacity of the cells, was particularly reduced in the population in apparently better nutritional condition.

Another interesting study involved the correlations, in a group of patients in hemodialysis, between free-amino acid plasma concentrations, anthropometric measurements, and other laboratory parameters [84]. It was found that valine concentration and mid-arm muscle circumference are the parameters that best correlate to other amino acids and anthropometric measurements. Further analysis of the variables, performed after ranking by plasma valine, showed that some parameters (VAL, ILE, LEU, THR, ASP, body weight, mid-arm muscle circumference) were interrelated and reflected calorie-protein malnutrition. Others, such as the fat mass, were correlated to calorie intake, while HIS and SER were correlated to protein intake. The alteration of other parameters which were lower in the low-valine group but still higher than normal (TAU, ASP, CYS, CITR, urea, creatinine, prealbumin, RBP) referred to the loss of nephron mass or to uremia itself. Others (SER, TYR, ARG, transferrin, C3 complement) were lower than normal, although this was unrelated to malnutrition. The glucogenic AA (GLY, ALA, PRO, ORN) were unaffected by malnutrition and were higher than normal due to uremia or loss in nephron mass.

Conclusions concerning the diagnostic value of low valine levels agree with data regarding uncomplicated malnutrition in which the depressed amino acids include leucine, lysine, and threonine [25] as well as valine; these conclusions are further reinforced by the simultaneous finding of low muscle

152

valine levels in hemodialysis patients [71]. Wolfson and associates [73] confirmed low valine levels, but did not find any correlation between them and anthropometric parameters.

Discrepancies in both the behavior and interpretation of the numerous parameters used to evaluate nutritional status and nitrogen metabolism are quite probably the result of the intermeshing of the patients' diverse clinical and alimentary histories (present, recent, and past). Thus for the present, evaluation of several parameters would seem most useful.

On the whole, patients in dialysis still present almost all of the calorie-protein indices seen in uremic patients in conservative treatment. There are some differences, however: (1) the average rate of weight-loss is considerably reduced; (2) anemia improves; (3) serum albumin increases; (4) glucose metabolism is normalized.

Dialysis can thus influence nitrogen metabolism indirectly by permitting increased and more varied food intake, and directly by improving water-electrolyte homeostasis and freeing the body of toxins.

Moreover, any kind of artificial treatment brings about an artificial equilibrium between the patient, his/her metabolic condition, and his/her eating habits. And treatment itself may be responsible for catabolism, as will be discussed later. The choice of type and amount of treatment can thus be decisive in conditioning nitrogen metabolism improvement as well.


**Dialysis prescription and nitrogen metabolism**

Early on, when dialysis was developing into a long-term therapeutic tool, the need for suitable clinical parameters to establish and monitor treatment became clear. Adequacy of treatment was evaluated in an extremely empirical way. In the mid-sixties, 18–24 hours per week (standard Kiil) were judged satisfactory to achieve blood pressure control and improve anemia and subjective well-being [85]. The state of the hematopoietic system [86], motor nerve conduction velocity [87], and certain neurobehavioral variables [88] were also considered reliable indices to evaluate the adequacy of dialysis prescription. However, these clinical paramaters were of little use in comparing different types of treatment and different dialysis populations.

Since uremia was defined as a clinical syndrome caused by the intoxication of waste products accumulated in the body, the substance responsible for clinical complications was actively sought: it was hoped that, once found, this substance or substances could be controlled by quantification of its/their accumulation rate and dialytic extraction. The best known substances, urea and creatinine, were not reliable parameters, inasmuch as their predialysis concentrations did not necessarily correspond to clinical condition. Moreover, it was not demonstrated that these substances were potential toxins, at least in the amounts commonly found in patients in chronic treatment. Although urea, in concentrations above 300 mg/dl, can induce uremic symptoms [89], it is also correlated to appetite loss in lower concentrations [90].

It was thus hypothesized that uremic toxins were substances (that even today have yet to be fully identified) of middle molecular weight, very few of which slowly diffuse across the common cuprophane membrane, and are more sensitive to convective forces [91, 92]. Vitamin $B_{12}$ was considered to be representative of this group of molecules, and its dialytic kinetics was used to create a mathematical model to quantify dialysis need precisely (the Dialysis Index) [93]. This hypothesis led to the prescription of increased dialysis time, especially for patients with very low to null residual renal function [94].

In the early seventies, in apparent contrast to the middle molecule hypothesis, Cambi demonstrated empirically that a 4-hour thrice-weekly dialysis schedule could be considered adequate [80, 81] despite less small and middle molecule removal than with standard Kiil.

The controversy over what substances are the most useful indicators of dialysis adequacy continues. However, the idea that urea and middle-molecular weight peptide metabolism is somehow interrelated has begun to take form, either because small molecule removal might facilitate the normal metabolic conversion of larger toxic products [90] and/or because the generation rate of both toxic peptides and urea might be correlated to dietary protein intake and endogenous protein catabolism [95]. Therefore, urea, though not in itself toxic, could be considered representative of the interrelationship of dialysis prescription, degree of waste-product intoxication, protein intake, and nitrogen metabolism.

The formulation of a kinetic model for urea and its utilization to guide dialysis treatment was first proposed by Gotch and associates [96, 97]. This model was used by the National Cooperative Dialysis study (NCDS) to prescribe and evaluate dialysis treatment carried out with two average BUN target levels (50 and 100 mg/dl) and two dialysis lengths (4.5–5.0 and 2.5–3.5 hours per session) in a wide-scale controlled trial [98]. Analysis of the clinical outcome of this study strongly suggested that either higher BUN levels or lower protein intake, as well as short dialysis length when concomitant with high BUN, were associated with increased morbidity [99].

At the same time, two studies only partially supporting the NCDS conclusions were published. Teshan and associates, who had taken part in the NCDS, analyzed changes in neurobehavior variables induced by switching the urea index (total urea clearance per week per ml of body urea space) from 3.0 to 2.5 [100]. They also observed clinical worsening when dialysis time was reduced and BUN levels increased, but denied any direct causal relationship between the 'common chemical moieties, BUN inclusive, in the concentration ranges measured in the study' and clinical outcome.

Acchiardo and associates evaluated the one-year incidence of morbidity and mortality in 120 dialysis patients and its correlation with the protein catabolism rate, BUN, the urea index, and dialysis frequency [74]. Seemingly

154

in contrast to the NCDS and Nashville groups, they found that the worst clinical outcome was associated with the lowest BUN levels and not with the urea index. They emphasized the role of malnutrition (indicated indirectly by the low protein catabolism rate) in morbidity and mortality.

In a retrospective study of 130 dialysis patients, Avram and associates have produced evidence that predialysis BUN and creatinine do not serve either as reliable indices of dialysis adequacy or as predictors of clinical outcome [101].

Furthermore, Gotch and Sargent made two criticisms of the statistical method adopted by the NCDS: first, dialysis prescription and nutritional indexes were considered independent variables, while they were in fact not, due to the study design; secondly, the prediction of failure was considered a continuous function of the protein catabolism rate and BUN [99], while its relationship to dialysis prescription resulted in two separate clusters [102].

The authors reelaborated the NCDS data by means of a 'mechanistic analysis' and, like Avram, Acchiardo, and Teshan, they concluded that BUN per se has no predictive value, but that PCR 0.8g/KgBW and KT/V 0.7 (i.e., urea index 2.1) indicate a high probability of failure. They also suggested that with the currently used cellulose dialyzers and a thrice-weekly treatment schedule, PCR = 1.0g/kg/day and KT/V = 1.0 provides a fully adequate dialysis prescription.

In conclusion, whatever the dialysis treatment, no absolute dialysis adequacy exists, but rather a dialysis need relative to the maintenance of good nutritional status.


**Dietary requirements**

Nitrogen balance studies of patients undergoing twice-weekly dialysis indicated that neutral or positive balance could be maintained with 0.75 g of high biological value protein/Kg BW/day [103–105]. When dietary intake was increased to 1.25 g protein/Kg BW/day, uremic symptoms began to appear [105] despite further improvement in nitrogen balance. This was not the case in Fish's study of patients in thrice-weekly maintenance dialysis: 80 g protein (1.4 g/Kg BW/day) improved nutritional status and rehabilitation without causing uremic symptoms [106]. Kopple, in a review of these data [107], has recommended a protein intake of 65–85 g/day (0.8–1.4 g/KgBW/day) for 6–8-hour thrice weekly dialysis treatments; his own studies [105] led to the recommendation of a minimum caloric intake of 35 Kcal/Kg of ideal BW/day. These figures, confirmed by further studies [108, 109], are generally considered adequate.

Our own studies, carried out on patients dialyzed 4 hours thrice weekly, indicate that an average of 1.1 g of protein and 35 Kcal/Kg DBW/day is needed to achieve neutrality of nitrogen balance [110] as judged by the ratio between the urea-nitrogen appearance rate to total dietary nitrogen (R) (figure 6–1).

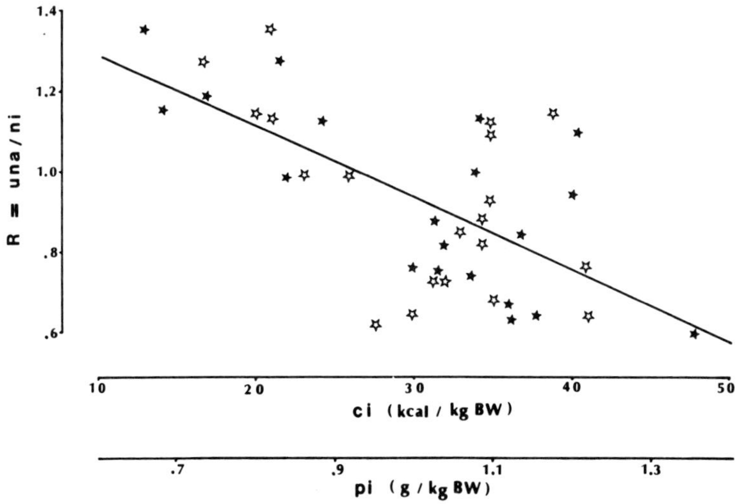


*Figure 6–1.* Correlation between urea nitrogen appearance-nitrogen intake ratio (R = UNA/NI) and protein (★) and caloric (☆) intake per kilogram body weight, in 20 patients on RDT.
★ $y = -0.878x + 1.824$ (p<0.01)
☆ $y = -0.017x + 1.462$ (p<0.05)

This index of nitrogen balance, different from others used to substitute the conventional one [111–114], indicates neutrality at around the 0.85 value. Interestingly, R does not correlate with the absolute value of nitrogen and caloric intake, but rather with intake relative to body weight.

It has been generally observed that a certain percent of the dialytic population does not take in recommended protein and especially caloric levels. In any case, it has been ascertained that the alimentary, and particularly protein, needs of patients in hemodialysis are decidedly higher than those of both normal subjects and patients in conservative tratment. This implies that dialysis treatment involves excessive nitrogen loss and/or the stimulus to protein catabolism.


**Nitrogen balance (NB)**

Nitrogen balance can be studied with one or more of the following aims in mind: to quantify protein and caloric needs, to verify adequacy of food intake, to evaluate metabolic effects brought about by different clinical conditions or dietetic or therapeutic changes. The accuracy required, which is difficult to verify even under normal conditions [115], varies according to the type of study and population considered. Nitrogen balance is influenced by various factors, aside from clinical and metabolic conditions, that must be kept in mind in order to guarantee accurate interpretation. These include: the subject's age, sex, size, weight, basal metabolism, mineral balance, and

156

perhaps race; the type of work he/she does; the environment (temperature, humidity, etc.) in which the subject lives and works; the food he/she eats, as well as how the food is cooked and stored and what its biological value is.

According to the mass conservation law, nitrogen balance equals the difference between the quantity of nitrogen taken in, represented chiefly by alimentary proteins, and nitrogen output.

*Nitrogen intake*

The methods commonly used to evaluate protein intake (PI) (24-hour recall, food history, food records) are frequently inaccurate. Accuracy increases when the patients are highly motivated, cooperative, and guided by skilled dietitians.

When the nitrogen content of foods cannot be directly measured, it is usually calculated using a multiplication factor (0.16) for protein, whose content in ingested food is found in tables of food composition. Actually, this factor is appropriate for meat and egg proteins, but it is different for milk proteins (0.157), vegetable, cereal, and nut proteins (0.160–0.193) [116]. The nitrogen content of drugs and food supplements should also be taken into account.

*Nitrogen output (Nout)*

After the suggestion of Munro, at the 1963 FAO/WHO Joint Expert Group Meeting [117], the concept of factorial analysis was introduced into nitrogen output calculation.

Nout = urinary nitrogen (UN) + fecal nitrogen (FN) + nitrogen content of integumental losses + nitrogen increment during growth, pregnancy, and lactation. Losses from fistulae, drains and blood drawn for analysis, or any other event can also be significant.

*Integumental losses*

The conventional NB does not measure nitrogen excreted through the skin as sweat, skin, and hair desquamation, etc., and assumes this to be constant under ordinary conditions at a rate of about 0.3 to 1.0 g/day [118–119] or 5 mg/KG BW/day [120].

It has been documented that urea concentration in the sweat of uremic subjects is increased and proportional to the plasma concentration of urea [121].

*Fecal nitrogen (FN)*

Nitrogen content in the stool varies widely. The following figures have been found in normal subjects with controlled dietary intake: 12 ± 5 mg/KG

BW/day during protein deprivation [120, 122], 0.24 g/day during fasting [123], 0.66 ± 0.15 g/day on minimal protein intake [124], 1.1 g/day on a mixed diet [125], up to 1.8 ± 0.2 g/day with 120 g of protein intake [126]. Aside from this clear relationship to protein intake, fecal nitrogen is chiefly correlated to dietary bulk [127]. Fecal nitrogen has been shown to be enhanced in uremia [128], and subclinical gastrointestinal disturbances [129] might be responsible for unrecognized losses. Blood losses may also be involved [130].

In patients in chronic renal failure on low protein diet (2.7 to 7.0 g/day of NI), FN was around 1 g/day ranging from 0.4 to 2.1 g/day, independent of NI [131–135]. FN shows the same variability in dialysis patients as in patients in conservative treatment [103, 136].

However, Maroni and associates recently studied the relationship between NI and FN in patients with highly varied protein intakes (range 5.4–15.1 g NI/day), and found FN increases of 56 mg per gram of NI. The same authors recalculated this ratio using data from other studies of patients in dialysis or conservative treatment, with a dietary intake ranging from 1.7 to 18.2 g NI/day) and found FN to increase 48 ± 7 mg/g NI. Values for normal subjects differed only slightly: an increase of 44 ± 7 mg/g NI was seen [137].

*Urinary and dialysate nitrogen*

Urinary and/or dialysate nitrogen form the highest portion of nitrogen output, and is made up of urea nitrogen to a great extent. On the other hand, urea is the nitrogen waste product which is most sensitive to variations in protein intake. Thus, the analysis of urinary and/or dialysate nitrogen is divided into two parts: (1) urinary nitrogen (UN) = urea urinary nitrogen (UUN) + nonurea urinary nitrogen (NUUN); and (2) dialysate nitrogen (DN) = urea dialysate nitrogen (UDN) + nonurea dialysate nitrogen (NUDN).

The basal NUUN in healthy subjects fed adequate calories without proteins is 1.16 g/day [138]; with adequate protein intake, NUUN changes only slightly (1.3 g/day), but with higher protein intake (80–120 g/day) it increases to 2.2 and 3.9 g/day, respectively [139].

In uremic patients in conservative treatment, NUUN averages 1.0–1.2 g/day [133–135, 137]. In analyzing the available data, especially that of Maroni [137], NUUN shows a wide range of variation (0.2–3.0 g/day). Moreover, single data are not correlated with GFR, body weight, or protein intake.

Protein, leukocytes, erythrocytes in the urine may also substantially increase NUUN.

Little data on NUDN are available. Saito and associates [140] compared nitrogen output during dialysis and hemofiltration and found a NUDN of 5 and 3 g/session, respectively: in both cases UDN consisted in 75% of total DN. On a thrice weekly schedule, these figures account for 1.5 to 2.1 g NUDN/day.

*Table 6–3.* Nitrogen output

| | Healthy subjects | | Uremic Patients | |
| | Average | Range | Average | Range |
| --- | --- | --- | --- | --- |
| Integumental Losses | 5mg/KgBW | 0.3–1.0g | not calculated (enhanced in sweat) | |
| Faeces* | 1.1g | 0.25–2.0g | 1.1g (enhanced?) | 0.4–2.1g |
| Urine UUN* | 10g | 1.2–42G | unchanged in stationary pre-dialysis state | |
| NUUN | 1.3g | 1.1–3.9g | 1.1g | 0.2–3.0g |
| Urine Faeces NUN | 30mg/KgBW | 2–3g | unchanged | |

| Dialysis | | Percentage of total nigrogen | |
| --- | --- | --- | --- |
| UDN* | 9.2g | Urea | 82% |
| NUDN | 2.0g | Creatinine | 6% |
| | | Uric acid | 3% |
| | | Free AA | 6% |
| | | Bound AA | 3% |

*In relation with nitrogen intake.

Table 6–3 reports our unpublished data on the distribution of total dialysate nitrogen, together with other components of nitrogen output in 15 patients on 4 hour thrice-weekly dialysis treatment. NUDN was 4.7 g/session on the average, or 2.0 g/day.

*Amino acid losses*

When dialysis losses of nitrogen compounds are considered, special concern must be addressed to the amino acids. In fact, the loss of these metabolically active substances might directly affect the still precarious conditions of nitrogen metabolism.

Early studies evidenced 0.1 to 3.5 grams of alpha-amino nitrogen losses [104, 141, 142] or 4 to 8 grams of free amino acids [10, 143]. Whereas amino acid loss involves an unquestionable loss of effective nutrient compounds, the nutritional meaning of the bound amino acids has yet to be clarified. Some authors grant them full metabolic dignity [144]; others more prudently simply distinguish the free from the bound form [8, 145]. In our opinion, most of the bound amino acids represent the end products of protein or of larger peptide degradation which have assuredly lost their nutritional properties. Comparison of the effects of different hemodialysis treatments on amino acid losses is difficult for a number of reasons: few studies exist, chromatographic

159

methods of analysis are not consistent, dialysis characteristics are often not fully described, and serum amino acid patterns are sometimes lacking.

Table 6–4 reports some data from the literature. Aside from total free and bound amino acids, the losses of 8 essential free amino acids are reported both to avoid interpretative difficulties due to different chromatographic patterns and to call attention to these major nutrient compounds.

Statistical analysis of these data did not evidence a significant relationship between AA losses and time or efficiency of dialysis. Nevertheless, in low-efficiency long dialysis (standard Kiil), a strikingly lower loss of EAA than in high-efficiency shorter dialysis [148, 149] was observed despite similar losses of total free amino acids. This suggests that factors in addition to dialysis kinetics are involved.

Our study demonstrated a significant correlation between the removal of each amino acid and its predialysis plasma concentration [148]. Furthermore, Kopple found increased AA losses when dialysis was carried out under nonfasting conditions, when plasma amino acid concentrations are higher [145]. It can thus be deduced that the time connection with meals influences quantitative and qualitative dialysis losses of amino acids.

Other related matters, such as blood amino acid behavior patterns during and after the dialysis session, are worth consideration. Despite substantial losses, inconsistent depression of plasma amino acids at the end of the dialysis session has been reported by some authors [143, 146]. More recent studies indicate an average reduction of 18–32%, most of which consists in nonessential amino acids [13, 148–150]. The 8 EAA decrease by 10–22% [148, 149], while red blood cell free amino acid concentrations change less [13, 150].

Variations of 17 AA related to dialysis time are reported in table 6–5. Some amino acids show a more or less consistent but in any case time-dependent reduction (HIS, MET, THR, VAL, TYR, ALA, GLY, PRO, SER) [26, 148–150]. Others do not significantly change or increase [ILE, LEU, GLUAc). Further insight can be gained from figure 6–2, where one intradialysis control is marked.

It is evident that after an early decrease, many amino acids appreciably slow their reduction rate by more than what dialysis kinetics would predict: this is the case for essential amino acids (in particular, branched-chain AA) and a few nonessential AA (SER). This behavior is consistent with major metabolic responses to dialysis treatment that are probably associated with observed protein hypercatabolism (see below).

After completion of the dialysis session, amino acid serum concentrations (except for that of CYS) reach or exceed their predialysis levels [13].

Dialysis fluid with a high glucose concentration is reported to counteract both free and bound amino acid losses [145]. This could be explained by the inhibitory effect of glucose on dialysis-induced protein hypercatabolism. Wathen and associates [151] indirectly confirmed that the glucose lose that occurs when glucose-free dialysis fluid is used may contribute to catabolic

160

Table 6–4. Amino acid losses during dialysis

| Reference | Dialysis Time (Hrs) | Dialysis Efficiency (Urea Clearance ml/m') | Number of Evaluations | Glucose in Dialysis Fluid | Number of AA Evaluated | AA losses (g) | | Free Essential |
|---|---|---|---|---|---|---|---|---|
| | | | | | | Free | Bound | |
| 8 | 6 | 100 | 3 | no | 20 | 6.9 | 10.3 | 2.7 |
| 146 | 8 | 74 | 9 | no | 25 | 6.6 | — | 1.6 |
| | 8 | 116 | 5 | no | 25 | 10.3 | — | 2.5 |
| 147 | 6 | 120* | 1 | ? | | | | 1.8 |
| 145 | 11 | 90* | 4 | no | 23 | 6.3 | 3.7 | 1.6 |
| | 11 | 90* | 3 | 4.5g/l | 23 | 3.3 | 1.9 | 0.8 |
| 148 | 4 | 153 | 6 | 1.0g/l | 17 | 5.5 | — | 2.6 |
| 149 | 5 | 160* | 8 | no | 24 | 8.2 | — | 2.3 |

* Presumed value.

*Table 6–5.* Percent post dialysis to predialysis changes in plasma free amino acid concentrations

| Reference<br>Dialysis Time (Hrs) | [26]<br>3–4 | [148]<br>4 | [149]<br>5 | [150]<br>6–7 | [13]*<br>11 | [13]<br>After 3 Hours |
|---|---|---|---|---|---|---|
| HIS | —— | −23 | −26 | −31 | −29 | −4 |
| ILE | +4 | −1 | −9 | −15 | +27 | +40 |
| LEU | +25 | +16 | +6 | +24 | +36 | +44 |
| LYS | —— | −25 | −36 | −32 | −17 | +6 |
| MET | −14 | −16 | −42 | —— | −17 | +8 |
| PHE | −10 | +1 | −19 | −22 | −10 | +40 |
| THR | −25 | −17 | −27 | −41 | −11 | +8 |
| VAL | −17 | −11 | −20 | −30 | −10 | +16 |
| CYS | −56 | −51 | −63 | —— | −53 | −51 |
| TYR | −19 | −19 | −36 | −37 | −4 | +42 |
| ALA | —— | −38 | −54 | −71 | −34 | +30 |
| ARG | —— | −35 | −43 | −37 | −10 | +6 |
| ASPAc. | —— | −32 | −64 | −63 | —— | —— |
| GLUAc. | —— | +15 | −14 | −3 | —— | —— |
| GLY | −39 | −24 | −34 | −53 | −18 | −10 |
| PRO | —— | −32 | −33 | −56 | —— | —— |
| SER | −19 | −19 | −19 | −42 | −9 | +7 |

* 1–2 meals were taken during the dialysis session.

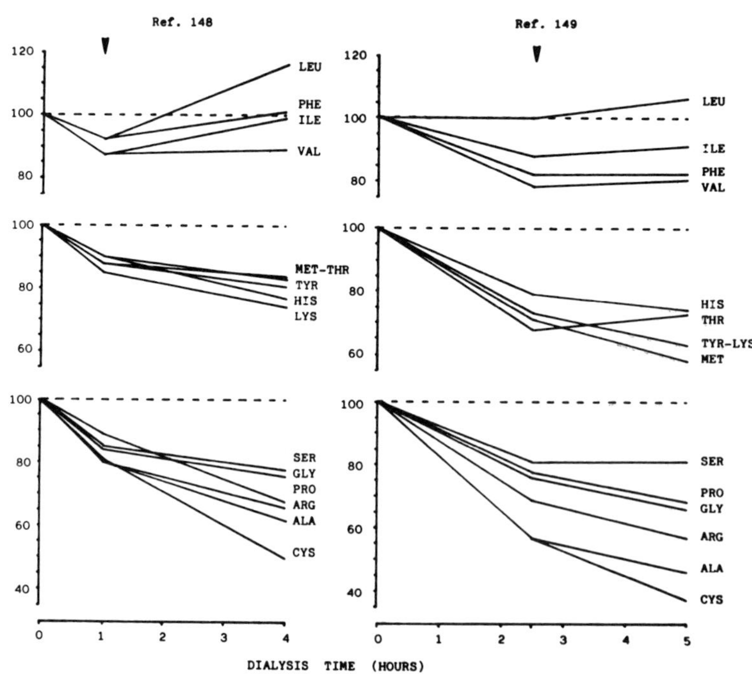


*Figure 6–2.* Serum free amino acid behavior during dialysis sessions of 4 (148) and 5 (149) hours. Arrow indicates the intradialysis control.

stress. Nevertheless, it has been reported that acetate metabolism introduced during dialysis can substantially supply needed calories [152].

*Non urea nitrogen (NUN)*

$$NUN = FN + NUUN$$

This expression combines two components of NB, only one of which (FN) has a direct relationship with NI. By means of this operation, there is no longer any correlation to NI; NUN is considered a relatively stable value and consequently urea is the only variable of the nitrogen balance that must be measured in relation to NI (see below).

NUN has been estimated at about 2–3 g/day [153, 114], 30 mg/KgBW/day [154] in both normal subjects and patients in renal failure. Maroni and associates have compared their data with the literature and conclude that 31 mg/kgBW/day of NUN leads, on the average, to a maximum NB estimation error of 1.3 g N/day [137]. They discourage adoption of these values in dialysis patients due to great NUN losses that can occur in this case; and yet the studies considered by these authors demonstrate an average NUN of 31 mg/kbBW/day (range 25.1–33.2).

*Urea nitrogen*

For a long time now it has been acknowledged that urea nitrogen is the most sensitive index of dietary protein intake [155]. For this and obviously practical reasons, it has often been the only value of nitrogen output monitored. In patients in renal failure, the net quantity of urea produced (unappearance UNA) must take into account possible variations in the body pool of urea as well as urinary urea. The changes in the urea body pool can be easily measured by multiplying the difference of the plasma urea concentration by the body distribution volume which under normal conditions of hydration can be quantified at 60% of body weight.

Some authors [114, 153] thus indicate that nitrogen balance can be expressed with the following equation:

$$NB = NI - (UNA + 2.5 \text{ g})$$

assuming that NUN is fixed at 2–3 g/day. Of identical significance to that of the nitrogen balance is the index utilized by other authors [111, 112] in which NUN is simply not considered: An index of NB = NI − UNA

After evaluating the following correlation between UNA and N out (UNA = 1.03 N out − 1.99), Kopple and Cianciaruso [156] propose values that are slightly different from the preceding, that is: NB = NI − (0.97 UNA + 1.93).

However, these authors obtained a rather different relationship between UNA and dietary nitrogen intake in clinically stable nondialyzed chronic uremic patients: UNA = 1.45 NI − 4.78.

In dialysis patients with poor or no residual renal function, urea removal takes place primarily or totally through the dialysis fluid; it can therefore be calculated by collection and measurement of the total dialysate. This procedure is both troublesome and inaccurate.

Alternatively, urea removal can be calculated as the difference in the urea body pool between the start and the end of the dialysis session. In this case, precise knowledge of the urea distribution volume is needed.

Although the urea space is very close to the water space in both normal [157–159] and uremic patients [1, 160, 161], the usual ratio to body weight (.6 × KgBW) leads to an additional degree of uncertainty in dialysis patients because their 'dry body weight' is determined on empirical grounds and their body water distribution is sometimes abnormal [162, 163]. Hence the urea space might be measured by means of dilution techniques using adequate tracers.

The introduction of a monocompartmental model of urea kinetics [95–98, 164] has solved the problem inasmuch as the iterative solution of two equations leads to finding two unknowns: urea generation rate and urea distribution volume (see chapter 9, 'Modeling Dialysis Therapy').

The term 'urea generation rate' coined by these authors is the exact equivalent of the more correct term 'urea appearance rate' adopted by other authors to define the net urea production in patients in conservative treatment. In fact, the total production or generation of urea exceeds the net production of a significant quota (20%) referred to the entero-hepatic recycling of urea itself [165].

In the frequently cited study of Cottini and associates [166], a significant direct relationship was established between nitrogen intake and urea appearance in patients in chronic renal failure who ate various amounts of protein or aminoacid mixtures:

$$\text{UNA (gN/day)} = 0.93 \text{ NI (gN/day)} - 1.21.$$

Similarly, when UNA obtained by the kinetic method in dialysis patients was related to simultaneously measured protein intake, a significant direct correlation was found: UNA (gN/day) = 0.69 NI (gN/day + 0.25) [96]. In this study, the calculated protein intake was between 0.5 and 2.0 g/KgBW and the average urea space was 54% of body weight. With the patients in stable condition, PI was also considered an estimate of protein catabolic rate (PCR).

With this method we were able to confirm that there are no significant differences between calculation of UNA with the kinetics method and total dialysate collection [167]. We have, moreover, obtained results very close to those cited regarding the relationship between UNA and PI: UNA (gN/day) = 0.67 NI (gN/day) + 0.65.

More detailed investigations of the meaning and value of UNA were carried out by Gotch and associates. UNA in particular, calculated with the kinetic method, was measured simultaneously with nitrogen balance, using the classical method [97].

Correction of data using results of the nitrogen balance gave a closer correlation between UNA and protein catabolism: UNA (gN/day) = 0.78 PCR (gN/day) − 0.55.

In subsequent studies, carried out with strict monitoring of the urea distribution volume and with diversified protein intake, an even closer correlation between UNA and PCR was obtained: UNA (gN/day) = 0.96 × PCR (gN/day) − 1.7 [109, 168, 169]. The last equation, further elaborated with the inclusion of the dry body weight variable [170] or the urea space variable [98], was considered conclusive and was utilized in the National Cooperative Dialysis Study: PCR (gN/day = 9.35 UNA (mg/m′) + 0.294 V (liters) or UNA (gN/day) = 0.96 PCR (gN/day) − 0.454 × V liters) [98].

These equations would indicate that in a patient weighing about 70 Kg in stable condition (PI = PCR), the UNA expresses 80% of protein intake with a dietary protein intake of 70 g (1 g/Kg), 85% with a protein intake of 100 g (1.45 g/Kg), and 69% for intakes of 40 grams (0.69 g/Kg). They give about a 10% increase in sensitivity over early equations.

By using the kinetics method, it is possible to measure dietary intake indirectly and the metabolic situation of the patient in dialysis: in fact, low calculated PCR values would indicate an anabolic situation or low protein intake, while high values would indicate excessive dietary intake or exaggerated catabolism [171].

However, there has always been considerable disagreement among outpatient studies comparing PCR to dietary protein intake, calculated by means of accurate food intake records [77, 132, 171, 172]. This has usually been interpreted as due to patient error in the estimation of dietary intake.

In the NCDS study [77], the concurrent findings of low caloric and protein intake is reported as evidence of patient tendency to underestimate dietary intake. When the graph referring to the DPI:PCR ratio is analyzed, aside from the great dispersion of data, in many cases PCR values very different from the average (63 g/day) are found: in fact, they exceed 83 g/day in 22% of the cases and are below 43 g/day in 5%. This casts some doubt on the accuracy of dietary records, as well as on the reliability of the method of measuring PCR. A possible source of error could be the less-than-perfect intercompartmental solute re-equilibrium during dialysis treatment.


*Postdialysis rebound and its implications in the evaluation of nitrogen balance*


Postdialysis rebound of plasma concentrations of some metabolites (urea, creatinine, uric acid, etc). has been recognized for a long time. Until about 10 years ago, it was thought to be exclusively due to solute reequilibrium between the unbalanced body compartments during dialysis due to trans-cellular transport coefficients generally lower than the efficiency of dialytic removal. The phenomenon was widely used to calculate transcellular trans-port coefficients of urea and creatinine [173–175]. Schindelm and Farrell [176] reflected on the meaning of the quite different values of the urea mass transport coefficient reported in the literature when different methods were used (postdialysis rebound sometimes gave a very low MTC, e.g., reference [173], whereas the off-dialysis radio-labelled urea dilution method gave a high MTC value [177]). They also onsidered the growing reports on the catabolic effect of dialysis and the clinical suitability of the single-pool model of urea kinetics, and concluded that 'post-dialysis plasma urea rebound is not due to post-dialysis transcellular reequilibration' but rather to an enhanced urea generation [176]. To date, there is general (but not unanimous) agreement with this statement, although direct evidence for it is still lacking.

Haas and associates [178] maintain that for urea, too, the rebound phenomen is, at least in part, due to intercompartmental imbalances. They cite the following: the presence of high concentration gradients between plasma and cerebrospinal fluid found immediately after dialysis [179]; urea distribution volume values, when calculated by using equilibrium concentra-tions 90 minutes after dialysis, are almost the same as generally accepted values (60% of body weight), while when they are calculated with immedi-ately postdialysis urea concentrations, they are significantly lower (50%) [180].

With this in mind, Haas and associates compared results from medium-efficiency and high-efficiency hemofiltration sessions (100 and 200 ml/m') and determined that a decrease in efficiency due to intracorporeal imbalance also exists with medium (5%) efficiency, and that it increases as efficiency is increased [178].

If urea rebound were chiefly due to a dialysis-induced intracompartmental imbalance, then: (1) it would be correlated to the length and efficiency of dialysis; (2) it would be resolved in less than an hour after dialysis.

While the data of Borah and associates, who demonstrate that accelerated urea generation continues for about 8 hours, confute point (2) [109], point (1) is supported by our nonpublished data (table 6–6) as well as those of Haas. Urea rebound effects 1 hour after the end of dialysis were studied in 5 patients in dialysis treatment at different levels of efficiency (by modifications of blood flow and session time). In order to avoid the predialysis BUN concentration and distribution volume variables, dialysis efficiency was measured as the total removal of urea with respect to the predialysis urea body pool.

Although the results are highly variable, they demonstrate a strict correla-tion between dialysis efficiency and 1-hour rebound ($p < 0.001$).

As far as other metabolites, such as creatinine, uric acid, and middle molecules, are concerned, it has been amply demonstrated that rebound is chiefly linked to the intercompartmental imbalance, since these metabolites

166

*Table 6–6.* One-hour urea rebound and dialysis efficiency

| Dialysis Parameters | % Urea Rebound After 1 Hour | Total urea removal. 100 Predialysis Pool |
|---|---|---|
| $Q_B$ = 280 ml/m′ Time = 4 hours | 27.2 ± 13.0 | 67.9 ± 3.4 |
| $Q_B$ = 150 ml/m′ Time = 4 hours | 13.9 ± 5.0 | 53.4 ± 6.1 |
| $Q_B$ = 280 ml/m′ Time = 3 hours | 12.9 ± 8.8 | 54.1 ± 10.1 |
| $Q_B$ = 150 ml/m′ Time = 3 hours | 6.7 ± 7.9 | 47.7 ± 7.4 |

Five patients were subsequently evaluated using different dialysis times and efficiencies.

have an MTC that is similar or actually below clearance values commonly in use. Their removal is thus influenced by dialysis time and efficiency.

## Dialysis-induced hypercatabolism

Another interesting result of kinetic urea evaluation concerns the postdialysis rate of urea appearance [109, 168, 170, 176, 181, 182].

In the study of Borah and associates [109] urea generation rates 28% higher on dialysis days than on nondialysis days (12.7 ± 3.1 g/24 hours versus 9.9 ± 3.2 g/24 hours) are reported in 5 patients with a protein intake of 1.4 g/ KgBW. The same patients again evaluated with a protein intake of 0.5 g/ KgBW showed UNA values about 40% higher on dialysis days than on non-dialysis days (5.6 ± 1.7 g/24 hours versus 4.0 ± 1.0 g/24 hours). Moreover, the nitrogen balance was constantly negative.

Another noteworthy finding reported in Borah's study is the course of urea generation in time: it was measured after 1.5, 3, 5, 8, and 20 hours after dialysis. Although the report does not specify if and when meals were taken during this period, UNA was still unequivocably higher than on the nondialysis day for at least 8 hours after the completion of the dialysis session, independent of food intake (1.4 g or 0.5 g protein/KgBW). In absolute terms, a 3.1 g increase in UNA with respect to the baseline when protein intake was 1.4 g/Kg (about 5.0 g/24 hours) was demonstrated; an increase of about half that amount (1.4 g/8 hours = 2.3 g/24 hours) was seen when protein intake was low (0.5 g/Kg). From the eighth hour on, urea generation values slowed down, then returned rapidly to average nondialysis day values.

These data are in keeping with the observations of Conley and associates [183] who studied protein turnover using C14-lysine. Aside from the main finding regarding the improvement but not complete correction by dialysis of the reduction of the protein turnover rate found in uremia, they demon-

167

strated that protein turnover rates were similar before and 16–19 hours after the dialysis session.

Most authors maintain that accelerated protein catabolism induced by dialysis is responsible for enhanced urea production. In fact, many indirect data contribute to this interpretation: increased antianabolic hormones such as cortisol, thyroxin, and glucagon or the reduction in GH [184], loss of nutritional substances [150, 151] and particularly amino acids [145] (but not of glucose) [182].

Interpretations of the meaning of these events are still inconclusive. For example, Farrel and Hone [170] measured UNA independently during both dialysis and the entire weekly cycle. They demonstrated that the acceleration of UNA occurs during dialysis and that it is directly correlated to predialysis urea concentrations. The first observation, though not unexpected, is rather striking because urea production is normally a direct function of serum amino acid concentration [185], whereas during dialysis it would increase concomitantly with a significant decrease in amino acid concentration. As far as the second observation is concerned, the authors reason that the phenomenon might be linked to a reactivation of the urea cycle which has been depressed because of high pre-dialysis BUN values [28]. This interpretation is not at variance with the data of Borah and associates who, as we have reported, found higher UNA values when protein intake was higher and therefore, presumably, when BUN levels were higher as well.

The recent finding of a direct stimulating effect of arginine-vasopressin on ureagenesis [186] would lead to the consideration that an increase of this hormone (presumably stimulated during dialysis by the reduction in plasma volume) might be responsible for the postdialytic increase in ureagenesis. However, in a recent report on ADH, PRA, and Aldosterone behavior during dialysis, it was demonstrated that ADH is reduced inasmuch as it is dialyzed [187].

In summary, postdialysis urea generation acceleration is characterized by the following: (1) it begins during dialysis; (2) it continues for 8 hours after dialysis; (3) the higher the predialytic urea concentrations, the more it is accentuated; (4) it is quantitatively correlated to dietary protein intake; and (5) it can be different in different types of depurative procedures; and finally, (6) it is followed by a period of depression of/in urea generation (presumably linked to anabolism).

Various hypotheses to interpret the mechanisms responsible for hyperureagenesis, aside from the loss of vital substances, could be suggested by observations of other hypercatabolic conditions (trauma, sepsis, ARF). One factor, in particular, concerns the release of granulocyte proteinase [188] into the circulation: since its activity is already sharply reduced at the end of dialysis, it should be unable to cause a UNA increase for several hours after dialysis.

An even more interesting factor involves the release of a peptide able to induce muscle proteolysis [189] or of the leukocyte pyrogen, interleukine 1

[190], able to stimulate muscular synthesis of prostalglandin $E_2$ which directly promotes proteolysis. According to Shaldon and associates [191], the monocytes adhering to the dialysis membrane are activated by the complement system, endotoxic substances and the acetate contained in the dialysis fluid: they produce and release interleukine 1 within 1–4 hours. Inteleukine 1 is responsible for fever, hypotension, and muscular hypercatabolism. According to the authors, the reduced monocyte activation found in hemofiltration with respect to hemodialysis due to the absence of contact with the dialysis liquid would explain the attenuation of hypotension and hypercatabolism seen in hemofiltration.

According to this hypothesis, a higher degree of catabolism and hypotension would be expected during hemodiafiltration because leukocyte contact with dialysis liquid across a more porous membrane is facilitated. However, this has never been demonstrated [75].

In hypercatabolic states in which interleukine 1 activation has been found, there is still a 'catabolic pattern' characterized by increased free (especially branched and aromatic) amino acids [192].

On the contrary, during ARF, plasma amino acids do not increase, but, as in the case of dialysis, decrease [193, 194]. This singular association calls attention to the particular clinical condition during the dialysis session that can be regarded as an acute 'reappearance' of ARF after dialysis has corrected some uremic imbalances.

The causes of reduced plasma amino acid concentrations of hypercatabolic ARF have not been clearly established, but increased hepatic utilization [195, 196] may be cited. Likewise, an increase in gluconeogenesis has been found in the postdialysis period [50].


**Final considerations**

The quantity of nitrogen-containing substances removed from the body by dialysis is the most consistent quota of total nitrogen *output*. Similar to what is seen in normal subjects, the principal component of this group is urea. When dialysis schedule, dietary intake, and metabolic conditions are constant, nitrogen balance is established by fixing the average levels of urea plasma concentrations and other nitrogenous waste products.

After years of study and debate, it has been demonstrated that the BUN concentration reasonably represents the degree of 'uremic intoxication,' and that average levels between 50 and 80 mg/dl are associated with less morbidity and mortality. It is equally important, however, that dietary intake be 'adequate.' Dietary intake and BUN concentration are linked by the amount of dialysis. The amount of dialysis is in turn a function of several factors: length, periodicity, filter efficiency, blood and dialysis fluid flows, and urea distribution. With a thrice-weekly schedule, and commonly used flows and filters, the required length of a dialysis session is between 3.5 and 5.0 hours.

An average of about 4 hours thrice weekly in dialysis thus seems to be adequate. Our dialysis unit has been using this schedule for about 15 years, and the nutritional indexes shown in table 6–2 can therefore provide a valid comparison to other dialysis schedules. They do not differ substantially from those of case series: this at least indicates that more prolonged dialysis sessions are unnecessary.

It has been confirmed that the need for nutritive substances in dialysis patients increases both with respect to normal subjects and with respect to patients with chronic renal failure in conservative treatment; moreover, in many dialysis patients, these levels are not reached (that is, the needs are not met). This could explain the appearance or persistence of a fair degree of malnutrition in these patients. The use of a mathematical model to measure UNA (though not totally accurate, as is emphasized in the section on nitrogen balance) can be a useful tool to measure dietary intake, although it does not furnish information regarding the actual state of nitrogen balance.

But what is the cause of the increased dietary need? The most logical explanation can be found in the nonselective nature of the dialytic membrane, causing the loss of fair amounts of amino acids with possible concomitant effects of antianabolic hormones.

Is it possible to limit the catabolic effect linked to dialysis through manipulation of dialytic parameters? The very similar incidence of malnutrition in dialysis units employing different dialysis schedules or the dissimilar incidence of malnutrition in units employing the same dialysis schedule has not substantiated this hypothesis. Nor has a crossover study between short and long dialysis times evidenced significant differences in protein catabolism [197].

At present, it would seem that the only available recourse is greater dietary control associated with amino acid supplements. However, if the activation of catabolism mediators through the dialysis procedure were confirmed, new technical and/or pharmacological approaches could be sought.

## References


1. Coles, G.A. (1972) Body composition in chronic renal failure. Quart, J. Med. 41: 25–47.
2. Blumenkrantz, M.J. and Kopple, J.D. (1976) Incidence of nutritional abnormalities in uremic patients entering dialysis therapy. Kidney Internat. 10: 514.
3. Blumenkrantz, M.J., Kopple, J.D., Gutman, R.A., Chan, Y.K., Barbour, G.L., Robert, C., Shen, F.H., Gandhi, V.C., Tucker, C.T., Curtis, F.K. and Coburn, J.W. (1980) Methods for assessing nutritional status of patients with renal failure. Am. J. Clin. Nutr. 33: 1567–1585.
4. Young, G.A., Keogh, J.B. and Parsons, F.M. (1975) Plasma aminoacids and protein levels in chronic renal failure and changes caused by oral supplements of essential amino acids. Clin. Chim. Acta 61: 205–213.
5. Bianchi, R., Mariani, G., Pilo, A., Toni, M.G. and Carmassi, F. (1976) Albumin depletion in uremic patients on conservative management. In *Plasma Protein Turnover*, R. Bianchi, G. Mariani and A.S. Mc Farlane (eds.). Baltimore: The Mac Millan Press L.T.D., pp. 237–250.

6. Holliday, M.A., Chantler, C., Mac Donnell, R. and Keitges, J. (1977) Effect of uremia on nutritionally-induced variations in protein metabolism. Kidney Internat. 11: 236–245.

7. Delaporte, C., Bergstrom, J. and Broyer, M. (1976) Variations in muscle cell protein of severely uremic children. Kidney Internat. 10: 239–245.

8. Giordano, C., De Pascale, C., De Cristofaro, D., Capodicasa, G., Balestrieri, C. and Baczik, K. (1968) Protein malnutrition in the treatment of chronic uremia. In *Nutrition in Renal Disease*, G.M. Berlyne (ed.). Edimburgh and London: E. and S. Livingstone LTD, pp. 23–34.

9. Czerniak, Z. and Burzynski, S. (1969) Free amino acids in serum of patients with chronic renal insufficiency. Clin. Chim. Acta 24: 367–372.

10. Mc Gale, E.H.F. Pickford, J.C. and Aber, G.M. (1972) Quantitative changes in plasma amino acids in patients with renal disease. Clin. Chim. Acta 38: 395–403.

11. Bergstrom, J., Furst, P., Norée, L.O. and Vinnars, E. (1978) Intracellular free aminoacids in muscle tissue of patients with chronic uremia: effect of peritoneal dialysis and infusion of essential aminoacids. Clin. Sci. Mol. Med. 54: 51–60.

12. Broyer, M., Jean, G., Dartois, A.M. and Kleinknecht, C. (1980) Plasma and muscle free aminoacids in children at the early stages of renal failure. Am. J. Clin. Nutr. 33: 1396–1401.

13. Jontofsohn, R., Trivisas, G., Katz, N. and Kluthe, R. (1978) Amino acid content of erythrocytes in uremia. Am. J. Clin. Nutr. 31: 1956–1960.

14. Metcoff, J., Dutta, S., Burns, G., Pederson, J., Matter, B. and Rennert, O. (1983) Effects of aminoacid infusions on cell metabolism in hemodialyzed patients with uremia. Kidney Internat. 24 (suppl. 16): S-87–S-92.

15. Maillet, C. and Garber, A.J. (1980) Skeletal muscle aminoacid metabolism in chronic uremia. Am. J. Clin. Nutr. 33: 1343–1353.

16. Tizianello, A., De Ferrari, G., Garibotto, G. and Robaudo, C. (1980) Amino acid metabolism and the liver in renal failure. Am. J. Clin. Nutr. 33: 1354–1362.

17. De Ferrari, G., Garibotto, G., Robaudo, C., Ghiggeri, G.M., Tizianello, A. (1981) Brain metabolism of aminoacids and ammonia in patients with chronic renal insufficiency. Kidney Internat. 20: 505–510.

18. Betts, P.R. and Green, A. (1977) Plasma and urine aminoacid concentrations in children with chronic renal insufficiency. Nephron 18: 132–139.

19. Fukuda, S. and Kopple, J.D. (1980) Uptake and release of aminoacids by the kidney of dogs made chronically uremic with uranyl nitrate. Mineral Electrolyte Metab. 3: 248–260.

20. Druml, W., Burger, V., Balcke, P., Kleinberger, G., Lenz, K., Zazgornik, J., Schmidt, P. and Laggner, A. (1983) Utilization of amino acids in renal failure. Kidney Internat. 24 (suppl. 16): S-328–S-328.

21. Sterner, G., Lindberger, T. and Demuberg, T. (1982) 'In vivo' and 'in vitro' absorption of amino acids and dipeptides in the small intestine of uremic rats. Nephron 31: 273–276.

22. Giordano, C., De Pascale, C., Pluvio, M., Se Santo, N.G., Fella, A., Esposito, R., Capano, G. and Pota, A. (1975) Adverse effects among amino acids in uremia. Kidney Internat. (7 suppl.) 3: S-306–S-310.

23. Tizianello, A., Deferrari, G., Garibotto, G., Robaudo, C., Saffioti, S., Salvidio, G. and Paoletti, E. (in press) Abnormal amino acid metabolism after the ingestion of amino acids in patients with chronic renal failure. Kidney Int.

24. Arroyave, G., Wilson, D., De Funes, C. and Behar, M. (1962) Free amino acids in blood plasma of children with kwashiorkor and marasmus. Am. J. Clin. Nutr. 11: 517–524.

25. Smith, S.R., Pozefsky, T., Chletri, M.K. (1974) Nitrogen and amino acid metabolism in adults with protein-caloric malnutrition. Metabolism 23: 603–618.

26. Wilcken, D.E.L. and Gupte, V.J. (1979) Sulphur containing amino acids in chronic renal failure with particular reference to homocystine and cysteine-homocysteine mixed disulphide. Eur. J. Clin. Invest. 9: 301–307.

27. Chan, W., Wang, M., Kopple, J.D. and Swendseid, M.E. (1974) Citrulline levels and urea cycle enzymes in uremic rats. J. Nutr. 104: 678–683.

28. Menyhart, J. and Grof, J. (1977) Urea as a selective inhibitor of argininosuccinate lyase.

Eur. J. Biochem. 75: 405–409.

29. Young, G.A. and Parsons, F.M. (1973) Impairment of phenylalinine hydroxylation in chronic renal insufficiency. Clin. Sci. 45: 89–97.

30. Letteri, J.M. and Scipione, R.A. (1974) Phenylalamine metabolism in chronic renal failure. Nephron 13: 365–371.

31. Jones, M.R. and Kopple, J.D. (1978) Valine metabolism in normal and chronically uremic man. Am. J. Clin. Nutr. 31: 1660–1664.

32. Saito, A., Niwa, T., Maeda, K., Kabayashi, K., Yamamoto, Y. and Ohta, K. (1980) Tryptophan and indolic tryptophan metabolites in chronic renal failure. Am. J. Clin. Nutr. 33: 1402–1406.

33. Cernacek, P., Becvarova, P., Gerova, Z., Valek, A. and Spustova, (1980) Plasma tryptophan level in chronic renal failure. Clin. Nephrol. 14: 246–249.

34. Blumenkrantz, M.J. (1979) Are low protein diets useful? In *Controversies in Nephrology*. Masson Publishing USA Inc., pp. 381–389.

35. Giordano, C. (1979) Are low protein diets useful? A critical approach. In *Controversies in Nephrology* Masson Publishing USA Inc., pp. 390–401.

36. Kampf, D., Fisher, H.C. and Kessel, M. (1980) Efficacy of an unselected protein diet (25gr) with minor oral supply of essential amino acids and keto analogues compared with a selective protein diet (40gr) in chronic renal failure. Am. J. Clin. Nutr. 33: 1673–1677.

37. Kopple, J.D., Jones, M., Fukuda, S. and Swendseid, M.E. (1978) Amino acid and protein metabolism in renal failure. Am. J. Clin. Nutr. 31: 1532–1540.

38. Wassner, S.J., Orloff, S. and Holliday, M.A. (1976) Protein catabolism in normal and uremic rats. Pediat. Res. 10: 445 (Abs. 861).

39. Young, G.A. and Parsons, F.M. (1970) Plasma and urine amino acid imbalance in chronic renal failure. Proc. Europ. Dial. Transpl. Ass. 7: 167–174. London: Pittman Medical.

40. Nadvornikova, H., Schuck, O., Maly, J., Pechar, J., Dobersky, P. and Tomkova, D. (1978) Renal clearance of amino acids in patients with severe chronic renal failure. Nephron 20: 83–89.

41. Tizianello, A., Ferrari, G.D., Garibotto, G., Cuneri, G. and Robaudo, C. (1980) Renal metabolism of amino acids and ammonia in subjects with normal renal function and in patients with chronic renal insufficiency. J. Clin. Invest. 65: 1162–1173.

42. Giordano, C., De Santo, N.G. and Senatore, R. (1978) Effects of catabolic stess in acute and chronic renal failure. Am. J. Clin. Nutr. 31: 1561–1571.

43. Grodstein, G.P., Blumenkratz, M.J. and Koppler, J.D. (1979) Effects of intercurrent illnesses on nitrogen metabolism in uremic patients. Trans. Am. Soc. Artif. Intern. Organs XXV: 438–441.

44. Casciani, C.U., De Simone, C. and Bonini, S. (1978) Immunologic aspects of chronic uremia. Kidney Internat. 13 (suppl. 8): S-49–S-54.

45. Drutz, D.J. (1979) Altered cell-mediated immunity and its relationship to infection susceptibility in patients with uremia. Dial. Transplant. 8: 320–368.

46. De Fronzo, R.A., Smith, D. and Alvestrand, A. (1983) Insulin action in uremia. Kidney Internat. 24 (suppl. 16): S-102–S-1014.

47. Bilbrey, G.L., Faloona, G.R., White, M.G. and Knochel, J.P. (1974) Hyperglucagonemia of renal failure. J. Clin. Invest. 53: 841–847.

48. Mondon, C.E., Marcus, R. and Reaven, G.M. (1982) Role of glucagon as a contributor to glucose intolerance in acute and chronic uremia. Metabolism 31: 374–379.

49. Rubenfeld, S. and Garber, A.J. (1978) Abnormal carbohydrate metabolism in chronic renal failure. The potential role of accelerated glucose production, increased gluconeogenesis and impaired glucose disposal. J. Clin. Invest. 62: 20–29.

50. Rubenfeld, S. and Garber, A.J. (1979) Impact of hemodialysis on the abnormal glucose and alanine kinetics of chronic azotemia. Metabolism 28: 934–942.

51. De Fronzo, R.A. (1978) Pathogenesis of glucose intolerance in uremia. Metabolism 27: 1866–1880.

52. Samaan, N.A. and Freeman, R.M. (1970) Growth hormone levels in severe renal failure.

172

Metab. Clin. Exp. 19: 102–113.

53. Holdsworth, S., Atkins, R.C. and De Krester, D.H. (1977) The pitnitary-testicular axis in men with chronic renal failure. N. Engl. J. Med. 296: 1245–1249.

54. Massry, S.G. (1977) Is parathyroid hormone a uremic toxin? Nephron 19: 125–130.

55. Massry, S.G. (1985) Current status of the role of parathyroid hormone in uremic toxicity. Contr. Nephrol. 49: 1–11.

56. Lim, V.S., Fang, V.S., Katz, A.I. and Refetoff, S. (1977) Thyroid disfunction in chronic renal failure. A study of the pituitary-thyroid axis and peripheral turnover kinetics of thyroxine and triodothyronine. J. Clin. Invest. 60: 522–534.

57. Kaptein, E.M., Feinstein, E.I., Nicoloff, J.T., Massry, S.G. (1983) Alterations of serum reverse triiodothyronine and thyroxine kinetics in chronic renal failure : role of nutritional status, chronic illness, uremia, and hemodialysis. Kidney Internat. 24, (suppl. 16): S-180–S-186.

58. Danforth, J.E., Horton, E.S. and Sims, E.A.H. (1981) Nutritionally induced alterations in thyroid hormone metabolism. In Beers, R.F. Jr. and Bassett, E.G. (eds) *Nutritional Factors: Modulating Effects on Metabolic Processes*, New York: Raven Press, pp. 139–153.

59. Blom an Assendelft, P.M. and Mees, E.J.D. (1970) Urea metabolism in patients with chronic renal failure. Influence of sodium bicarbonate or sodium chloride administration. Metabolism 19: 1053–1063.

60. Papadoyannakis, N.J., Stefanidis, C.J. and Mc Geown, M. (1984) The effect of the correction of metabolic acidosis on nitrogen and potassium balance of patients with chronic renal failure. Am. J. Clin. Nutr. 40: 623–627.

61. Spergel, G., Bleicher, S.J., Goldberg, M., Adesman, J. and Goldner, M.G. (1967) The effect of potassium on the impaired glucose tolerance in chronic uremia. Metabolism 16: 581–585.

62. Delaporte, C., Gros, F. and Anagnostopoulos, T. (1980) Inhibitory effects of plasma dialysate on protein synthesis in vitro: influence of dialysis and transplantation. Am. J. Clin. Nutr. 33: 1407–1410.

63. Schreiner, G.E. (1975) The search for uremic toxin(s). Kidney Internat. 7 (suppl. 3): S-270–S-271.

64. Brenner, B.M., Meyer, T.W. and Hostetter, T.H. (1982) Dietary protein intake and the progressive nature of kidney disease: the role or hemodinamically mediated glomerular injury in the pathogenesis of progressive glomerular sclerosis in aging, renal ablation and intrinsic renal disease. N. Engl. J. Med. 307: 652–659.

65. Barsotti, G., Morelli, E., Giannoni, A., Guiducci, A., Lupetti, S. and Giovannetti, S. (1983) Restricted phosphorus and nitrogen intake to slow the progression of chronic renal failure: a controlled trial. Kidney Inter. 24 (suppl. 16): S-278–S-284.

66. Rosman, J.B., Ter Wee, P.M., Meijer, S., Piers-Becht, T.P.M., Sluiter, W. and Donker, A.J.M. (1984) Prospective randomised trial of early dietary protein restriction in chronic renal failure. Lancet II: 1291–1296.

67. Kopple, J.D., Swendseid, M.E. (1975) Protein and amino acid metabolism in uremic patients undergoing maintenance hemodialysis. Kidney Internat. 7 (supp. 2): S-564–S-572.

68. Kluthe, R., Luttgen, F.M., Capetianu, T., Heinze, V. and Katz, N., Sudhoff, A. (1978) Protein requirements in maintenance hemodialysis. Am. J. Clin. Nutr. 31: 1812–1820.

69. Knochel, J.P. (1983) Endocrine changes in patients on chronic dialysis. In *Replacement of Renal Function by Dialysis*, W. Drukker, F.M. Parsons and J.F. Maher (eds.). Boston: Martinus Nijhoff Pub., pp. 712–723.

70. Thunberg, B.J., Swami, A.P. and Cestero, R.V.M. (1981) Cross-sectional and longitudinal nutritional measurements in maintenance hemodialysis patients. Am. J. Clin. Nutr. 34: 2005–2012.

71. Alvestrand, A., Furst, P. and Bergstrom, J. (1983) Intracellular amino acids in uremia. Kidney Internat. 24 (suppl. 16): S-9–S-16.

72. Guarnieri, G., Toigo, G., Situlin, R., Faccini, L., Coli, U., Landini, S., Bazzato, G., Dardi, F., Campanacci, L. (1983) Muscle biopsy studies in chronically uremic patients:

evidence for malnutrition. Kidney Internat. 24 (suppl. 16): S-187–S-193.

73. Wolfson, M., Strong, C.J., Minturn, D., Gray, D.K. and Kopple, J.D. (1984) Nutritional status and lymphocyte function in maintenance hemodialysis patients. Am. J. Clin. Nutr. 39: 547–555.

74. Acchiardo, S.R., Moore, L.W., Latour, P.A. (1983) Malnutrition as the main factor in morbidity and mortality of hemodialysis patients. Kidney Internat. 24 (suppl. 16): S-199–S-203.

75. Arisi, L., Riggio, P., Bignardi, L., Mancuso, S., Corradi, A., Garini, G., Gatti, G., Rossi, E., Bacchi, M. and Cambi, V. (1983) Evoluzione naturale del peso corporeo dal primo riscontro di nefropatia alla fase uremica. Rapporti con lo stato nutrizionale in corso di trattamento dialitico prolungato. In *Nefrologia, Dialisi, Trapianto 1983*, Milano: Wichtig, pp. 295–298.

76. Van Itallie, T.B. and Yang, M. (1977) Diet and weight loss. N. Engl. J. Med. 297: 1158–1161.

77. Schoenfeld, P.Y., Henry, R.R., Laird, N.M. and Roxe, D.M. (1983) Assessment of nutritional status of the national cooperative dialysis study population. Kidney Internat. 23 (suppl. 13): S80–S88.

78. Kopple, J.D., Henry, D.A., Roberts, C.E., Goodman, W.G. and Blumenkrantz, M.J. (1981) Relationship between nutritional status of patients undergoing maintenance hemodialysis and duration of dialysis therapy. In *Uremia: Pathobiology of Patients Treated for Ten Years Or More*, C. Giordano and E.A. Friedman (eds.) Milano: Wichtig Editore, pp. 26–32.

79. Arisi, L., Bignardi, L., Cambi, V., David, S., Garini, G., Manari, A., Rossi, E. and Savazzi, G.M. (1981) Clinical and statistical evaluation of chronic hemodialysis treatment after 10 years. In *Uremia: Pathobiology of Patients Treated for Ten Years Or More*, C. Giordano and E.A. Friedman (eds.) Milano: Wichtig Editore, pp. 60–63.

80. Cambi, V., Dall'Aglio, P., Savazzi, G., Arisi, L., Rossi, E., Migone, L. (1972) Clinical assessment of hemodialysis patients with reduced small molecule removal. Proc. Eur. Dial. Transpl. Ass. 9: 67–73.

81. Cambi, V., Savazzi, G., Arisi, L., Bignardi, L., Bruschi, G., Rossi, E. and Migone, L. (1974) Short dialysis schedule (S.D.S.) Finally ready to become a routine? Proc. Eur. Dial. Transpl. Ass. 11: 112–119.

82. Buzio, C., Dall'Aglio, P., Scarpioni, L., Arisi, L., David, S., Del Monte, G. (1978) Le proteine sieriche come indici delle condizioni di nutrizione nei pazienti in trattamento emodialitico periodico. Minerva Nefrologica 25: 199–212.

83. Baker, J.P., Detsky, A.S., Wesson, D.E, Wolman S.L., Stewart, S., Whitewell, J., Langer, B. and Jeejeebhoy, K.N. (1982) Nutritional assessment. A comparison of clinical judgement and objective measurements. N. Engl. J. Med. 306: 969–972.

84. Young, G.A., Swanepoel, C.R., Crofo, H.R., Hobson, S.M. and Parsons, F.M. (1982) Anthropometry and plasma valine, amino acids, and proteins in the nutritional assessment of hemodialysis patients. Kidney Internat. 21: 492–499.

85. Eschbach, J.W., Wilson, W.E., People, R.W., Wakefield, A.W., Babb, A.B., Scribner, B.H. (1966) Unattended overnight home hemodialysis. Trans. Ar. Soc. Artif. Intern. Organs 12: 346–356.

86. Gotch, F., Lipps, B., Weaver, J., Brandes, J., Rosin, J., Sargent, J. and Oja, P. (1969) Chronic hemodialysis with the hollow fiber artificial kidney. Trans. ASAIO 15: 87–96.

87. Christopher, T.G., Cambi, V., Harker, L.A., Hurst, P.E., Popovich, R.P., Babb, A.L. and Scribner, B.H. (1971) A study of hemodialysis with lowered dialysate flow rate. Trans. ASAIO 17: 92–95.

88. Ginn, H.E., Teschan, P.E., Freeman, M., Bourne, J., Ward, J.W., McLain, W. (1973) Neurobehavioral and clinical responses to hemodialysis. Proc. 6th Am. Contractors Conference D.H.E.W. Publication No. (NIH) 74–248, pp. 15–17.

89. Johnson, W.J., Hagge, W.W., Wagoner, R.D., Dinapoli, R.P. and Resevear, J.W. (1972) Effects of urea loading in patients with far-advanced renal failure. Mayo Clin. Proc.

47: 21–29.

90. Lowrie, E.G., Stenberg, S.M., Galen, M.A., Gagneux, S.A., Lazarus, J.M., Gottlieb, M.N. and Merrill, J.P. (1976) Factors in the dialysis regimen which contribute to alterations in the abnormalities of uremia. Kidney Internat. 10: 409–422.

91. Babb, A.L., Popovich, R.P., Christopher, T.G. and Scribner, B.H. (1971) The genesis of the square-meter-hour hypothesis Trans. Am. Soc. Artif. Intern. Organs 17: 81–91.

92. Babb, A.L., Farrel, P.C., Uvelli, D.A. and Scribner, B.H. (1972) Hemodialyzer evaluation by examination of solute molecular spectra. Trans. Am. Soc. Artif. Intern. Organs 18: 98–103.

93. Milutinovic, J., Strand, M., Casaretto, A., Follette, W., Babb, A.L., Scribner, B.H. (1974) Clinical impact of residual glomerular filtration rate (GFR) on dialysis time. A preliminary report. Trans. ASAIO 20: 410–416.

94. Milutinovic, J., Cutler, R.E., Hoover, P., Meijsen, B. and Scribner, B.H. (1975) Measurement of residual glomerular filtration rate in the patient receiving repetitive hemodialysis. Kidney Internat. 8: 185–190.

95. Gotch, F.A., Sargent, J.A., Keen, M.L., Seid, M.A. and Foster, R. (1972) Comparative treatment time with Kiil, Gambro and Cordis Dow Kidney. Proc. Dialysis Transplant. Forum 3: 217.

96. Gotch, F.A., Sargent, J.A., Keen, M.L. and Lee, L. (1974) Individualized quantified dialysis therapy of uremia. Proc. Dialysis Transplant Forum 4: 27–37.

97. Gotch, F.A., Sargent, J.A., Keen, M.L., Lam, M.A., Prowitt, M. and Grady, M. (1976) Clinical results of intermittent dialysis therapy (IDT) guided by ongoing kinetic analysis of urea metabolism. Trans. Am. Soc. Artif. Intern. Organs 22: 175–189.

98. Sargent, J.A. (1983) Control of dialysis by a single-pool urea model: the National Cooperative Dialysis Study. Kidney Internat. 23 (suppl. 13): S-19–S-25.

99. Laird, N.M., Berkey, C.S. and Lowrie, E.G. (1983) Modeling success or failure of dialysis therapy: the National Cooperative Dialysis Study. Kidney Internat. 23 (suppl. 13): S-101–S-106.

100. Teshan, P.E., Ginn, H.E., Bourne, J.R., Ward, J.W., Schaffer, J.D. (1983) A prospective study of reduced dialysis. ASAIO Journal 6: 108–122.

101. Avram, M.M., Slater, P.A., Gan, A., Iancu, M., Pahilan, A.N., Okanya, D., Rajpal, K., Paik, S.K., Zouabi, M. and Fein, P.A. (1985) Predialysis BUN and creatinine do not predict adequate dialysis, clinical rehabilitation, or longevity. Kidney Internat. 28 (suppl. 17): S-100–S-104.

102. Gotch, F.A. and Sargent, J.A. (1985) A mechanistic analysis of the National Cooperative Dialysis Study (NCDS). Kidney Internat. 28: 526–534.

103. Shinaberger, J.H. and Ginn, H.E. (1968) A low protein, high essential amino acid diet for nitrogen equilibrium in chronic dialysis In *Nutrition in Renal Disease*, G.M. Berlyne (ed.). Edimburgh and London: E.&S. Livingstone LDT, pp. 55–65.

104. Ginn, H.E., Frost, A., Lacy, W.W. (1968) Nitrogen balance in hemodialysis patients. Am. J. Clin. Nutr. 21: 385–393.

105. Kopple, J.D., Shinaberger, J.H., Coburn, J.W., Sorenson, M.K. and Rubini, M.E. (1969) Optional dietary protein treatment during chronic hemodialysis. Trans. Am. Soc. Artif. Intern. Organs 15: 302–308.

106. Fish, J.C., Remmers, AR., Jr., Lindley, J.D. and Sarles, H.E. (1972) Albumin kinetics and nutritional rehabilitation in the unattended home-dialysis patient. N. Engl. J. Med. 287: 478–481.

107. Kopple, J.D. (1976) Dietary requirements. In *Clinical Aspects of Uremia and Dialysis*, S.G. Massry and A.L. Sellers (eds.) Springfield: Charles C. Thomas Publisher, pp. 453–489.

108. Schaeffer, G., Heinze, V., Jontofsohn, R., Katz, N., Rippich, Th., Schafer, B. and Sudhoff, A. (1975) Amino acid and protein intake in RDT patients. A nutritional and biochemical analysis. Clin. Nephrol. 3: 228–233.

109. Borah, M.F., Schoenfeld, P.Y., Gotch, F.A., Sargent, J.A., Wolfson, M., Humphreys,

MH. (1978) Nitrogen balance during intermittent dialysis therapy of uremia. Kidney Internat. 14: 491–500.

110. Arisi, L., Bacchi, M., Bignardi, L., Bizzi, S., Corradi, A., David, S., Mancuso, S., Riggio, P. and Cambi, V., (1982) Significato e limiti della generazione dell'urea (Gu) nella valutazione dei pazienti in trattamento dialitico cronico. In *Nefrologia, Dialisi, Trapianto*. Milano: Wichtig SRL, pp. 275–278.

111. Abitbol, C.L. and Holliday, M.H. (1978) The effect of energy and nitrogen intake upon urea production in children with uremia and undernutrition. Clinical Nephrology 10: 9–15.

112. Attman, P.O., Bucht, H., Isaksson, B. and Uddebom, G. (1979) Nitrogen balance studies with amino acid supplemented low-protein diet in uremia. Am. J. Clin. Nutr. 32: 1033–2039

113. Abitbol, C., Jean, G. and Broyer, M. (1981) Urea synthesis in moderate experimental uremia. Kidney Internat. 19: 648–653.

114. Kelly, A.R. and Mitch, W.E. (1984) Nutrition. In *The Systemic Consequences of Renal Failure*, G. Eknoyan and JP. Knochel (eds.). New York. Grune & Stratton, pp. 461–500.

115. Hegsted, D.M. (1976) Balance studies. J. Nutr. 106: 307–311.

116. (1981) Composition of foods. In *Geigy Scientific Tables*, Vol. 1, C. Lentner (ed.), Basle: Ciba-Geigy Ltd, pp. 241.

117. WHO Tech., Rep. Ser. 301. (1965) Protein requirements: report of a joint FAO/WHO Expert Group. Geneva, October 8–17, 1963.

118. Mitchell, H.H. and Hamilton, T.S. (1949) The dermal excretion under controlled environmental conditions of nitrogen and minerals in human subjects, with particular reference to calcium and iron. J. Biol. Chem. 178: 345–361.

119. Colloway, D.H., Odell, A.C.F., Margen, S. (1971) Sweat and miscellaneous nitrogen losses in human balance studies. J. Nutr. 101: 775–786.

120. W.H.O. Tech Rep. Ser. 522. (1973) Energy and protein requirement: report of a joint FAO/WHO Ad hoc expert committee.

121. Koralnik, O. and Scholz, H. (1968) Le gradient de l'azote ureique entre le sueur et le plasma. In *Proc. 4th Conf. Europ. Dial. Transpl. Ass.*, D.N.S. Kerr (ed.). Amsterdam: Excepta Medica Foundation.

122. Uavy, R., Schrinshaw, N.S., Rand, W.M. and Young, V.R. (1978) Human protein requirements: obligatory urinary and fecal nitrogen losses and the factorial estimation of protein needs in the elderly males. J. Nutr. 108: 97–103.

123. Krzywanek, Flashentrager. (1957) In *Physiologische Chemie*, Vol. 2, Flashentrager and Lehnartz (Eds.). Berlin: Springer, p. 202.

124. Schrimshaw, N.S., Hussein, M.A., Murray, E., Rand, W.M. and Young, V.R. (1971) Protein requirements of man: variations in obligatory urinary and fecal nitrogen losses in young man. J. Nutr. 102: 1595–1604.

125. Tremolieres, J., Santier, C., Faudemay, F., Flament, C. and Farquet, J (1961) The effect of various fats on the nature and composition of human feces. Nutr. et diete (Basel) 3: 17–39.

126. Pimparker, B.D., Tuloky, E.G., Kalser, M.H. and Bockus, H.L. (1961) Correlation of radioactive and chemical fecal fat determinations in the malabsorption syndrome. I. Studies in normal man and in functional disorders of the gastrointestinal tract. Am. J. Med. 30: 910–926.

127. Peters, J.P. and Van Slyke, D.D. (1946) *Quantitative Clinical Chemistry Interpretations*, Baltimore: Williams & Wilkins, Vol. 1. (2nd ed.). p. 641

128. Wilson, D.R., Ing, T.S., Metcalfe-Gibson, A. and Wrong, O.M. (1968) The chemical composition of faeces in uraemia, as revealed by in vivo faecal dialysis. Clin. Sci. 35: 197–209.

129. Gilbert, R.J. and Goyal, R.K. (1984) The gastrointestinal system. In *The Systemic Consequences of Renal failure*, G., Eknoyan and J.P. Knochel (eds.). New York: Grune & Stratton, pp. 133–175.

130. Rosenblatt, S.G., Drake, S., Fadem, S., Welch, R., Lifschitz, M.D. (1982) Gastrointestinal blood loss in patients with chronic renal failure. Am. J. Kid. Dis. 1: 232–236.

176

131. Hyne, B.E., Fowell, E. and Lee, H.A. (1978) The effect of caloric intake on nitrogen balance in chronic renal failure. Clin. Sci. 43: 679–688.

132. Bergstrom, J., Furst, P. and Norée, L.P. (1975) Treatment of chronic uremic patients with protein-poor diet and oral supply of essential amino acids. I Nitrogen balance studies. Clin. Nephrol. 3: 187–194.

133. Mitch, W.E., Abras, E., Walser, M. (1982) Long-term effects of a new ketoacid amino acid supplement in patients with chronic renal disease. Kidney Internat 22; 48–53.

134. Mitch, W.E. and Walser, M. (1977) Effects of oral neomycin and kanamycin in chronic uremic patients: II. Nitrogen balance. Kidney Internat. 11: 123–127.

135. Mitch, W.E. (1978) Effects of intestinal flora on nitrogen metabolism in patients with chronic renal failure. Am. J. Clin. Nutr. 31: 1594–1600.

136. Mitch, W.E. and Sapir, D.G. (1981) Evaluation of reduced dialysis frequency using nutritional therapy. Kidney Internat. 20: 122–126.

137. Maroni, B.J., Steinman, T.I. and Mitch, W.E. (1985) A method for estimating nitrogen intake of patients with chronic renal failure. Kidney Int. 27: 58–65.

138. Jourdan, M., Margen, S., Bradfield, RB. (1974) Protein-sparing effect in obese women fed low caloric diets. Am. J. Clin. Nutr. 27: 3–12.

139. Bortz, W.M., Howat, P. and Holmes, W.L. (1968) Fat, carbohydrate, salt and weight loss. Further studies. Am. J. Clin. Nutr. 21: 1291–1301.

140. Saito, A., Asada, H., Maeda, K. and Ohta, K. (1980) Urea and nitrogen metabolism in patients treated with haemofiltration. Proc. EDTA 17: 341–346.

141. Young, G.A. and Parsons, F.M. (1966) Amino $N_2$ loss during hemodialysis, its dietary significance an replacement. Clin. Sci. 31: 299–307.

142. Lubash, G.D., Stenzel, K.H., Rubin, A.L. (1964) Nitrogenous compounds in hemodialysate. Circulation 30: 848–852.

143. Rubini, M.E. and Gordon, S. (1968) Individual plasma free amino acids in uremics: effect of hemodialysis. Nephron 5: 339–351.

144. Tepper, T., Van Der Hem, G.K., Tuma, G.J., Arisz, L. and Donker, A.J.M. (1978) Loss of amino acids during hemodialysis: quantitative and qualitative investigations. Clinical Nephrology 10: 16–20.

145. Kopple, J.D., Swendseid, M.E., Shinaberger, J.H. and Umezawa, C.Y. (1973) The free and bound amino acids removed by hemodialysis. Trans. Amer. Soc. Artif. Int. Organs 19, 309–313.

146. Aviram, A., Peters, J.H. and Gulyassy, P.F. (1971) Dialysance of amino acids and related substances. Nephron 8: 440–454.

147. Noree, L.O., Bergstrom, J., Furst, P., Hallgren, B.O. (1971) The effect of essential amino acid administration on nitrogen metabolism during dialysis. Proc. Europ Dial. Transpl. Ass. 8: 182–187.

148. Arisi, L., Rossi, E., Bignardi, L., David, S., Garini, G., Savazzi, G., Cambi, V. and Migone, L. (1979) Analisi del porfilo plasmatico degli amino acidi liberi, delle loro clearances e rimozioni in corso di dialisi brevi. Minerva Nefrologica 26: 49–54.

149. Wolfson, M., Jones, M.R. and Kopple, J.D. (1982) Amino acid losses during hemodialysis with infusion of amino acids and glucose. Kidney Internat. 21: 500–506.

150. Ganda Om, P., Aoki, T.T., Soeldner, J.S., Morrison, R.S. and Cahill, G.F. (1976) Hormone-fuel concentrations in anephric subjects. Effect of hemodialysis (with special reference to amino acids). J. Clin. Invest. 57: 1403–1411.

151. Wathen, R.L., Keshaviah, P., Hommeyer, P., Cadwell, K. and Comty, C.M. (1978) The metabolic effects of hemodialysis with and without glucose in the dialysate. Am. J. Clin. Nutr. 31: 1870–1875.

152. Sigler M.H., Skutches, C.L., Teehan, B.P., Cooper, J.H., Reichard, G.A. (1983) Acetate and energy metabolism during hemodialysis Kidney Internat. 24 (suppl. 16): S-97–S101.

153. Walser, M. (1980) Determinants of ureagenesis, with particular reference to renal failure. Kidney Internat 17: 709–721.

154. Waterlow, J.C. and Alleyne, G.A.D. (1971) Protein malnutrition in children. Advances in

knowledge in the last 10 years. Adv. Protein. Chem. 25: 177–241.

155. Folin, O. (1905) Laws governing the chemical composition of urine. Am. J. Physiol. 13: 67–115.

156. Kopple, J.D. and Cinaciaruso, B. (1984) The role of nutrition in acute renal failure. In *Acute Renal Failure: Pathophysiology, Prevention and Treatment*, V. Andreucci (ed.). Boston: Martinus Nijhoff, pp. 421–446.

157. Steffenson, K.A. (1947) Some determinations of the total body water in man by means of intravenous injections of urea. Acta Physiol Scand. 13: 282–290.

158. San Pietro, A. and Rittenberg, D. (1953) A study of the rate of protein synthesis: I. Measurement of the urea pool and urea space. J. Biol. Chem. 201: 445–473.

159. Bradbury, M.W.B. (1961) Urea and deuterium-oxide spaces in man Br. J. Nutr. 15: 177–182.

160. Scholz, A. (1968) Investigation on distribution and turnover rate of 14-C urea and tritiated water in renal failure In *Proc. 4th Conf. European Dialysis and Transplant Association*, Kerr D.N.S. (ed.). Amsterdam: Excepta Medica Foundation.

161. Walser, M. (1974) Urea metabolism in chronic renal failure J. Clin. Invest. 53: 1385–1392.

162. Oh, O.M., Levison, S.P. and Carroll, H.J. (1975) Content and distribution of water and electrolytes in maintenance hemodialysis. Nephron 14: 421–432.

163. Brennan, B.L., Yasumura, S., Letteri, J.M., Cohn, S.H. (1980) Total body electrolyte composition and distribution of body water in uremia. Kidney Internat. 17: 364–371.

164. Farrell, P.C. and Gotch, F.A., (1977) Dialysis therapy guided by kinetic modelling: applications of a variable volume single pool model for urea kinetics. Second Australasian Conference on Heat and Mass Transfer, The University of Sydney, February, pp. 29–37.

165. Walser, M. and Bodenlos, L.J. (1959) Urea metabolism in man. J. Clin. Invest. 38: 1617–1626.

166. Cottini, E.P., Gallina, D.L. and Dominiquez, J.M. (1973) Urea excretion in adult humans with varying degrees of kidney malfunction fed milk, egg, or an amino acid mixture: assessment of nitrogen balance. J. Nutr. 103: 11–19.

167. Arisi, L., Biasini, A., Bono, F., David, S., Garini, G., Savazzi, G.M., Cambi, V. and Migone, L. (1982) Generazione dell'urea (Gn) nel trattamento dialitico. Confronto fra due metodi. Minerva Nefrologica 29: 37–42.

168. Gotch, F.A., Borah, M.F., Keen, M., Sargent, J., Ayns, C. and Hunphreys, M.H. (1977) The solute kinetics of intermittent dialysis therapy. Proc. Ann. Contractors Conf. Artif. Kidney Program NIAMDD 10: 105–107b.

169. Sargent, J., Gotch, F., Borah, M., Piercy, L., Spinozzi, N., Schoenfeld, P. and Humphreys, M. (1978) Urea kinetics: a guide to nutritional management of renal failure. Am. J. Clin. Nutr. 31: 1696–1702.

170. Farrell, P.C. and Hone, P.W. (1980) Dialysis induced catabolism. Am. J. Clin. Nutr. 33: 1417–1422.

171. Sargent, J.A., Gotch, F.A., Henry, R.R. and Bennett, N. (1979) Mass balance: a quantitative guide to clinical nutritional therapy II the dialyzed patient. J. Amer. Dietetic Ass. 75: 551–555.

172. Wineman, R.J., Sargent, J.A. and Piercy, L. (1977) Nutritional implications of renal disease. J. Amer. Dietetic Ass. 70: 483–487.

173. Bell, R.L., Curtis, F.K. and Babb, A.L. (1965) Analog simulation of the patient artificial kidney system. Trans. Am. Soc. Artif. Intern. Organs 11: 183–188.

174. Rastogi, S.P., Frost, T., Anderson, J., Ashcroft, R. and Kerr, D.N.S. (1968) The significance of disequilibrium between body conpartments in the treatment of chronic renal failure. Proc. Europ. Dial. Transplant. Assoc. 5: 102–115.

175. Abbrecht, P.H. and Prodany, N.W. (1971) A model of patient-artificial kidney system. IEEE Trans. Biomed Eng. 18: 257–264.

176. Schindhelm, K. and Farrell, P.C. (1978) Patient-hemodialyzer interactions. Trans. Am. Soc. Artif. Intern. Organs 24: 357–365.

178

177. Popovich, R.P., Hlavinca, D.J., Bomar, J.B., Moncrief, J.W. and Decherd, J.F. (1975) The consequences of physiological resistence on metabolite removal from the patients-artificial kidney system. Trans. Am. Soc. Artif. Intern. Organs. 21: 108–115.

178. Haas, T., Dongradi, G., Willeboeuf, F., de Viel, E., Fournier, J.F. and Duruy, D. (1983) Plasma kinetics of small molecules during and after hemofiltration: decrease in hemofiltration efficiency related to increase in ultrafiltration rate. Clinical Nephrology 19: 193–200.

179. Kennedy, A.C., Linton, A.L., Eaton, J.C. (1962) Urea levels in cerebrospinal fluid after haemodialysis. Lancet 1: 410–411.

180. Lawrie, E. and Sargent, J. (1980) Clinical example of pharmacokinetic and metabolic modeling: quantitative and individualized prescription of dialysis therapy. Kidney Internat. 18 (suppl 10): S-11–S-16.

181. Ward, R.A., Shirlow, M.J., Hayes, J.M., Chapman, C.V. and Farrell, P.C. (1979) Protein catabolism during hemodialysis. Am. J. Clin. Nutr. 32: 2443–2449.

182. Gotch, F.A., Sargent, J.A., Keen, H.L., Lam, M., Prowitt, M.M., Grady, M., Schoenfeld, P., Borah, M., Wolfson, M., Humphreys, M. and Leddy, E. (1976) Solute kinetics in intermittent dialysis therapy. Proc. Am. Contractors Conf. Artif. Kidney Program. NIAMDD 9: 98–101.

183. Conley, S.B., Rose, G.M., Robson, A.M. and Bier, D.M. (1980) Effects of dietary intake and hemo-dialysis on protein turnover in uremic children. Kidney Internat. 17: 837–846.

184. Alfred, H., Kirkwood, G., Kunitomo, I., Williams, G., Emanuel, R. and Lowrie, E. (1979) Acute hormone changes with conventional (CD) and high flux dialysis (HFD).

185. Raforth, R.J. and Onstad, G.R. (1975) Urea synthesis after oral protein loading in man. J. Clin. Invest. 56, 1170–1174.

186. Drew, P.J.T., Monson, J.P., Metcalfe, H.K., Evans, S.J.W., Iles, R.A., Cohen, R.d. (1985) The effect of arginine vasopression on urea genesis in isolated rat hepatocytes. Clin. Sci. 69: 231–233.

187. Iitake, K., Kimura, I., Matsui, K., Ota, K., Shoji, M., Inove, M., Yoshinaga, K. (1985) Effect of haemodialysis on plasma ADH levels, plasma renin activity and plasma aldosterone levels in patients with end-stage renal disease. Acta Endocrinol 110: 207–213.

188. Horl, W.H., Heidland, A. (1984) Evidence for the partecipation of granulocyte proteinases on intradialytic catabolism. Clin. Nephrol. 21: 314–322.

189. Clowes, G.H.A., Jr., George, B.C., Villee, C.A., Jr., Saravis, C.A. (1983) Muscle proteolysis induced by circulating peptide in patients with sepsis or trauma. N. Engl. J. Med. 308: 545–552.

190. Baracos, V., Rodemann, H.P., Dinarello, C.A., Goldberg, A.L. (1983) Stimulation of muscle protein degradation and prostaglandin $E_2$ release by leukocytic pyrogen (interlekin-1) A mechanism for the increased degradation of muscle proteins during fever. N. Engl. J. Med. 308: 553–558.

191. Schaldon, S., Deschodt, G., Branger, B., Granolleras, C., Baldamus, C.A., Koch, K.M., Lysaght, M.J. and Dinarello, C.A. (1985) Haemodialysis hypotension: the interleukin hypothesis restated Proc. EDTA-ERA, vol. 22: 229–243.

192. Askanazy, J., Furst, P., Michelsen, C., Elwin, D.H., Vinnairs, E., Gump, F.E., Stinchfield, M.D. and Kinney, J.M. (1980) Muscle and plasma amino acids after injury. Hypocaloric glucose vs amino acid infusion. Ann. Surg. 191: 465–472.

193. Feinstein, E.I., Blumenkrantz, M.J., Healy H., Koffler, A., Silberman, H., Massry, S.G. and Kopple, J.D. (1981) Clinical and metabolic responses to parenteral nutrition in acute renal failure. A controlled double blind study. Medicine 60: 124–137.

194. Salusky, I.B., Flugel-Link, R.M., Jones, M.R., Kopple, J.D. (1983) Effect of acute uremia on protein degradation and amino acid release in the rat hemicorpus. Kidney Internat. 24 (suppl. 16): S-43–S-47.

195. Lacy, W.W. (1969) Effect of acute uremia on amino acid uptake and urea production by perfused rat liver. Am. J. Physiol. 216: 1300–1305.

196. Frohlich, J. Scholmerich, J., Hoppe-Seyler, G., Maier, KP., Talke, H., Schollmeyer, P.

and Gerok, W. (1974) The effect of acute uremia on gluconeogenesis in isolated perfused rat liver. Eur. J. Clin. Invest. 4: 453–458.

197. Chapman, G.V., Mahony, J.F., Farrell, P.C., (1980) A crossover study of short time dialysis. Clin. Nephrol. 13: 78–84.

# 7. Nutrition in dialysis patients

Giuseppe Maschio and Giovanni Panzetta

In patients on regular hemodialysis treatment (RDT) the daily intake of fluids and solutes is critical in modulating the production of uremic toxins and the homeostasis of water, electrolytes, and minerals, with resultant effects on the clinical conditions, including hydration, nutrition, and function of several organs.

Regardless of the relative importance of low and/or higher molecular weight solutes in the pathogenesis of the uremic syndrome, a proper dietary prescription may keep relatively symptomless most patients with advanced renal failure. For instance, dietary protein restriction reduces nitrogen production and load, improves acid-base balance by reducing metabolic hydrogen ions generation, and retards the progression of osteodystrophy by avoiding hyperphosphatemia.

From a theoretical point of view, dialysis patients might be periodically treated in such a way to overcome any dietary excess. Actually, this is not easily performed if relatively short and well-tolerated dialysis sessions are to be planned in these patients. Adequate dietary restrictions must be prescribed if a dialysis schedule of 4 hours 3 times a week is to be performed with few side effects. With no dietary control, patients on this schedule will present unacceptably high BUN levels, acid-base imbalance, hyperkalemia, poor control of body fluids, and hyperphosphatemia with progressive worsening of osteodystrophy.

In addition, the basic rules of dietary management in dialysis patients should be individually tailored according to the various clinical settings that may be observed in these patients.

## Clinical setting of patients on RDT

### Adaption to dialysis

During the first months of treatment patients are expected to change their dietary regimen, especially by increasing protein and reducing fluid intakes. A sizable percentage of patients may experience dialysis-related symptoms,

*Vincenzo Cambi (editor) Professor of Nephrology*
© *1987 Martinus Nijhoff Publishing, Boston. ISBN 0-89838-858-9. Printed in The United States.*

such as nausea and vomiting, which may limit food ingestion. Infectious diseases, febrile illnesses, and catabolic stresses, which are frequently observed in this phase, may induce negative caloric and protein balances. In addition, aminoacid losses in the dialysate add further to the negativity of nitrogen balance. As a consequence, malnutrition may still be observed up to 18 months after starting RDT [1].

This adaptation phase is critical in determining the long-term clinical status, or even the survival probability of dialysis patients [2]. On the other hand, this phase is also influenced by the clinical conditions prior to dialysis [2, 3]. In our experience, too, those patients who start RDT after uncontrolled dietary intakes do have the most severe clinical and biochemical evidence of osteodystrophy, anemia, and malnutrition. During the adaptation phase these patients experience an uncommonly high frequency of infections, cardiac failure, peripheral neuropathy, and sometimes progression of protein-energy malnutrition.

A careful evaluation of dietary habits and nutritional and clinical parameters should be made in all patients at the start of RDT.

Dietary intakes should be regularly checked by means of interviews and written diaries. The net protein catabolic rate (PCR), evaluated from the net rate of urea nitrogen generation, is a good index of nitrogen balance [4] and can be used to estimate dietary protein intake, provided that it is obtained in 'stable' patients. In patients whose clinical conditions suggest nitrogen imbalance, the simultaneous determination of PCR and dietary nitrogen intake provides an estimation of the degree of nitrogen imbalance.

*Intercurrent catabolic episodes*

As previously noted, several superimposed illnesses may induce metabolic abnormalities in dialysis patients. A reduced caloric and protein intake is to be expected in many serious conditions such as systemic infections, GItract bleeding, pericarditis, or major surgery. In some other less dramatic, circumstances, however, minor reductions in caloric and protein intakes, if prolonged, may be followed by a subtle degree of malnutrition. In addition, an inadequate dialysis therapy may contribute to anorexia and limit food consumption.

In all these situations a correct nutritional evaluation is of great importance and should be done.

*The steady state phase of dialysis patients*

Several biochemical abnormalities are observed in dialysis patients, which at the same time may affect nutritional status and result from malnutrition.

Plasma amino acid pattern may be similar to that described in calorie-protein malnutrition [3, 5, 6]; it improves after nutritional supplementation, though not completely [7]. The amino acid imbalance probably results from predialysis protein depletion, inadequate protein intake, altered amino acid uptake and release by the kidney, and endocrine abnormalities found in uremia. Whatever its cause, the amino acid imbalance is usually more evident in patients with malnutrition, and a close relationship exists between plasma amino acid concentrations, plasma proteins, and body composition [3].

The carbohydrate intolerance is well known in uremic patients and is associated with peripheral resistance to insulin [8]. Interestingly the impaired glucose metabolism has been attributed, at least in part, to a disorder in the tricarboxylic acid cycle function, due to an excess of amino acids, which undergo massive transamination with TCA cycle intermedia [9]. On the other hand, glucose production has been found increased in liver, due to stimulated neoglucogenesis from amino acids such as valine [10]. Apparently, then, the abnormality in carbohydrate metabolism could be linked to that of amino acids, even though the interrelationship between these substances in the liver is still controversial [11, 12].

Alterations in lipid metabolism include high serum triglyceride levels, due to an increase of very low-density lipoproteins (VDDL), intermediate-density lipoproteins (ILP), and low-density lipoproteins (LDL) [13, 14]. Normal serum cholesterol levels may be observed, though its content in high-density lipoproteins is reduced [15].

These abnormalities may be due both to increased synthesis and, more likely, to a reduced catabolism of lipoproteins [16, 18]. A prominent role in determining hyperlipidemia can be probably attributed to some endocrine disturbances found in uremia, such as thyroid dysfunction, insulin resistance, glucagon hypersensitivity, and hyperparathyroidism. Among these, secondary hyperparathyroidism seems worthful.

This hormone not only affects calcium metabolism and bone morphology, but also affects lipid metabolism by increasing plasma levels and reducing the catabolism of triglycerides [19, 20]. In addition, PTH stimulates protein catabolism in muscle tissue and neoglucogenesis in liver [21], and impairs insulin secretion and peripheral glucose utilization [22]. It is of interest that both biochemical suppression and surgical removal of hyperparathyroidism are followed by significant improvement in insulin resistance and glucose metabolism [22] and by correction of hyperlipidemia [20].

The clinical importance of metabolic abnormalities in dialysis patients and their relationship to nutritional status and survival are not fully elucidated. No definite relationship between metabolic abnormalities and cardiovascular risk has also been established [23].

An adequate alimentation in well-dialyzed patients seems to allow good nutritional status and survival for a long time.

Dialysis has been regarded as an intermittent catabolic stress [24], and it has been suggested that essential aminoacid and protein supply should be higher than normal in these patients. However, the estimated nitrogen requirement for balance was only 2.0 g/day in a group of undialyzed uremic patients fed by continuous nasogastric infusion with a caloric intake of 34 kcal/kg [25], and the biochemical consequences of prolonged fasting are not different in dialysis patients and in controls [26]. These observations seem to suggest that the metabolic requirements of dialysis patients may not be too different from normals.

It should be stressed, however, that this conclusion only applies to stable patients treated with adequate dialysis. When factors such as episodic illnesses, inadequate dialysis, or insufficient dietary intake supervene, then the costellation of metabolic and endocrine disorders may play an important role in promoting malnutrition. The consequences may persist for long time and should be adequately prevented or treated.


**Caloric intake**

Dialysis patients may display several alterations of body composition [1, 27] including losses of body fat and muscle tissue, and body weight is lower in these patients than in controls, matched for age and sex.

Whether these abnormalities result from uremia or from a reduced caloric and protein intake is still matter of discussion, as well as the optimum energy intake to keep a neutral nitrogen balance.

Several studies have shown that there is a close relationship between caloric intake and nitrogen balance both in patients on dietary treatment [28] and in those on RDT [4].

Dialysis patients tend to underestimate food intake [27], and hence dietary interviews may not be completely true.

Therefore, patients should be carefully instructed on how to collect dietary information, and written diaries should be obtained periodically.

In a previous study we observed a close relationship between energy intake and body weight with respect to ideal parameters [29] (figure 7–1). Most patients had adequate values of both parameters, but a substantial percentage of them were either undernourished or overnourished, due to inappropriately low or high caloric intakes. An energy intake of about 35 kcal/kg b.w. seems to be critical in maintaining an ideal body weight, in keeping with other reports [30, 31].


**Protein intake**

It is now accepted that a protein intake of about 0.6 g/kg b.w. is adequate to maintain a nitrogen balance in patients with chronic renal failure [32, 33]. Patients on RDT are usually prescribed 1.0 to 1.2 g/kg b.w. [30, 31] of protein, provided that an adequate caloric intake is also given. However, others have suggested a wider range of protein intakes (1.1 + 0.3 g/kg b.w.) [27].

Two different goals should be achieved in dialysis patients: (1) to provide a

184

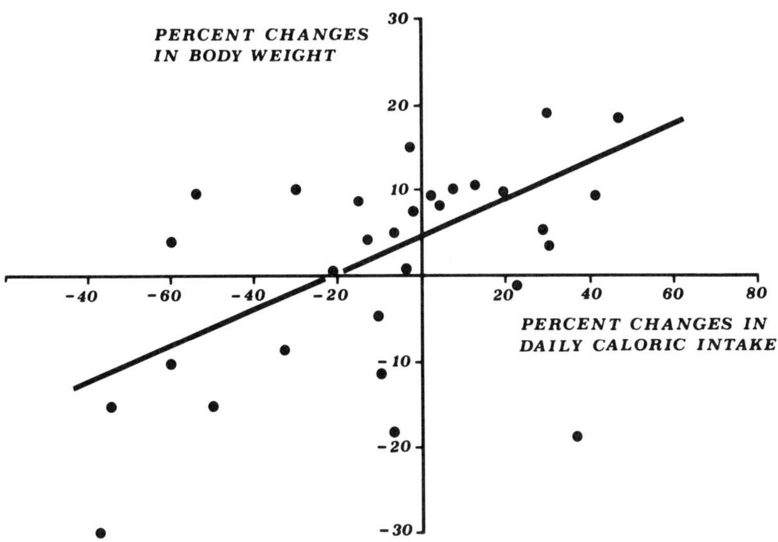


*Figure 7–1.* The relationship between percent changes in daily caloric intake and body weight. The 0 point represents the correspondence between the observed and the predicted parameters. Percent changes are indicated by numbers. Patients ingesting 35 kcal/kg bw had body weight close to the ideal one.

protein intake sufficient to keep a nitrogen balance; (2) to avoid a nitrogen overload due to excessive protein ingestion.

The nitrogen intake may become inadequate for several reasons: protein losses due to blood rest in filters and routine analysis, amino acid losses (up to 8 g each 5 hours dialysis) in the dialysate, urinary protein losses in patients with residual diuresis and proteinuria. Moreover, as previously noted, some patients may develop anorexia as a side effect of dialysis treatment or as a consequence of intercurrent illnesses. Under these circumstances a negative nitrogen balance may occur.

An excessive nitrogen intake, on the other hand, increases the generation of nitrogen-containing waste products, which are responsible for the uremic syndrome [34, 35]. Evidence has been obtained that high levels of BUN are associated with increased need for hospitalization and high mortality rate in dialysis patients [36]. High BUN levels have been obtained by modulating the time of dialysis and the clearances of dialyzers in patients kept on constant protein intake ranging from 0.8 to 1.4 g/kg b.w. [37]. The effects of increased BUN levels due to excessive protein intake on patients kept on constant dialysis therapy is still unknown.

In our population of patients dialyzed 4 hours 3 times a week, a close relationship exists between predialysis midweek BUN levels and protein catabolic rate obtained by direct determination of urea nitrogen in dialysate (figure 7–2). The statistical analysis showed that a BUN level of 80 mg/dl (the

185

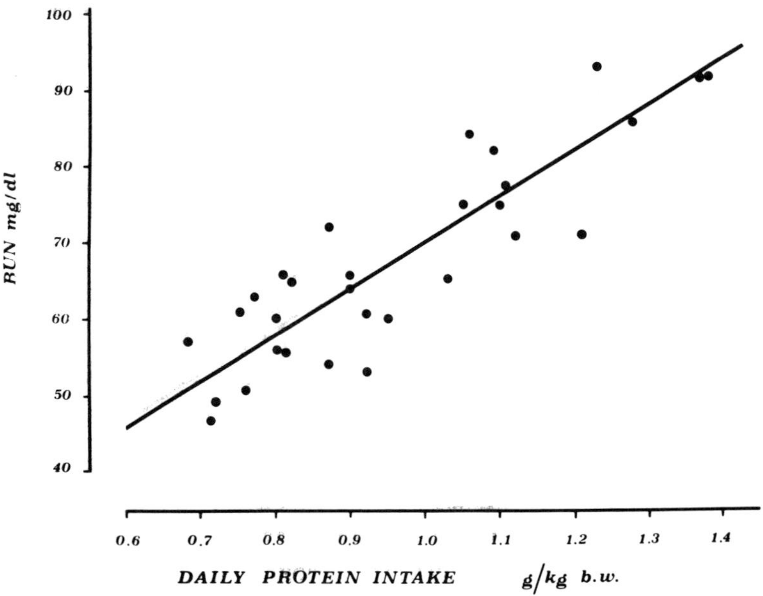


*Figure 7–2.* A close relationship exists between daily protein intake (derived from net protein catabolic rate) and predialysis midweek BUN in 30 patients on RDT. r = 0.878 p<0.001; y = 12.04 + 57.74 ×.

upper safe limit according to the National Cooperative Study) corresponds to a daily protein intake of 1.17 g/kg b.w.

These results may not apply to all dialysis patients, but are expecially suitable to patients like ours dialyzed 4 hours 3 times a week with a mean in vitro urea clearance of 190 ml/min.

Moreover, they show that with this modality of treatment protein intake must be carefully checked if the critical levels of BUN 80 mg/dl are not to be overcome. The BUN value is affected by the dietary proteins and also by the efficiency of dialysis therapy. Thus, BUN values may not represent the ideal index of protein intake in dialysis patients. The BUN-to-creatinine ratio could better reflect dietary protein intake, as shown in patients with chronic renal failure on dietary and dialysis treatment [38]. A disproportionate increase in the BUN concentration as compared to the serum creatinine value should indicate an excess in the quantity of dietary protein intake.

In dialysis patients this ratio has been found lower than in nondialyzed uremic patients at the same degree of protein intake [38], due to more efficient removal of urea with respect to creatinine.

In our patients the BUN-to-creatinine ratio is directly related to protein intake obtained from PCR. Values ranging from 6 and 7.5 mg/dl indicate protein intakes ranging from 0.8 to 1.2 g/kg b.w. (figure 7–3).

However, in keeping with Kopple and Coburn [38], our data show that the best relationship is that relating daily protein intake to blood urea nitrogen.

186

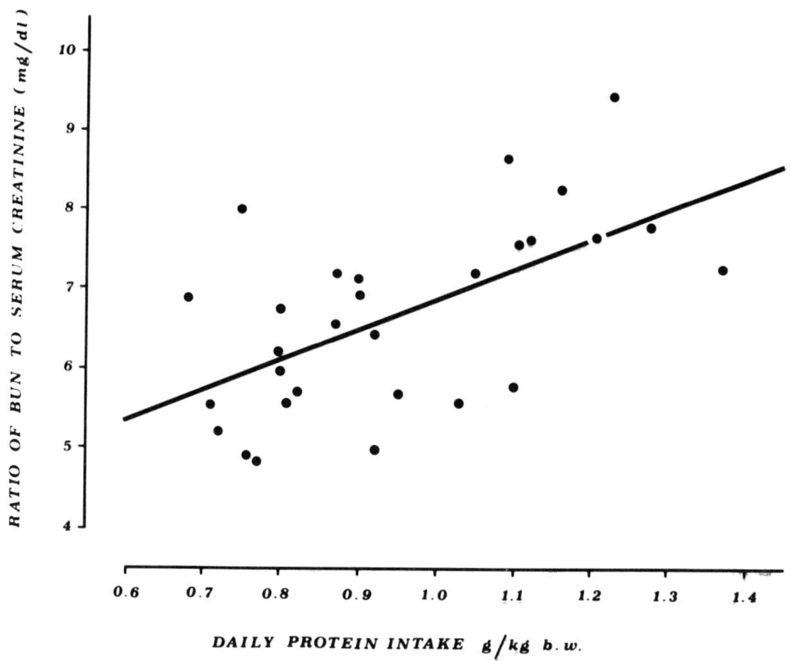


*Figure 7–3.* A direct relationship between daily protein intake and the BUN: serum creatinine is shown. r = 0.577 p<0.001; y = 3.13 + 3.74 ×.


## Carbohydrate and lipid intakes

Although abnormalities of carbohydrate and lipid metabolism are well known in patients with chronic renal failure, there is no clearcut evidence that these may result from inadequate dietary intakes. Diet composition in uremic patients may be excessively high in carbohydrates and lipids, with relatively low amounts of protein. Excessive ingestion of monomere carbohydrates and saturated lipids might play a role in the pathogenesis of hyperlipemia. Abnormal proportions of dietary intakes of saturated and polyunsaturated fatty acids may be responsible for the increment of oleic acid as compared to linoleic acid in cholesterol esters, phospholipids, and triglycerides of some uremic patients. [39].

Elevated insulin levels may result in increased synthesis of triglycerides [40] although a relationship between insulin secretion and serum triglycerides has not been regularly observed [41].

In a previous study we found no relationship between serum lipids and total amount of calories, calories supplied by carbohydrates and lipids, and dietary intake of satured fatty acids [42]. Similar results have been reported by Pierides and associates [43]. Our data showed that mean plasma levels of

187

triglycerides were higher in patients having a body weight higher than the ideal value, although the difference was not satistically significant, due to scattered distribution of values. In male patients a positive correlation was found between the percentage of body fat/body weight and serum triglycerides.

These data, in addition to those concerning the correlation between triglycerides and the observed/ideal body weight ratio [44], indicate that overweight affects serum lipids in dialysis patients, as well as in normal population [45].

It should be stressed, however, that patients with normal body fat may have elevated serum triglycerides. As a possible implication, only the reduction of fat body mass below the normal range should normalize serum triglycerides.

Conflicting views exist concerning the possibility of changing serum lipids through changes in diet composition. Yet, Sanfelippo and associates [46] have obtained a significant reduction in serum triglyceride turnover rate and serum triglyceride levels by 15% lowering of carbohydrate intake in dialysis patients. Similar results on serum lipids have been obtained by Gokal and coworkers [47] and Cottran and associates [48] by increasing the polyunsaturated to saturated fatty acid ratio. On the contrary, Wass and colleagues [49] were not able to observe significant changes in serum lipids of dialysis patients with a 43% of caloric intake been supplied by lipids and with an increased polyunsaturated to saturated fatty acid ratio.

Despite these apparently conflicting results, and considering that the carbohydrate and lipid composition of the diet affects serum lipid levels in normal subjects [50–53], the dietary content of carbohydrate and lipids should be controlled in dialysis patients.

The ideal diet to prevent or to correct hyperlipidemia is unknown at the moment. As general rule, a correct diet for dialysis patients should contain carbohydrates as 45–50% of total calories, with strict limitation of monomere carbohydrates. The lipid intake should represent the 35–40% of total calories, and the polyunsaturated to saturated fatty acid ratio should be about 0.8.


**Relationship between protein intake and acid-base balance**

The catabolism of ingested protein results in generation of metabolic hydrogen ions, due to $SO_4$ ion production by neutral amino acids (cysteine and methionine) and hydrochloric acid production by cationic amino acids (lysine and argynine).

The net $H^+$ production in normal subjects on free diet ranges from 20 to 120 mEq/24 hours, and this acid load is completely excreted through the kidney [54]. In patients with chronic renal failure, despite the respiratory mechanism of compensation, a reduction in plasma bicarbonate and blood pH is usually observed. Some evidence has been obtained that the bone buffers participate in the neutralization of dietary-related $H^+$ production in chronic renal failure. In fact, experimental chronic renal acidosis is associated with a significant loss of both mineral and organic components of bone tissue [55, 56]. In our dialysis patients we have observed no relationship between $H^+$ production, indirectly assumed from PCR, and acid-base status of the blood. Yet in dialysis patients the acid-base balance is regulated by several factors, including the amount of dietary-related production of acids, buffer capacity of extracellular fluids, buffer capacity of intracellular compartment (bone, muscle cells), amount of buffer supplied by the dialysate, and amount of bicarbonate and other anions lost during dialysis.

In our experience, the higher serum PTH levels, the higher the acetate concentration in dialysate must be in order to keep blood pH within normal limits [57]. Moreover, the administration of vitamin D is usually followed by an increase in blood pH without any further increment in acetate concentration in the dialysate. These observations can be interpreted as indirect evidence of the involvment of bone tissue metabolism in buffering acidosis in dialysis patients. Hyperparathyroidism seems to reduce this capacity, and vitamin D supplementation seems to improve it.


**Relationship between dietary protein and calcium and phosphate metabolism**

The dietary intake of protein and phosphate are directly and mutually correlated, 100/g of protein containing 1,000–1,500/mg of phosphate.

Dietary phosphate plays an important role in the pathogenesis of uremic osteodystrophy [58]. Therefore, dietary phosphate intake should be carefully monitored in dialysis patients in order to prevent the development of hyperphosphatemia and minimize the amount of aluminum containing antiacids.

Our experience shows that a controlled dietary phosphate intake, associated with an adequate removal of phosphate during dialysis, is very important in maintaining normal serum phosphate levels.

The average removal of phosphate during a single dialysis is 1,000 mg [59]. In our patients, the mean phosphate loss measured in the dialysate was 730/mg per session, equivalent to a daily removal of 312/mg. Since nearly 70% of dietary phosphate is absorbed, 450/mg of phosphate intake is the critical value above which positive balance may ensue. This dietary phosphate content is invariable associated with a protein content that is too low to make the diet palatable to patients. Therefore, most dialysis patients must be prescribed phosphate binders. The aluminium-containing binders may be very effective in reducing phosphate absorption, but the long-term administration may be followed by side effects, such as constipation and bone and brain disturbances [60–61].

Therefore, dietary phosphate and protein intakes should be carefully prescribed and controlled in dialysis patients in order to avoid the metabolic consequences of hyperphosphatemia.

This dietary manipulation should also include calcium supplements, taking into account that dialysis patients are still in negative calcium balance, which may not be completely corrected by the calcium assumed from the dialysate. Our previous study showed that the calcium transfer during a 4-hours dialysis ranges from 338 to 893/mg (mean 600 ± 191/mg) [62]. However, this amount must be curtailed by the calcium lost with ultrafiltration. The net calcium uptake, therefore, is much lower, and oral calcium supplements are required.

Calcium supplements have been shown to increase plasma calcium with a consequent reduction in serum PTH [63, 64].

When calcium supplements are given, serum phosphate levels must be maintained within normal limits, since a $Ca \times Pi$ product above 55 may be associated with an increased incidence of soft tissue calcification [65]. Even more carefully should phosphate intake be checked when vitamin D metabolites, which are known to increase intestinal absorption of both calcium and phosphate, are administered to dialysis patients.


**Potassium intake**

Although an adequate urinary potassium excretion can be maintained in advanced renal failure, with the start of dialysis treatment the inability of the kidney to eliminate potassium may lead to an overall increase in body potassium stores.

Fecal potassium output increases when creatinine clearance drops below 5 ml/min [66], but its contribution to potassium balance is of minor significance.

Dietary restrictions and low potassium concentrations in dialysis fluid are required in order to maintain potassium homeostasis.

Isotopic determination of exchangeable [67, 68] and total body potassium [69], however, have demonstrated normal or reduced potassium pool in patients dialyzed against a dialyzate with low potassium content. Similar results have been obtained with muscle tissue analysis [70]. On the contrary, plasma potassium concentrations are generally higher than normal, when measured before the dialysis session. These data seem to suggest that the cell capacity for potassium is reduced in uremic patients. Accordingly, a low tolerance to potassium administration has been demonstrated both in patients with renal failure [71] and in animal models [77].

Among the factors responsible for hyperkalemia and decreased cellular potassium stores, acidosis must be taken into account because its practical importance in dialysis patients. Acidosis results in a redistribution of potassium across cell membranes, every 0.1 U change in extracellular pH inducing an inverse 0.6 mEq/l change in serum potassium concentration [66].

Therefore, if hyperkalemia in acidotic patients is corrected through a dialysis fluid with a low potassium content, a true potassium deficiency may be induced. These patients may be erroneously recommended to limit dietary potassium intake, by reducing the ingestion of vegetables and fruit, with negative effects on the palatability of the diet and vitamin introduction.

As general rule, however, dialysis patients must limit potassium ingestion at about 60–80 mEq/day, because the risk of potassium intoxication.

The consequence of hyperkalemia on the electrophysiology of the heart are too well known to be discussed. Cardiac arrhythmias due to the acute variation in plasma potassium concentration during dialysis represent an additional complication in the maintenance of potassium balance [73]. It has been shown that the use of a dialysate potassium concentration higher than 1.5 mEq/l can reduce the incidence of cardiac arrythmias in susceptible patients [74]. This useful measure, however, may lead to hyperkalemia if patients cannot properly regulate their potassium intake. Generally this can be quite easily made by avoiding unnecessary foods rich in potassium, such as cocoa and nuts, and by limiting some vegetables and fruits. Milk, which contains potassium in the amount of 142 mg/100 ml, may be a neglected source of potassium. Patients must be provided with a list of potassium-rich foods.


**Vitamins**

Vitamin supplementation is a widely accepted measure in dialysis patients. Water-soluble vitamins are lost into the dialysis fluid, although many of the B group vitamins are bound to blood proteins. Low plasma levels of several water-soluble vitamins have been shown in dialysis patients [75]. Vitamin $B_{12}$ stores seem to be adequate [76], while folic acid deficiency has been reported [76, 77], although not invariably [78]. Both these vitamins are dialysable.

Vitamins A, D, and K are not lost with dialysis. With the exception of active vitamin D metabolites, these vitamins are not prescribed to dialysis patients. Moreover, vitamin A supplementation may be followed by toxic effects [79].

Beyond vitamin losses with dialysis, the poor dietary intake constitutes an additional reason for prescribing vitamin supplements to dialysis patients. Small doses of vitamins are generally suggested, the recommended dose of folic acid being 1 mg after each dialysis [77] in order to avoid possible toxic symptoms [78].

We regularly prescribe vitamins in patients ingesting a poor diet, and only periodically in well-nourished patients.


**Practical suggestions**

Table 7–1 summarizes the basic recommendations for a correct dietary composition in dialysis patients.

*Table 7–1.* Recommended dietary intakes for dialysis patients

| | |
|---|---|
| Calories | : 30–35 kcal/kg of ideal body weight |
| Proteins | : 1–1.2 g/kg bw, most of them of high biological value |
| Carbohydrates | : 45–50% of total caloric intake, monomere carbohydrates must be limited. |
| Lipids | : 35–40% of total caloric intake; polyunsaturated to saturated fatty acid ratio should about 1.0 |
| Phosphate | : not higher than 900–1,200 mg |
| Calcium | : supplements are required to increase total intake up to 1,500 mg |
| Potassium | : 60–80 mEq. |

During the catabolic phases, which may occur as a consequence of febrile illnesses, systemic infections, and many other complications with inadequate food consumption, the caloric and nitrogen intakes should be increased to meet the increased needs of the patients. The administration of essential synthetic amino acids intravenously has proved to be useful when performed together with hypertonic glucose during dialysis [80]. When this procedure is not sufficient to ameliorate nitrogen balance, a role for total parenteral nutrition may be advocated. We sometimes administer lipids as 30% of total calories and regularly add amino acids 0.8 g/kg b.w. The amount of insulin should be carefully determined in each patient to avoid hyperglycemia or hypoglycemia. When lipid are used, and glucose content is limited, insulin may be omitted. Phosphate should be added (20–30 mg/kg b.w.) if hypophosphatemia develops due to increased cell uptake of phosphate.

Enteral nutrition by nasogastric infusion is not usually performed in catabolic dialysis patients, but since it has been shown to result in highly efficient utilization of nitrogen [25], this procedure might also be considered.

Needless to say that these nutritional indications must be accompanied by adequate dialysis, effective treatment of infections and other complications, and attempt to correct anemia, if present.


## Acknowledgments

The authors wish to express their appreciation to Mrs. Teresa Zamboni for her secretarial assistance.


## References

1. Thunberg, B.J., Swamy, A.P. and Cestero, R.V.H.: Crossectional and longitudinal nutritional measurements in maintenance hemodialysis patients. Am. J. Clin. Nutr.34: 2005–2012. (1981)
2. Kluthe, R., Luttgen, F.N., Heinze, V. and Findeisen, M. (1979) Predialysis strategy and long term prognosis of RDT-patients. Proc. 2nd Prague Symposium on Renal Failure. Lund, Sweden. Gambro Publ.
3. Young, G.A., Swanepoel, C.R. Croft, M.R., Hobson, S.M. and Parsons, F.M. (1982)

Anthropometry and plasma valine, amino acids, and proteins in the nutritional assessment of hemodialysis patients. Kidney Int. 21: 492–49.

4. Sargent, J., Gotch, F., Borah, M., Percy, L., Spinozzi, N., Schoenfeld, P. and Humphreys, M (1978). Urea kinetics: a guide to nutritional management of renal failure Am. J. Clin. Nutr. 31: 1696–1702.

5. Peters, J.H., Gulyassy, P.F. and Lin, C. (1968) Amino acid patterns in uremia: comparative effects of hemodialysis and transplanation. Trans. Am. Soc. Artif. Intern. Organs 14: 405–410.

6. Kopple, J.D., Jones, M. Fukuda, S. and Swendseid, M.E. (1978) Amino acid and protein metabolism in renal failure. Am. J. Clin. Nutr. 31: 1532–1540.

7. Kleinknecht, C., Salusky, I., Broyer, M. and Bubler, M.C. (1979) Effect of varius protein diets on growth, renal function and survival of uremic rats. Kidney Int. 15: 534–541.

8. De Fronzo, R.A., Andres, R., Edgar, P. and Walker, W.G. (1978) Carbohydrate metabolism in uremia: a review. Medicine (Baltimore) 52: 469–480.

9. Campanacci, L., Guarnieri, G.F., Siliprandi, N. and Fiaschi E. (1968) Metabolic studies of acetoacetate, pyruvate, lactate and citrate in uremic acidosis. Clin. Chim. Acta 20: 341–347.

10. Rubenfeld, S. and Garber, A.J. (1978) Abnormal carbohydrate metabolism in chronic renal failure. J. Clin. Invest. 62: 20–27.

11. De Fronzo, R.A., Alvestrand, A., Smith, D., Hendler, R., Hendler, E., Wahren, J. (1981). Insulin resistance in uremia. J. Clin. Invest. 67: 563–568.

12. Robaudo, C., Deferrari, G., Garibotto, G., Canepa, A., Salvidio, G., Gurreri, G. and Tizianello, A. (1982) L'intolleranza glucidica nell'insufficienza renale cronica dipende da una aumentata produzione epatica di glucosio? Nefrologia, Dialisi e Trapianto: 239–242.

13. Daubresse, J.C., Lerson, G., Plomteux, G., Rorive, G., Luyckx, A.S., Lefebvre, P.J. (1976). Lipids and lipoproteins in chronic uremia: a study of the influence of regular hemodialysis. Eur. J. Clin. Invest. 6: 159–166.

14. Nestel, P.J., Fidge, N.H. and Tan, N.H. (1982) Increased lipoprotein-remnan formation in chronic renal failure. N. Engl. J. Med. 307: 329–333.

15. Chan, M.K., Varghese, Z., Persaud, J.M., Baillod, R.A. and Moorhead, J.F. (1982) Hyperlipidemia in patients on maintenance hemo-and peritoneal dialysis: The relative pathogenetic roles of triglyceride production and triglyceride removal. Clin. Nephrol. 17: 183–190.

16. Ibels, L.S., Reardon, M.F. and Nestel, P.J. (1976) Plasma post-heparin lipolytic activity and triglyceride clearance in uremic and hemodialysis patients and renal allograft recipients. J. Lab. Clin. Med. 87: 648–658.

17. Chan, M.K., Varghese, Z., Persaud, J.W., Baillod, R.A. and Moorhead, J.F. (1980) HDL cholesterol and intravenous fat tolerance in dialysis patients. Proc. EDTA 17: 247–252.

18. Cattran, D.C., Fenton, S.S.A., Wilson, D.R. and Steiner, G. (1976) Defective triglyceride removal in lipemia associated with peritoneal dialysis and hemodialysis. Ann. Intern. Med. 85: 29–33.

19. Lacour, B, Basile, C., Drueke, T, Funck-Brentano, J.L. (1982). Parathyroid function and lipid metabolism in the rat. Mineral Electrolyte Metab. 7: 157–165.

20. Drueke, T., Lacour, B., Roullet, J.B., Funck-Brentano, J.L. (1983) Recent advances in factors that alter lipid metabolism in chronic renal failure. Kidney Int. 24, (suppl. 16): 134–138.

21. Stenzel, K.H. (1977). Nutritional supplements in renal failure. Am. J. Med. 62: 548–553.

22. Mak, R.H.K., Turner, C., Haycock, G.B., Chantler, G. (1983) Secondary hyperparathyroidism and glucose intolerance in children with uremia. Kidney Int. 24, (suppl. 16): 128–133.

23. Rostand, S.G., Kirk, K.A. and Rutsky, E.A. (1982) Relationship of coronary risk factors to hemodialysis-associated ischemic heart disease. Kidney Int. 22: 304–308.

24. Farrell, P.C. and Hone, P.W. (1980) Dialysis-induced catabolism. Am. J. Clin. Nutr. 33: 1417–1422.

25. Abras, E., Walser, M. (1982) Nitrogen utilization in uremic patients fed by continuous

nasogastric infusion. Kidney Int. 22: 392–397.

26. Dumbauld, S.L., Rutsky, E.A. and McDaniel, H.G. (1983) Carbohydrate metabolism during fasting in chronic hemodialysis patients. Kidney Int. 24: 222–226.

27. Shoenfeld, P.Y. Henry, R.R., Laird, N.M., Roxe, D.M. (1983). Assessment of nutritional status of the National Cooperative Dialysis Study Population. Kidney Int. 23 (suppl. 13): 80–88.

28. Hyne, B.B., Fowell, E., Leed, H.A. (1972) The effect of caloric intake on nitrogen balance in chronic renal failure. Clin.Science 43: 679.

29. Panzetta, G., Mioni, G., Cristinelli, L., Broccoli, R., Mombelloni, S., Zanotto, E., Prandini, G. and Maiorca, R. (1978) Indagine dietetica e valutazione dello stato di nutrizione in pazienti emodializzati. Rapporti con l'ipertrigliceridemia. Min. Nefrol. 25: 179–182.

30. Kluthe, R.K.A. (1983) Nutrition in dialysis patients. In: *Replacement of Renal Function by Dialysis*, W. Druckker, M. Parsons and J. Maher (eds.). Boston: Martinus Nijhoff.

31. Wolfson, M. (1984) Nutrition in hemo- and peritoneal dialysis patients. A.R. Nissesson, R.N. Fine and D.E. Gentile. In *Clinical Dialysis*, (eds.). Norwalk: Appleton.

32. Kopple, J.D. and Coburn (1973) J.W. Metabolic studies of low protein diets in uremia. I: nitrogen and potassium. Medicine 52: 583–595.

33. Maschio, G., Oldrizzi, L., Tessitore, N., D'Angelo, A., Valvo, E., Lupo, A., Loschiavo, C., Fabris, A., Gammaro, L., Rugiu, C. and Panzetta, G. (1983) Early dietary protein and phosphorus restriction is effective in delaying progression of chronic renal failure. Kidney Intern. 24 (suppl. 16): s273–277.

34. Giovannetti, S. and Maggiore, Q. (1964) A low nitrogen diet with proteins of high biological value for severe chronic uraemia. Lancet 1: 1000.

35. Kopple, J.D., Sorensen, M.K., Coburn, J.W., Gordon, A. and Rubin, M.E. (1968) Controlled comparison of 20 g and 40 g protein diets in the treatment of chronic uremia. Am. J. Clin. Nutr. 21: 553.

36. Parker, T.F., Laird, N.M., and Lowrie, E.G. (1983) Comparison of the study groups in the National Cooperative Dialysis Study and a description of morbidity, mortality, and patient withdrawal. Kidney Int. 23, (suppl. 13): 42–49.

37. Lowrie, E.G., Laird, N.M. and Henry, R.R. (1983) Protocol for the National Co-operative Dialysis Study. Kidney Int. 23, (suppl. 13): 11–18.

38. Kopple, J.D. and Coburn, J.W. (1974) Evaluation of chronic uremia. Importance of serum urea nitrogen, serum creatinine, and their ratio. J.A.M.A. 277: 41–44.

39. Hirsch, J., Farquhar, J.W., Ahrens, E.H., Jr., Peterson, N.L. and Stoffel, W. (1960) Studies of adipose tissue in man. A microtechnique for sampling and analysis. Am. J. Clin. Nutr. 8: 499.

40. Norbeck, H.E. and Walldius, G. (1982) Fatty acid composition of serum and adipose tissue lipids in males with chronic renal failure. Acta Med. Scand. 211: 75–85.

41. Bagdade, J.D., Porte, D., Jr. and Biernan, E.L. (1968) Hypertriglyceridemia: a metabolic consequence of chronic renal failure. N. Engl. J. Med. 279: 181–185.

42. Ponticelli, C., Barbi, G.L., Cantaluppi, A., Donati, C., Annoni, G., Brancaccio, D. (1978) Lipid abnormalities in maintenance dialysis patients and renal transplant recipients. Kidney Int. 13 (suppl. 8): 72–78.

43. Pierides, A.M., Weightmann, D., Goldfinch, M., Tsoukantas, A. and Kerr, D.N. (1975) Serum lipid in uraemic patients on regular haemodialysis. Proc. E.D.T.A. 12: 397.

44. Shirlow, M.J., Savdie, E. and Mahony, J.F. (1977) Hemodialysis, diet, and hyperlipidemia. Dial. and Transplant. 12: 36.

45. Sailer, S., Sandhofer, F. and Braunsteiner H. (1966) Overweight and triglyceride level in normal persons and patients with diabetes mellitus. Metabolism 15: 135.

46. Sanfelippo, M.L., Swenson, R.S. and Reaven, G.M. (1977) Reduction of plasma triglicerides by diet in subjects with chronic renal failure. Kidney Int. 11: 54–61.

47. Gokal, R., Mann, J.I., Oliver, D.O., Ledingham, J.G. and Carter, R.D. (1978) Treatment of hyperlipidemia in patients on chronic hemodialysis. Br. Med. J. 1: 82–83.

48. Cattran, D.G., Steiner, G., Fenton, S.S.A. and Ampil, M. (1980) Dialysis hyperlipemia:

194

response to dietary manipulations. Clin. Nephrol. 13: 177.

49. Wass, W.J., Jarrett, R.J., Meilton, V., Start, M.K., Mattock, M., Ogg, C.S. and Cameron, J.C. (1981) Effect of a long-term fat-modified diet on serum lipoprotein levels of cholesterol and trigliceride in patients on home haemodialysis. Clinical Science 60: 80.

50. Keys, A. (1970) Coronary heart disease in seven countries. Circulation 41 (4, suppl. 1).

51. Mc Gill, H.C. (1968) The geographical pathology of atherosclerosis. Lab. Invest. 18: 498.

52. Chait, A., Onitri, A., Nicoll, A., Rabaya, E., Davies, J. and Lewis, B. (1974) Reduction of serum triglyceride levels by polyunsaturated fat. Studies on the mode of action and very low density lipoprotein composition. Atherosclerosis 20: 347.

53. Kinsell, L.W., Partidge, J., Boling, L., Margen, S. and Michaels, G. (1952) Dietary modification of serum cholesterol and phospholipid levels. J. Clin. Endocrinol. 12: 909.

54. Lennon, E.J., Lemann, J. Jr., Litzow J.R. (1966) The effect of diet and stool composition on the net external acid balance of normal subjects. J. Clin. Invest. 45: 1601–1607.

55. Barzel, U.S. and Jowsey, J. (1969) The effects of chronic acid and alkali administration on bone turnover in adults rats. Clin. Science 36: 517–524.

56. Burnell, J.M. (1971) Changes in bone sodium and carbonate in metabolic acidosis and alkalosis in the dog. J. Clin. Invest. 50: 327–331.

57. Castellani, A., Cristinclli, L., Gozzi, G., Miletti, M., Cannella, G., Mioni, G., Panzetta, G., Cecchettin, M., Mombelloni, S. and Maiorca, R. (1975) Short dialysis or personalized dialysis? Opuscola medico-technica lundensia 16: 69–8.

58. Rutherford, W.E., Bordier, P., Marie, D., Hruska, K., Harter, H., Greewalt, A., Blondin, J., Haddad, J., Bricker, N., Staopolsky, E. (1977) Phosphate control and 25-hydroxychole-calciferol administration in preventing experimental renal osteodystrophy in the dog. J. Clin. Invest. 60: 332–343.

59. Bishop, M.C., Ledingham, J.G.G., Oliver, D.O. (1971) Phosphate deficiency in hemo-dialyzed patients. Proc. E.D.T.A. 8: 106–110.

60. Fleming, L.W., Stewart, W.K., Fell, G.S., Halls, D.J. (1982) The effect of oral aluminium therapy on plasma aluminium levels in patients with chronic renal failure in an area with low water aluminium. Clin. Nephrol. 17: 222–227.

61. Masselot, J.P., Adhemar, J.P., Jandon, M.C., Kleinknecht, D., Galli, A. (1978) Reversible dialysis encephalopathy: role for aluminium-containing gels. Lancet 11: 1386.

62. Panzetta, G., Adami, S., Fabris, A., Tessitore, N., Solero, P., Cocco, C., Tartarotti, D. and Maschio, G. (1982) Calcium fluxes and calciotropic hormone changes during hemodialysis with Secon 133 Dialyzer. Proc. First SIFRA Meeting on New Dialysis trends. Wichtig, Milano,

63. Clarkson, E.M., Eastwood, J.B., Koutsaimanis, K.G. and De Wardener, H.E. (1973) Net gastrointestinal absorption of calcium in patients with chronic renal failure. Kidney Int. 3: 258–265.

64. Meyrier, A., Marsac, J. and Richet, G. (1973) The influence of a high calcium carbonate intake on bone disease in patients undergoing hemodialysis. Kidney Int. 4: 146–153.

65. Parfitt, A.M. (1967) Soft tissue calcification in uremia. Arch. Int. Med. 124: 544–549.

66. Van Ypersele De Strihou, C. (1977) Potassium homeostasis in renal failure. Kidney Int. 2: 491–504.

67. Seedat, Y.K. (1969) Exchangeable potassium study in patients undergoing chronic hemodialysis. Br. Med. J. 2: 344–345.

68. Rettori, V., Grai, T., Massry, S.G., Villamil, M.F. (1972) Exchangeable potassium content and distribution in normal subjects and uraemic patients on chronic haemodialysis. Clin. Sci. 42: 673–684.

69. OH, M.S., Levison, S.P., Carrol, H.J. (1975) Content and distribution of water and electrolytes in maintenance hemodialysis. Nephron 14: 421–428.

70. Butkus, D.E., Alfrey, A.C. and Miller, N.L. (1974) Tissue potassium in chronic dialysis patients. Nephron 13: 314–324.

71. Gonick, H.C., Maxwell, M.H., Cutler, R.E., Dowling, J.T. and Kleeman, C.R. (1961) Potassium excretion in renal disease. J. Clin. Invest. 40: 1044.

72. Schon, D.A., Silva, P. and Hayslett, J.P. (1974) Mechanism of potassium excretion in renal insufficiency. Am. J. Physiol. 227: 1323–1330.

73. Edson, J., Avram, M., Gan, A. and Edson, J.N. (1977) Cardiac arrhythmias in hemodialysis patients. Proc. Dial. Transplant Forum 7: 82–86.

74. Comty, C.M. and Shapiro, F.L. (1983) Cardiac complications of regular dialysis therapy. In *Replacement of Renal Function by Dialysis*, W. Drukker, M. Parsons, and J. Maher (eds.). Boston: Martinus Nijhoff.

75. Lasker, N., Harvey, A. and Baker, H. (1963) Vitamin levels in hemodialysis and intermittent peritoneal dialysis. Trans ASAIO 9: 51–56.

76. Hampers, C.L., Streiff, R., Nathan, D.C., Snyder, D. and Merril, J.P. (1967) Megaloblastic hematopoiesis in uremia and in patients on long-term hemodialysis. New Engl. J. Med. 276: 551–554.

77. Skoutakis, V.A., Acchiardo, S.R., Meyer, M.C. and Hatch, F.E. (1975) Folic acid dosage for chronic hemodialysis patients. Clinical Pharmacology and Therapeutics 18: 200–204.

78. Sharman, V.L., Cunningham, J., Goodwin, F.J., Marsh, F.P., Chaput de Saintonge, D.M. and Evans, S.W.J. (1982) Do patients receiving regular hemodialysis need folic acid supplements? Br. Med. J. 285: 86–87.

79. Werb, R., Clark, W.F., Lindsay, R.M., Jones, E.O.P. and Linton, A.L. (1979) Serum vitamin A levels and associate abnormalities in patients on regular dialysis treatment. Clin. Nephrol. 12: 63.

80. Wolfson, M., Jones, M.R. and Kopple, J.D. (1982) Amino acid losses during hemodialysis with infusion of aminoacids and glucose. Kidney Int. 21: 500–506.

# 8. Acid-base metabolism in short dialysis

Giuseppe Mioni, Antonino Favazza, and Piergiorgio Messa

Clinical application of short dialysis has become feasible since the introduction of the high efficiency type of dialyzer, which has enabled high rates of water and solute exchange between the blood and the dialysate to be obtained [1, 2]. The side effects of this aggressive dialysis technique, such as symptomatic hypotension, muscolar cramps, plasma bicarbonate dissipation, etc., were the price that had to be paid for a more rapid and intensive metabolic waste product elimination [1–5]. Besides the problem of dialysate sodium concentration, which was progressively increased from 132–135 to 140 mmol/l or more [2, 3, 6, 7], the following problems had to be faced: the high performance of the dialyzers; the kind of buffers in the dialysis bath; the choice of the single-pass (SP) or the recirculating dialysate delivery system (RS); the rate of body weight loss, i.e., water ultrafiltration rate ($Q_f$). The solution of these new problems appeared strictly connected with the dialysis correction of A-B status.

## Metabolic Aspects of A-B Correction

### General considerations

Correction of metabolic acidosis is one of the goals we endeavor to achieve with dialysis therapy. Metabolic acidosis is characterized by low plasma bicarbonate concentration and by reduced nonbicarbonate buffers availability in their dehydrogenated form. Conversely the titrable $H^+$ ion pool appears to be expanded. At any expansion level of this pool, an equilibrium tends to be reached between the $H^+$ ion generation and elimination rate. To obtain this result in patients lacking any residual renal function, acetate or bicarbonate must be delivered, that neutralize the excess of $H^+$ ion generation. If an acetate containing dialysate is chosen together with a highly efficient dialyzer in an SP dialysis system, more acetate must enter the EC space than bicarbonate, disodium phosphate, and organic metabolizable anions leave it in order that not only can the intradialytic buffer dispersion be counterbalanced

*Vincenzo Cambi (editor) Professor of Nephrology*
© *1987 Martinus Nijhoff Publishing, Boston. ISBN 0-89838-858-9. Printed in The United States.*

but also the weekly $H^+$ ion generation and accumulation rate can be buffered. The higher the filter performance, the higher the acetate concentration in the bath and the lower the predialysis plasma bicarbonate values must be so as to obtain a positive buffer balance, if an SP dialysis is chosen. The second very important point concerns the rate of acetate utilization, which normally ranges from 2.5 to 4.5 mmol/min. [8–11]. It is well known that high acetate dialysance also means high bicarbonate dialysance: consequently, if acetate delivery is greater than bicarbonate from acetate generation, the only result obtained at the end of dialysis is bicarbonate depletion, compensated for by a more or less important acetate accumulation. It is only after the end of dialysis that a rapid acetate metabolization can restore, at least in part, the excess of bicarbonate lost. In this way, from a condition of metabolic acidosis, the patients shift to one of steep metabolic alkalosis, only partially mitigated by compensatory hypoventilation [9–13]. The last aspect to be considered regards the rate of weight loss ($Q_f$), which in some patients can reach even 30–50 ml/min during a 4-hour dialysis time. When ultrafiltration rates of such values are induced, the acetate into blood transfer is strongly reduced [14–16], bicarbonate dispersion equally potentiated and extracellular volume (ECV) contracted even by 7–12 liters [12–16]. If a patient begins dialysis with plasma bicarbonate of 20 mmol/l and an extracellular pool of 400 mmols his/her pool will reduce to 350 mmol at the end of dialysis, given a plasma bicarbonate concentration of 19 mmol/l, an acetate concentration of 6 mmol/l, and extracellular volume of 14.1. It appears that during the course of this dialysis bicarbonate generation has been about 0.56 mmol/min slower than that of bicarbonate dispersion. We shall discuss this important aspect when the relationship between the RQ (respiratory quotient) and the ventilatory exchange ratio, R, are examined. Lastly, the net loss of extracellular bicarbonate, which can be found in amounts as high as 100 mmols, must be taken into account when acid-base balance is calculated, because an equivalent amount of dialysis-regenerated nonextracellular buffers must be consumed to restored bicarbonate to ECV, when it expands again [15] (figure 8–1). In order to obviate the excessive bicarbonate dispersion and the steep A-B variations in acetate SP dialysis (ASPD), the substitution of bicarbonate for acetate has been suggested [4, 5, 9, 16, 17]. Alternatively the recirculating dialysate delivery system has been suggested whether containing acetate or bicarbonate [12, 18, 19]. It is obvious that the dialysate concentration of bicarbonate must be sufficiently high with respect to plasma concentration, so as to induce a net gain of the buffer. Conversely in acetate recirculating system (ARSD) bicarbonate concentration increases with time in the dialysate, so that its dispersion rate from the blood to the box progressively reduces, while its generation from acetate remains constant [12]. It is interesting to note that in both bicarbonate SPD and acetate or bicarbonate RSD, a certain amount of dissolved $CO_2$ is given off in the dialysate, which not only opposes bicarbonate precipitation but also has interesting respiratory and metabolic implications [12, 19, 20].

198

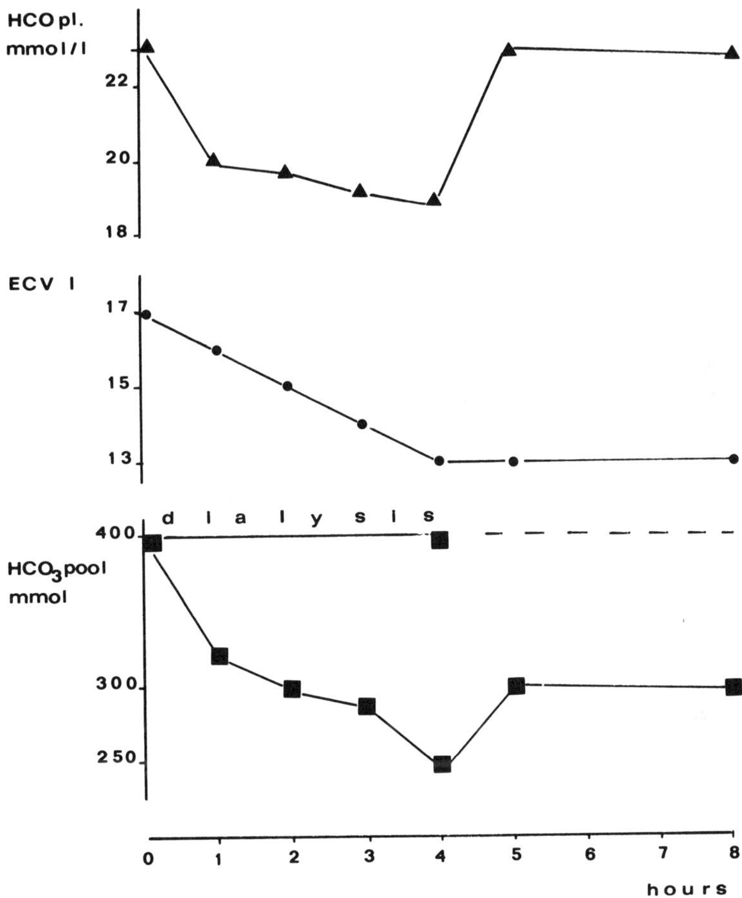


*Figure 8–1.* Dialysis-induced variations of plasma bicarbonate concentration, ECV and bicarbonate pool. During dialysis a reduction of plasma bicarbonate concentration takes place together with extracellular volume(ECV) and bicarbonate pool contraction, due to the imbalance between acetate gain and buffers dispersion that prevails. In spite of the rapid acetate activation to acetyl-CoA after the end of dialysis — which allows plasma bicarbonate concentration to be restored — the pool of extracellular bicarbonate is kept lower by around 100 mmol, as compared with the predialytic values. The pool will be restored at the expense of the dialysis-regenerated nonbicarbonate buffers (180 mmol) during the interdialytic period, allowing plasma bicarbonate to be maintained constant while ECV is expanding again. Consequently the residual 80 mmols of buffers gained per dialysis are not sufficient to counterbalance the metabolic generation of $H^+$ ions (buffer regenerated and retained per week ~240 mmol vs. ~350 mmol of $H^+$ ions produced per week). It is concluded that other mechanisms must operate that are able to neutralize the excess of the metabolically generated $H^+$ ions. This indicates that a nonrenal-nondialysis controlled setpoint for extracellular bicarbonate concentration is operating.

199

*Acetate as a buffer: the kinetics of acetate metabolism*

Once acetate enters the blood, at a rate ranging from 2.5 to 4.3 mmol/min
[8–12] only a very small amount of it is reduced to acetic acid. Since the pKa
of acetate/acetic acid buffer pair is 4.73, only 3.4% of all the acetate salts
present in the acetate distribution volume will be converted to acetic acid if
the blood pH is 7.35. For example, given a distribution volume for acetate
equal to 19% of bw [9] and a pool of 53 mmols in a 70 kg subject, only 0.13
mmols of $H^+$ ions will be eliminated and an equivalent amount of buffers
regenerated. Moreover, the reaction is reversible [22]. Of much greater
importance is the reaction, which activates the acetic acid to acetyl-CoA:

$$\text{acetate}^- \text{ Na}^+ + \text{Buffer}^- \text{ H}^+ \rightarrow \text{Acetate}^- \text{ H}^+ + \text{Buffer}^- \text{ Na}^+$$

$$\text{Acetate}^- \text{ H}^+ + \text{HS CoA} \xrightarrow{\text{ATP}} \text{Acetyl CoA} + \text{H}_2\text{O} + \text{P} \sim \text{P} + \text{AMP}.$$

It is only after $P \sim P$ is split to 2 Pi by the pyrophosphatase activity that the
reaction becomes irreversible [8, 21]. The reaction of acetate to acetyl CoA
activation is an energy-consuming process, that operates as the true driving
force transporting $H^+$ ions from their titratable pool into the $H_2O$ molecule
[8, 12, 13, 21]. It has been calculated that ~85% of the exchangeable $H^+$ ions
consumed in this reaction are compensated for by dissociation of $H_2CO_3$ to
$HCO_3$, while ~15% is supplied by the other 'nonvolatile buffers' [12]. With
respect to bicarbonate generation, 0.85 mmol of dissolved $CO_2$ is converted
to the nonvolatile hydrosoluble form of $HCO_3$, when 1 mmol of acetate is
converted to acetyl-CoA. In this way dissolved $CO_2$ is diverted from
pulmonary ventilation, increasing the amount of total $CO_2$ in the body, but in
the form of bicarbonate. Since the pool of $H_2CO_3$ in a 60 kg BW person is
about 43 mmols, the shifting of ~3 mmols/min of dissolved $CO_2$ to hydrosoluble bicarbonate reduces this pool by 50% [15, 22] within ~10 minutes.
Given a constant $CO_2$ generation rate by the Krebs cycle of 11 mmol/min [4,
22], some 30% of this production will not be eliminated by the lungs, being
shifted to bicarbonate by acetate to acetyl CoA activation. As a consequence,
a double alkalosis situation is produced, metabolic, due to bicarbonate generation and accumulation excess, hypocapnic, of the same value, due to
metabolic, nonventilatory, $CO_2$ elimination [12, 17]. A small amount of dissolved $CO_2$ is also lost from the blood into the dialysis bath: 0.12–0.2 mmol/
min versus ~3 mmol/min, due to the metabolic process. This loss is therefore
of little importance as far as ventilation is concerned [22]. If bicarbonate from
dissolved $CO_2$ were generated at a rate of about 2 mmol/min in a 60 kg man,
his plasma bicarbonate being 20 mmol/min, $PCO_2$ 35 mmHg, pH 7.38, then
~15 min after the beginning of dialysis, the expected plasma bicarbonate
would have to be ~22 mmol/l, $pCO_2$ 17 mmHg and pH 7.71, with his $HCO_3$/
$H_2CO_3$ buffer pair shifting from the initial ratio of 20/1.05 = 19/1 to that of
21.7/0.5 = 41/1. It immediately appears evident that a ventilatory inhibition is
needed to compensate for this important reduction of $CO_2$ availability in

order to reduce the $HCO_3/H_2CO_3$ ratio from ~40/1 to as near as possible to 20/1. However, it should be stressed that during the first minutes of dialysis the increment of plasma bicarbonate is too small to play any important role by itself. On the contrary, at the end of a 4-hour dialysis, about 800 mmols of $HCO_3$ entered the E.C.V. [12]. In the same 60 kg person this enormous amount of $HCO_3$ should determine an increment in plasma bicarbonate from 20 to 78 mmol making pH vary from 7.38 to 7.91, although hypoventilation keeps $PaCO_2$ at 40 mmHg. Fortunately bicarbonate is lost across the dialyzer at a rate quite similar, but generally greater than that of its generation. It is only by the cooperation between the lungs, that compensate for the metabolic $CO_2$ removal and the dialyzer, which opposes bicarbonate accumulation, that the $HCO_3/H_2CO_3$ ratio can be kept near normal values. It is quite strange, therefore, that hypoventilation is attributed to loss of $CO_2$ by dialyzer [23–25], since it is just bicarbonate that is dissipated in large amounts and not the dissolved $CO_2$. The hypothesis of hypoventilation, due to bicarbonate dissipation, is based on the assumption that an amount of $H_2CO_3$, of the same magnitude as bicarbonate lost, splits to $HCO_3$ and $H^+$, the latter being at first taken up by the intra red-cell buffers and thereafter irreversibly eliminated by the acetate to acetyl CoA activation [24]. This hypothesis is untenable because: (1) the red cells of the arterialized blood flowing through the filter act as a $CO_2$ source, when $CO_2$ is leaving the plasma [24], and not like a $CO_2$ sink, as would be expected if bicarbonate were generated [24]; (2) hemoglobin of the arterialized red cells is in its oxygenated form, with a pKa of 6.8, that is too low as compared with the blood pH and its buffer activity too weak to generate bicarbonate at lower than normal $PaCO_2$; (3) the $HCO_3/H_2CO_3$ ratio, at the blood pH, is strongly umbalanced (20/1) with respect to what the mass action equation dictates. This umbalance is kept at a constant value by an irreversible, energy-consuming, $H^+$ ion disposition activity. The spontaneous tendency of the in vivo reaction:

$$CO_2 + H_2O \rightleftharpoons H_2CO_3 \rightleftharpoons H^+ + HCO_3 \qquad (8.2)$$

with $H_2CO_3 \ll HCO_3$, is that of running to the left, so as to equate $H_2CO_3$ and $HCO_3$ (equilibrium condition), unless a $CO_2$ excess is produced (see later) in the presence of high pKa buffers (pKa $\gg$ blood pH). For all the above mentioned reasons we do not agree that bicarbonate can be generated while the blood is flowing through the filter [26] and $CO_2$ is spreading out of it into dialysate. It is interesting to note that, according to this theory, the acetate to acetyl CoA activation would eliminate an amount of $H^+$ ions exactly equal to the quantity of bicarbonate lost via the dialyzer. In fact, it has been stated that the amount of dissolved $CO_2$, which is shifted from ventilatory elimination to bicarbonate generation, is just equal to the amount of bicarbonate eliminated across the filter [23–25]. However, it is easy to demonstrate that the generation and dispersion rates of these substances are seldom of the same magnitude, the latter being higher, so that an extra-cellular bicarbonate depletion is generally found at the end of dialysis [4, 5, 9,

11, 12]. Just as $CO_2$ production can be measured from respiratory $CO_2$ elimination on condition that $PaCO_2$ values are kept constant, in the same way bicarbonate generation during dialysis can be evaluated from the dispersion rate of bicarbonate across the filter, but only if its extracellular pool is not changing during dialysis. If the latter does change, appropriate corrections must be introduced in the calculation in order to avoid either an overstimation, if the pool is reducing, or an understimation if the pool is expanding. This kind of mistake has been systematically made when the intradialytic RQ ($\dot{V}CO_2$ + amount of bicarbonate generated + amount of dissolved $CO_2$ lost via the filter/$\dot{V}O_2$), is calculated from the respiratory exchange ratio R ($\dot{V}CO_2/\dot{V}O_2$), using bicarbonate loss instead of the bicarbonate generation rate. As a consequence an RQ even greater than 1 can be found, falsely suggesting lipids synthesis [27, 28] or as low as to indicate that the excess of acetate infused is not entering the Krebs cycle.

*Acetate utilization kinetics in SP and recirculating delivery system (Redy)*

When acetate concentration in the plasma is low, the rate of activation to acetyl-CoA follows a first order kinetics, which becomes a zero order kinetics when concentration increases over 3–5 mmol/l [9, 12, 22]. In ASPD using $CO_2$ free dialysates a mean km of 1.14 ± 0.19 mmol/l and a mean Vmax of 5.01 ± 0.27 mmol/min may be found, the mean peak of acetate activation rate being 3.5 ± 0.27 mmol/min (mean ± s.d.) (table 8–1 and figure 8–2) [12]. Of most interest is the metabolic effect on acetate utilization induced by the dissolved form of dialysate $CO_2$, as can be studied with the recirculating regenerative dialysis system (ARSD) [12]. In fact, the rate of acetate

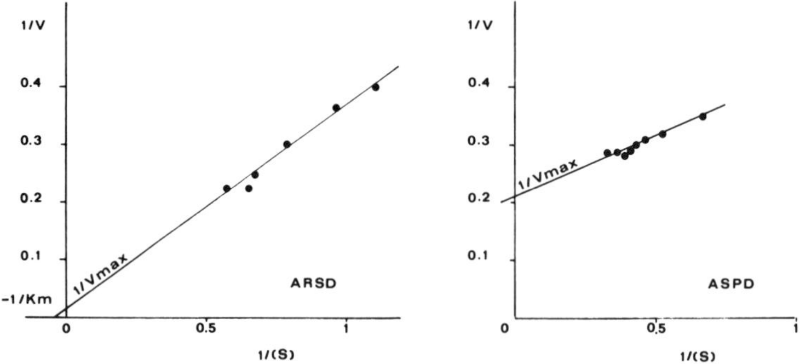


*Figure 8–2.* The Michaelis constants of acetate to acetyl-CoA activation rate during ASPD and ARSD. The lefthand side of the diagram represents the Lineweaver-Burk transformation of acetate to acetyl-CoA activation rate (I/V) as a function of the plasma acetate concentrations (I/[S]) in ARSD: values for Vmax and Km as high as 61±17.4 mmol/min and 21±6.7 mmol/l (m ± sd) are found. At the right side, the ASPD values for Vmax and Km appear to be 5.01±0.27 mmol/min and 1.14±0.19 mmol/l; i.e., significantly lower than those observed in ARSD. ARSD: 1/V as a function of 1/[s]; r = 0.9977; ASPD: 1/V as a function of 1/[S]; r = 0.9924.

202

*Table 8–1.* Parameters of acetate-bicarbonate balance

| Cases N. 10 | | ASPD<br>m ± sd | ARSD<br>m ± sd |
|---|---|---|---|
| Acetate delivery to ECV | mmol/4 h | 2.808 ± 288*** | 1.226 ± 212 |
| Acetate entered the blood | mmol/4 h | 848 ± 84** | 703 ± 121 |
| Peak of plasma acetate | mmol/l | 2.73 ± 0.9* | 1.71 ± 0.35 |
| Acetate to acetyl-Coa activ. | mmol/4 h | 792 ± 144 | 693 ± 117 |
| Vmax of acetate activ. | mmol/min. | 5.01 ± 0.27*** | 61 ± 17 |
| Km of acetate activ. | mmol/l | 1.14 ± 0.19*** | 21 ± 7 |
| Peak of acetate activ. | mmol/min. | 3.5 ± 0.27** | 4.33 ± 0.86 |
| $HCO_3$ generation | mmol/4 h | 671 ± 52*** | 198 ± 88 |
| Peak of $HCO_3$ generation | mmol/min. | 3.16 ± 0.18 | 2.01 ± 0.48 |
| $HCO_3$ from box-$CO_2$ generation | mmol/min. | / | 216 ± 58 |
| Dialyzer loss of $HCO_3$ | mmol/4 h | 728 ± 102*** | 246 ± 39 |
| Non — $HCO_3$ buffer generation | mmol/4 h | 120 ± 15*** | 311 ± 83 |
| Dialyzer loss of box-$CO_2HCO_3$ | mmol/4 h | / | 216 ± 58 |
| Neutralization of box-$CO_2H^+$ | mmol/4 h | / | 216 ± 58 |
| Box accumulation of $HCO_3$ | mmol/4 h | / | 137 ± 27 |
| $H_2CO_3$ to $HCO_3$ shifting | mmol/4 h | 671 ± 52*** | 198 ± 88 |
| Dialyzer loss of $H_2CO_3$ | mmol/4 h | 25 ± 12 | / |
| Total $H_2CO_3$-balance | mmol/4 h | −696 ± 62 | ± 0 |

ASPD versus ARSD: $p < 0.05$ *; $p < 0.01$ **; $p < 0.001$ ***
ASPD = Acetate Single Pass Dialysis; ARSD = Acetate Redy System Dialysis.
ECV = Extracellular Volume.

disappearing from the extracellular fluids appears to be far greater in ARSD than in ASPD, with values for km of 21.5 ± 6.7 mmol/l and Vmax of 61 ± 17.4 mmol/min, the mean peak of acetate activation rate being as high as 4.33 ± 0.86 mmol/min (table 8–1; figure 8–2) [12]. During dialysis, $PCO_2$ progressively increases in the dialysate up to 200 mmHg or more, its source being bicarbonate that comes from the blood. In fact, bicarbonate is reduced to carbonic acid when it passes through the cartridge, which releases $H^+$ ions in exchange for calcium, magnesium, potassium, and ammonium [18]. Ammonium is produced by the urea-splitting activity of the cartridge according to the following simplified reactions:

$$CO(NH_2)_2 + H_2O \rightarrow CO_2 + 2\ NH_3 \tag{8.3}$$

$$2\ Na\ Cl + 2NH_3 + 2\ H_2CO_3 \rightarrow 2\ Na\ HCO_3 + 2\ NH_4\ Cl \tag{8.4}$$

Even if these reactions can generate bicarbonate, the amount of $H^+$ ions released from the cartridge is far greater, so as to titrate not only all the amount of urea splitting-dependent bicarbonate but also part of that coming from the blood. In fact, much more bicarbonate enters the cartridge than leaves it. On the contrary, carbonic acid leaves the cartridge at a much higher rate than it enters: the result is that both bicarbonate and dissolved $CO_2$ accumulate in the box (table 8–2) [12]. ARDS therefore presents some

*Table 8–2.* Regenerating cartridge effects on acetate-bicarbonate balance in ARSD

| Cases N. 10 | Acetate<br>m ± s.d. | $HCO_3$<br>m ± s.d. | $H_2CO_3$<br>m ± s.d. |
|---|---|---|---|
| Cartridge inlet<br>mmol/4 h | 520 ± 156 | 807 ± 128 | 96 ± 22 |
| Cartridge outlet<br>mmol/4 h | 1.224 ± 212 | 506 ± 137 | 289 ± 90 |
| Balance<br>mmol/4 h | +704 ± 116 | −301 ± 41 | +193 ± 83 |
| Outlet versus inlet | p < 0.001 | p < 0.01 | p < 0.001 |

interesting features [12]: (1) it prevents bicarbonate from being dissipated, as in ASPD, by reducing its plasma-dialysate concentration gradient; (2) it allows a large part of dissolved $CO_2$ (70%), converted to bicarbonate by acetate to acetyl CoA activation, to be recovered thanks to the $H^+$ ion donation activity of the regenerating cartridge; (3) when dialysate $PCO_2$ is sufficiently high it spreads into the blood, at first opposing hypoventilation, thereafter causing hyperventilation; (4) when $CO_2$ enters the arterialized blood that is flowing through the filter, the oxygenated hemoglobin releases $O_2$, changing its pKa from 6.68 to 7.93, which allows a fraction of carbonic acid to become bicarbonate due to the increased $H^+$ ion buffering capacity of deoxygenerated hemoglobin. These events are well documented by a sharp increase in $PO_2$ at both blood and dialysate outlets of the filter with respect to the blood and dialysate $PO_2$ at the filter inlets (figure 8–3) [12]. However, bicarbonate generated in this manner spreads again into dialysate so that a net gain of $H^+$ ions of about 200 mmols per dialysis takes place, which will be released from hemoglobin, when the latter loads with $O_2$ passing through the lungs [12] (table 8–1).

*Bicarbonate as a buffer: the kinetics of bicarbonate utilization*

The intradialytic kinetics of bicarbonate utilization appears to be less complicated than that of acetate. Like the latter, bicarbonate influx from the dialysate depends on the concentration gradient between dialysate and blood water on the one hand and the filter dialysance on the other, which is given by the algebraic sum of the diffusive and convective dialysances [14,16,17]. It is important to stress that besides Bicarbonate, dialysate often contains acetate in concentrations generally ranging from 5 to 10 mmol/l. With acetate dialysance in the range of 100–120 ml/min, amounts of this buffer varyging from 0.5 to 1.2 mmol/min gain the extracellular space. Since this flux is far slower than the maximum rate of acetate metabolization [9, 12, 22] even in the most acetate-intolerant patients, it does not accumulate in the plasma, so that its delivery will not reduce with time. In fact, if a dialysis bath is chosen, where 30 mmols of bicarbonate and 10 of acetate are dissolved, and a patient,

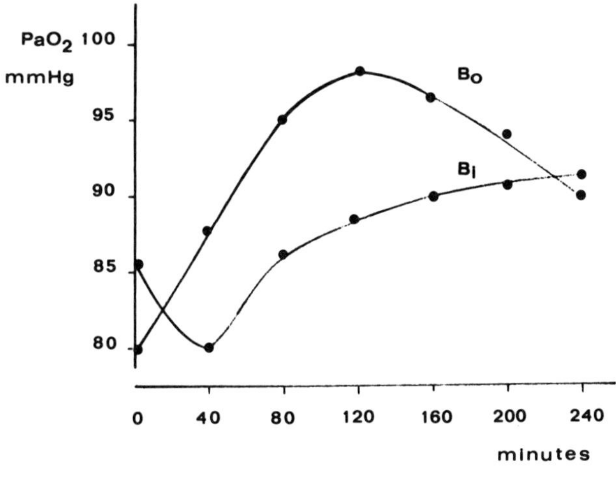

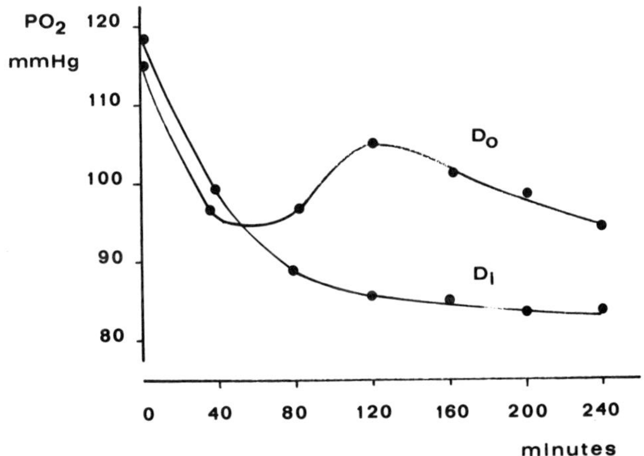



*Figure 8–3.* Blood and dialysate variations of $PO_2$ caused by ARSD (acetate Redy system dialysis). During ARSD the dialysate $CO_2$ spreads into the blood across the filter, making the oxygenated form of hemoglobin release $O_2$ that diffuses in the blood and back to the dialysate. Consequently $PO_2$ appears higher, at both the dialysate (Do) and blood (Bo) outlets of the filter, as compared with the $PO_2$ values at the blood (Bi) and dialysate (Di) inlets of the dialyzer. Each point represents the mean of 10 observations [12].

whose plasma bicarbonate concentration is 20 mmol/l and acetate 0.3, the same gradient for both buffers develops, which will reduce with time only for bicarbonate. If operational parameters exist for bicarbonate and acetate, respectively, such as: dialysance = 0.14 and 0.11 l/min; end-dialysis plasma concentrations = 26 and 1 mmol/l; mean plasma-dialysate concentration gradient = 6 and 9.7 mmol/l, then mean fluxes of 0.84 mmol/m′ for bicarbonate and 1.0 for acetate will occur from dialysate to the blood, with a gain of 200 and 250 mmoles for a 240-minute dialysis. It can be seen how

205

important even small amounts of acetate in bicarbonate containing dialysate are. This is a still neglected aspect, that has been introduced as a technical measure to improve bicarbonate solubility [20] by making acetic acid react with bicarbonate. In fact, if acetic acid is used so that final dialysate concentrations between 5–10 mmol/l may be obtained, proportional amounts of dissolved $CO_2$ develop, ranging from 60 to 80 mmHg, i.e., 30–50 mmHg higher than the plasma $PaCO_2$. This means that significant variations of total $CO_2$ content are induced in the blood, that leaves the dialyzer flowing toward the lungs [12, 29–31]. When only 2 mmol of acetic acid are dissolved per liter of dialysate, $PCO_2$ values around 30–35 mmHg are given off, i.e., of the same order of magnitude as plasma $PaCO_2$. We had the opportunity to investigate the effect on A-B status of 5 types of dialysates, the composition of which were as follows: bic. 25 + ac. 2; bic. 27 + ac. 5; bic. 35 + ac. 5; bic. 27 + ac. 10; bic. 31 + ac. 10 mmol/l; these are commercially available in Italy. Each kind of dialysis bath was used in 5 groups of 35 patients, so that every group could be dialyzed against only 1 of the 5 different baths. After an equilibration period of at least 3 months, the predialytic, intradialytic, and postdialytic A-B parameters were studied in both the blood and dialysate, at the inlets and outlets of the dialyzer. Bicarbonate concentration of dialysate was calculated from $PCO_2$ and total $CO_2$ (Astra method [32]). The mean predialytic and postdialytic concentrations of plasma bicarbonate are illustrated in figure 8–4, as a function of the total buffers in the dialysate (Bic + Ac). When the predialytic plasma bicarbonate values, measured after a 68-hour interval, were considered as the dependent variable in a multiple linear regression analysis, where the dialysate concentrations of bicarbonate and acetate were the independent variables, it was found that 11% of the total plasma bicarbonate concentration variability (deviance) was controlled by the dialysate acetate; 33% by the dialysate bicarbonate; the remaining 56% of deviance by factors not taken into consideration (the set-point factors: see later) (r = 0.451; D.F. 173; p < 0.001). Moreover, when the effects of the same dialysate compositions on postdialysis plasma bicarbonate levels were investigated after a standard 4-hour dialysis, acetate was found to influence deviance by 14%, bicarbonate by 59%, while 27% appeared unexplained by the factors considered (r = 0.856; D.F. 173; p < 0,001). Lastly, when also the predialytic values of plasma bicarbonate concentration were considered as independent variables besides the dialysate acetate and bicarbonate, it appeared that 61% of postdialytic plasma bicarbonate concentration deviance was dependent on its predialytic values, 22% on total buffer delivery, only 7% being unexplained. Using the mean predialytic and postdialytic values of the plasma bicarbonate in the 5 groups, the following equation was obtained:

$$\text{A.D.} \bar{m}[HCO_3] = 1.7 + 0.42 \text{ [total buffer]} + 0.39 \text{ B.D.} \bar{m}[HCO_3]$$
$$\text{with } r = 0.975; \text{ D.F. 5}; p < 0.01 \tag{8.5}$$

A.D. = after dialysis; B.D. = before dialysis; $\bar{m}$ = mean. This equation allows us to choose the dialysate total buffer concentration necessary to

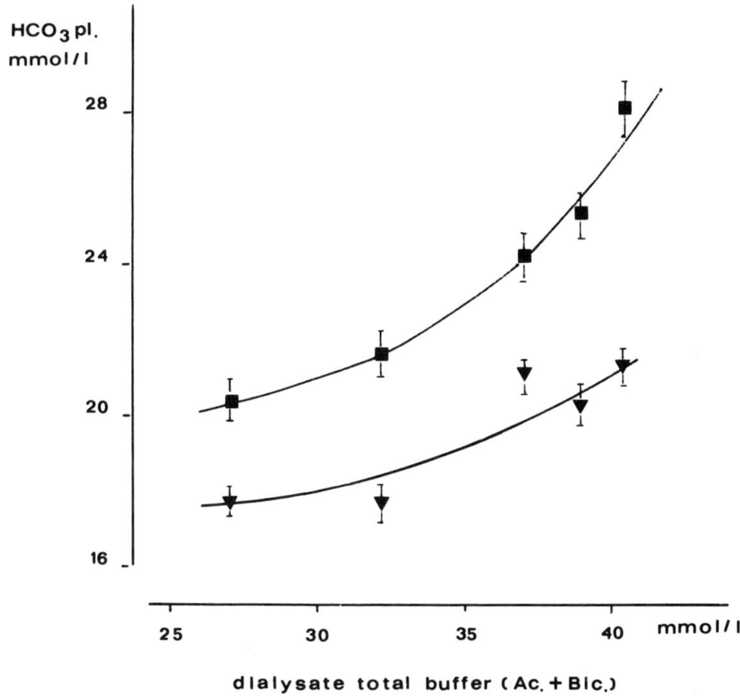


*Figure 8–4.* Predialysis and postdialysis plasma bicarbonate concentrations as a function of dialysate buffer supply. Predialysis and postdialysis plasma bicarbonate increase as a function of total buffer (bicarbonate + acetate) concentration in the dialysate. The increment of predialysis bicarbonate is far slower than the postdialytic one and follows the equation: $BD[HCO_3]\,pl = 21.5 - 0.4\,[\text{total buffer}] + 0.0102\,[\text{total buffer}]^2$; $r = 0.8906$; D.F. 3; $p<0.05$. The post dialytic bicarbonate concentration rises according to the equation: $AD[HCO_3]\,pl = 42 - 1.7\,[\text{total buffer}] + 0.033\,[\text{total buffer}]^2$; $r = 0.996$; D.F. 3; $p<0.001$. Each point represents the mean of 35 determinations (m ± s.e.).

increase the postdialysis plasma bicarbonate to the values required, if the predialytic concentration is known:

$$[\text{Total buffer}] = A.D.[HCO_3] - 1.7 - 0.39\,B.D.[HCO_3]/0.42. \quad (8.6)$$

We tested the reliability of this approximation by comparing the postdialytic values of plasma bicarbonate calculated using equation 8.5 with experimental data reported by others [33], and we found it very good (expected versus measured, $r = .966$; D.F. = 16; $p < .001$). When the different buffer concentrations used were investigated more fully as far as their effects on predialysis and postdialysis acid-base correction were concerned, only in a minority of patients were the predialytic bicarbonate concentrations found to be above 18 mmol/l, when dialysate buffers lower than 35 mmol/l were used (figure 8–5). Moreover, the extracellular pools of bicarbonate decreased from predialytic values of $277 \pm 77$ and $285 \pm 67$ ( m ± sd) to values of 258

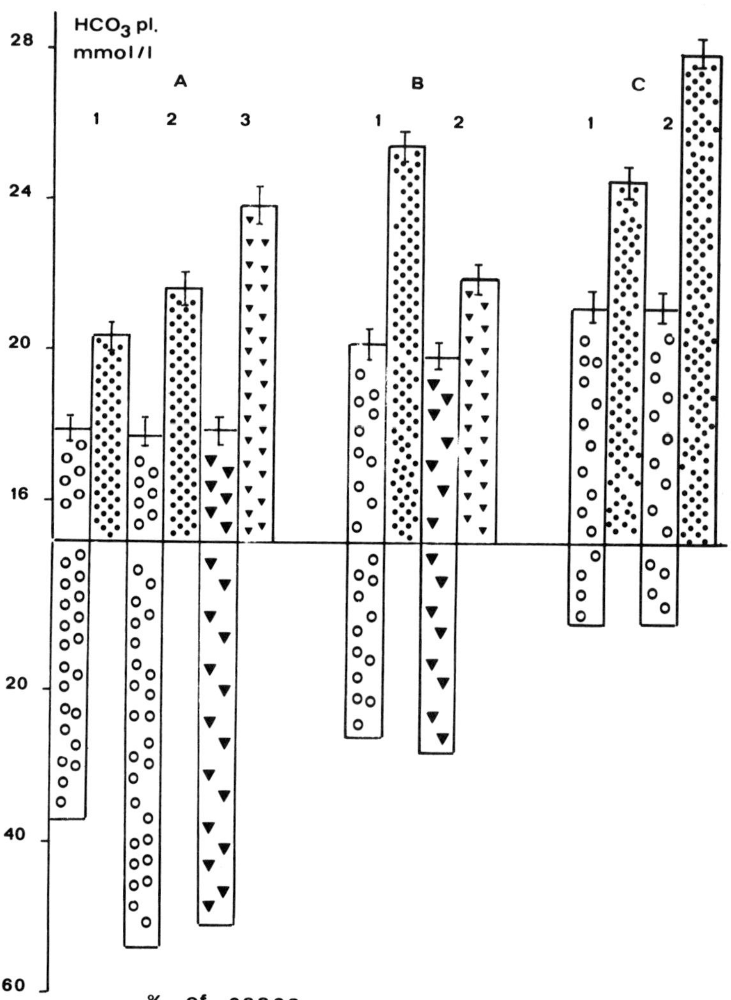


*Figure 8–5.* Predialysis and postdialysis values of plasma bicarbonate concentration during acetate and bicarbonate single pass dialysis. *Upper part:* three groups (A-B-C) of predialysis and postdialysis bicarbonate concentrations are shown (m ± s.e.). The first group (A) is represented by three pairs of predialysis and postdialysis bicarbonate values (1–2–3). It is evident that in group A, predialysis plasma bicarbonate concentrations are not different, while a clear difference exists among the postdialysis values. The dialysate buffers are: Bic 25 + Ac 2 mmol/l (A1), Bic 27 + Ac 5 mmol/l (A2), and Ac 38 mmol/l (A3). The group B is represented by two pre–postdialysis pairs (1–2) of bicarbonate concentrations. Also in this group, the predialysis values are not different from each other but are significantly higher than the corresponding values of the group A. On the other hand, the postdialysis concentrations appear quite different. The dialysate buffers are: Bic 35 + Ac 5 mmol/l (B1) and Ac 38 mmol/l (B2). The group C demonstrates not different predialysis values for plasma bicarbonate, that are higher than the corresponding values in groups A and B. Also in the C group the postdialysis bicarbonate concentrations are significantly different from each other. In this C group the dialysate buffers are: Bic 27 + Ac 10 mmol/l (C1) and Bic 31 + Ac 10 mmol/l (C2). As a whole, if the ASPD and BSPD patients are

208

± 65 and 257 ± 67, with buffers in the dialysis baths of 27 and 32 mmol/l. In these cases the intradialytic increase of plasma bicarbonate was solely due to the extracellular volume contraction. Moreover, the A–B parameters modification was quite similar to that obtained using acetate containing dialysates (figure 8–5). The mean rates of bicarbonate transport into the blood and the fraction of them, that regenerate the nonextracellular buffers, are shown in table 8–3. Using filters with bicarbonate dialysance of around 0.14 liters and patients whose mean extracellular volume was 14.5 liters, transport rates ranging from 1.1 to 2.43 mmol/min have been found, the fractions of which capable of regenerating the nonextracellular buffer varying from 70% to 61% as a function of the dialysate buffer concentrations. It is also interesting to note that the greater the buffer inputs, the greater both predialysis and postdialysis bicarbonate concentrations. However, the post-dialysis plasma values increased much more than the predialysis ones, the regression coefficient being at least 3 times greater for postdialysis concentrations (figure 8–4). The following interdialytic drop of plasma bicarbonate was of the same extent as the intradialytic increment, since the mean values of plasma bicarbonate reported here represent an equilibrium situation for each type of dialysate buffer concentration. In order to explain the different increments of predialytic and postdialytic plasma bicarbonate as a function of buffers donation, it has been suggested that after regenerating the very large pool of titratable (reduced) buffers, bicarbonate tends to accumulate in the extracellular space [16, 33–35]. Moreover, during the intradialytic time, the extracellular compartment behaves as if it were secluded from a second intracellular and bony line of defence, the buffering capacity of which might seem affected by an inertness condition, secondary to an excessive depletion of the titratable $H^+$ ion pool. When acid-base balance is estimated in bicarbonate-dialysis-treated patients, negative values of the $H^+$ ion balance are always found [16, 17, 33–35] in spite of extracellular bicarbonate, disodium phosphate, and metabolizable anion depletion (table 8–3). When buffer concentrations are used in the dialysate as low as 27–32 mmol/l, this result is obtained even if the predialysis and postdialysis plasma bicarbonate concentrations are maintained in the range of acidosis (17–21 mmol/l. table 8–3). Surprisingly, in acetate Redy system dialysis sufficiently high amounts of buffers enter the vascular space to neutralize all the $H^+$ ions given off by protein intakes as high as 1–1.2 g/kg/day, in spite of the acidifying effect of

---

considered together, no correlation can be found between the predialysis and postdialysis values of plasma bicarbonate concentrations. The two subgroups of patients treated with acetate-containing dialysate (A3, B2) were differentiated on the ground of their $PaO_2$ behavior, which sistematically decreased in the A3 group but increased in the B2 group. In the ASPD patients the postdialysis plasma bicarbonate was measured at 1 hour after the end of dialysis. The lower part of the diagram shows the percentage of patients for each group presenting themselves to next dialysis with plasma bicarbonate concentrations under 18 mmol/l. Differences exist only among the percentage of the 3 groups.

*Table 8–3.* Effects of bicarbonate and acetate SPD and RSD on acid-base balance

| | Bicarbonate | | | | | Acetate | |
| --- | --- | --- | --- | --- | --- | --- | --- |
| | SPD | | | | | SPD | RSD |
| $C_{Di}$ mmol/l | 27 | 32 | 37 | 39 | 41 | 38 | 38 |
| $C_{B(o)}$ mmol/l | 17.9 | 17.7 | 21 | 20.2 | 21.2 | 19.0 | 20.5 |
| $C_{B(t)}$ mmol/l | 20.4 | 21.6 | 25.0 | 25.4 | 28 | 23.40 | 22.70 |
| $MH^+$ mmol/min | 0.75 | 1.14 | 1.35 | 1.53 | 1.49 | 0.50 | 1.30 |
| $JHCO_3$ mmol/min | 1.10 | 1.68 | 1.92 | 2.25 | 2.43 | $-3.03$ | $-1.02$ |
| $MH^+/JHCO_3$ | 0.68 | 0.68 | 0.70 | 0.68 | 0.61 | 0.14 | 0.30 |
| $GH^+$ mmol/week | 350 | 350 | 350 | 350 | 350 | 350 | 350 |
| Net $JHCO_3$ mmol/week | 570 | 987 | 1,214 | 1,452 | 1.582 | 240 | 420 |
| $H^+$ balance mmol/week | $-220$ | $-637$ | $-864$ | $-1.102$ | $-1.232$ | $+110$ | $-70$ |

$C_{Di}$ = dialysate buffer concentration at the inlet of the filter; $C_{B(o)}$ = plasma [$HCO_3$] at the beginning of dialysis; $C_{B(t)}$ = plasma [$HCO_3$] at the end of dialysis; $MH^+$: $H^+$ ion neutralization. $JHCO_3$ = $HCO_3$ gain or loss; $MH^+/JHCO_3$ = $H^+$ ion neutralization as a fraction of $HCO_3$ gain or net buffer generation; net $JHCO_3$ = difference between bicarbonate gain and buffer dispersion per week. All the data are expressed as mean values. $MH^+$ and $JCO_3$ have been calculated according to reference [34], for a 65 kg bw patient with a mean ECV of 14.5 and a dialysance for $HCO_3$ of 0.12 l/min., $GH^+$ has been calculated considering the same BW patient on protein diet of 1 g/kg B.W. per day $\times$ 0.77 (34).
SPD = Single pass dialysis; RSD = Redy sistem dialysis.

the regenerative cartridge, in addition to the other aforementioned factors of buffer depletion (table 8–3). On the contrary, acetate single pass dialysis proves unequal to facing $H^+$ ion accumulation, even at protein intakes as low as 0.16 g/kg BW per day. Nevertheless the level of predialytic acidosis in these subjects is not different from that found in patients treated with dialysate buffer concentrations under 35 mmol/l. (table 8–3; figure 8–5).

*Respiratory aspects of acetate and bicarbonate short dialysis: general considerations*

Acetate dialysis can be considered as a $CO_2$ consuming process, since acetate to acetyl CoA activation causes the dissolved form of carbon dioxide to become bicarbonate [8, 12] thanks to titratable $H^+$ ion pool depletion; moreover, in the single pass delivery system not only is the newly generated bicarbonate lost but also dissolved $CO_2$ is dissipated, even if in small amounts (0.12–0.2 mmol/min) [12, 22, 24], because the acetate-containing dialysate is

210

not provided with dissolved $CO_2$. On the contrary, bicarbonate dialysis can be considered a $CO_2$ donor process, not only because $\sim 70\%$ of bicarbonate which enters the extracellular space is converted to $CO_2$ as a consequence of $H^+$ ions titration [17, 34] but also because $CO_2$ is present in the dialysis bath at sufficiently high concentration so as not only to oppose $CO_2$ dispersion from the blood, but also to spread into the plasma from the dialysate [12, 29–31, 36–39]. Both acetate and bicarbonate dialysis tend to increase plasma bicarbonate concentration, causing a more or less important amount of alkalosis that is able by itself to cause hypoventilation [5, 32, 36]. The consequence of these various factor interactions on ventilatory activity cannot be easily foreseen. It is well known that $PaO_2$ decreases during ASPD, but is kept constant or increases during ARSD [12, 18, 23, 25, 31, 37]. Moreover, contradictory effects on $PaO_2$ are reported with BSPD, but not with BRSD, where $PaO_2$ necessarily increases with time [5, 12, 29, 31, 33, 36]. We have investigated the $PaO_2$ variations in 6 groups of patients treated with BSPD using different dialysate buffer and $CO_2$ concentrations and 3 groups of patient under ASPD with dialysate containing 38 mmol/l of acetate, without $CO_2$. At the same time pH, $HCO_3$, and $PaCO_2$ were measured in arterial blood. In all, 514 measurements of these parameters were randomly performed, half before and half at the end of dialysis. When the mean values for $PaO_2$ were considered as the dependent variable in a multiple linear regression analysis, in which a.pH, a.[$HCO_3$] and $PaCO_2$ were the independent variables, the following equation was found:

$$PaO_2 = 0.87\ PaCO_2 + 49\ pH - 2.37\ a[HCO_3] - 260 \qquad (8.7)$$

where $F = 6.63$; D.F. 3/14; $p < 0.01$. The standardized coefficients demonstrated the following values: a[$HCO_3$] = 1.51; $PaCO_2$ = 0.57; a.pH = 0.004. It was also calculated that 37% of the total $PaO_2$ variability (deviance) was explained by [$HCO_3$]; 22% by $PaCO_2$; 41% was explained by other unknown factors. It was also evident that arterial blood pH had no independent effect on the $PaO_2$ variations. A clear effect of the dialysate $CO_2$ variations on $PaO_2$ is obtained in ARSD, where $PaO_2$ drops during the first 30 minutes of dialysis, when $CO_2$ concentration in the recirculating dialysate is very low, but increases thereafter together with the dialysate $PCO_2$ values [12, 18, 31]. If $CO_2$ is bubbled into the dialysis bath of ASPD, so that $PCO_2$ may be obtained as high as 160 mmHg, high $PaO_2$ is also found [39] without any drop during dialysis, if dialysate $PCO_2$ is kept high too [12, 29–31, 36–40]. It has been demonstrated that high $PaO_2$ values in patients treated with $CO_2$ containing dialysates are hyperventilation-mediated effects [12, 31, 40]. On the contrary, when $PaO_2$ decreases during dialysis (a well-known finding in ASPD and in low $CO_2$ − high bicarbonate − SPD), lower than normal minute ventilation is always found [23, 25, 36, 38, 41–44]. *Ventilatory activity and acetyl CoA utilization during dialysis.* After exogenous acetate to acetyl-CoA activation, the pool of acetyl-CoA expands [21]. At the same time acetate generation from the endogenous sources is slowed down [21], unless it enters the Krebs cycle [KC] to be oxydized to $H_2O$ and $CO_2$, or is alternatively utilized by other metabolic pathways [21]. If acetyl CoA enters the KC an increase in $O_2$ consumption ($\dot{V}O_2$) and $CO_2$ generation ($\dot{V}CO_2$) of the same magnitude takes place, since acetate RQ is 1. Of course, the possibility of acetate entering the Krebs cycle depends on the energy balance of the patient in that moment, i.e., on the Pi + AMP/ATP ratio [21]. It is worth noting that during dialysis the high dialysate $CO_2$-dependent hyperventilation is also accompanied by a significant increase in $\dot{V}O_2$ [31, 38, 40, 43, 44], that is generally not evident when dialysate is lacking in $CO_2$ [36, 38, 40, 43, 44]. It has also been shown that $O_2$ consumption is greater when acetate rather than bicarbonate is used in the dialysate [31, 37, 45]. In condition of acetate repletion, an increment of $O_2$ consumption must be referred to a consensual increase of KC activity [21]. The intradialytic rising of $\dot{V}O_2$ therefore suggests a greater performance of the Krebs cycle, causing a larger production of $CO_2$ that opposes dissolved $CO_2$ depletion due to bicarbonate generation. Since 1 mol of acetyl CoA gives rise to 2 mol of $CO_2$ in the KC, only 1.6 mmol must enter the KC of the 3.5 produced per unit time, for amounts of $CO_2$ to be generated, able to compensate not only for the dissolved $CO_2$ shifted to bicarbonate (3.0 mmol/min) but also for the amount of $CO_2$ lost through the dialyzer (0.2 mmol/min). If this manner of reasoning is correct, then one cannot understand how an increased consumption of $O_2$ during dialysis may be considered as a cause of hypoxemia, as is generally said [30, 37, 41, 46]. The relation between ventilatory and metabolic activity is expressed by the respiratory quotient RQ ($\dot{V}CO_2/\dot{V}O_2$), when an equilibrium situation is operating. However, when a condition of nonequilibrium exists, only a respiratory exchange ration, R, can be measured ($\dot{V}CO_2 \pm \triangle \dot{V}CO_2/\dot{V}O_2$). It is evident that during dialysis a condition of $-\triangle \dot{V}CO_2$ is operating, due to dissolved $CO_2$ both shifting to bicarbonate and diffusing out of the blood [12]. Therefore, when acetate to acetyl CoA conversion is taking place and, at the same time, hyperventilation is induced, one would expect the RQ to increase, due to acetyl-CoA oxydation, but the R ratio to decrease with respect to the predialytic values due to bicarbonate from $CO_2$ generation. In fact, it can be observed that $\dot{V}O_2$ may change from 10 to 16 mmol/min and $\dot{V}CO_2$ from 8.6 to 10 mmol/min after the beginning of dialysis, while ventilatory exchange ratio reduces from 0.86 to 0.63 [31]. Given an RQ of 1 for acetate, $\dot{V}CO_2$ would have increased from 8.6 to 14.6 mmol/min. if we admit that $\dot{V}O_2$ has increased for only acetate to be oxydized. The difference in $\dot{V}CO_2$ (14.6 − 10 = 4.6 mmol/min) between the expected and the actual value, is given by bicarbonate generation plus $CO_2$ elimination with dialyzer. Hyperventilation, therefore, can be attributed to the absolute increment in dissolved $CO_2$ delivered to the lungs equal to 1.4 (10 − 8.6) mmol/min) [47, 48]. An interesting relationship between the rate of $O_2$ consumption and the kinetics of acetate utilization is suggested by the higher values of Vmax observed in ARSD-treated patients, when compared with the same parameter in ASPD-treated subjects (table 8−1). This difference in Vmax values can be attributed to an increased performance of

212

tricarboxylic acid cycle, that opposes the acetyl CoA pool expansion, making free coenzyme A available for a swifter acetate to acetyl CoA activation [21]. It is known, in fact, that the limiting step in the rate of acetate activation is the amount of free coenzyme A available for the reaction [21]. This effect can be inferred from the very small or absent increment of bicarbonate concentrations, measured at one hour after the end of dialysis: which suggests that very low acetate concentrations are attained in the plasma even during ASPD, provided high $CO_2$ tension is present in the dialysate and high levels of $PCO_2$ in venous blood are found, together with high $PaO_2$, $\dot{V}O_2$ and $\dot{V}CO_2$ values [12, 40]. It has been stated that the level of KC performance depends on the energy balance for each subject at a particular moment, which explains why in some patients $\dot{V}O_2$ goes up under acetate load, while in others $\dot{V}O_2$ remains constant or is even reduced [25, 36, 38, 40, 43, 44]. However, what is really worth noting is that even small amounts of dissolved $CO_2$, that gain the plasma from the dialysis bath and are not able to compensate for its metabolic consumption, are able to cause hyperventilation. In fact in cases of ASPD, where $PCO_2$ as high as 140–160 mmHg was present in the dialysate, bicarbonate was lost through the dialyzer at a rate of 3 mmol/min, while only 1 mmol/min of dissolved $CO_2$ spread from the dialysate into the blood. This notwithstanding, the patients were hyperventilating from the beginning of dialysis (preliminary obstervations). The problem of hyperventilation, there-fore, cannot be solved only in terms of $CO_2$ balance, but also of distrectual $CO_2$ concentration [12, 31, 38, 40]. In conditions of negative balance of dissolved $CO_2$ the increased tension of $CO_2$ in the venous blood coming from the dialyzer operates as an exciting factor for hyperventilation that persists thereafter due to the excess of endogenous $CO_2$ production. Faced with a near zero total $CO_2$ balance at the level of dialyzer, the ventilatory elimina-tion of $CO_2$ increased from $182.7 \pm 48.4$ to $246.7 \pm 72.7$ ml/min after the beginning of dialysis in a group of ASPD patients treated with $CO_2$ enriched dialysates [39]. Leaving aside the delivery of exogenous $CO_2$ able to induce hyperventilation, one asks why patients who, a few minutes before, did not demonstrate the need to have their own energy supply restored, must increase oxygen consumption and what fate awaits the energy given off.

*Relationship between ventilatory variations and functional integrity of the lungs*

If it is accepted that dialysis hypoxemia is caused by pulmonary diffuse microembolization due to nonbiocompatible dialyzer membranes [37, 49], an increment of minute ventilation would be expected [25] as a compensatory mechanism for $AaDO_2$ gradient increase [37, 50]. In fact, an increment in alveolar-arterial $O_2$ diffusion gradient ($AaDO_2$) has seldom been found when cellulosic nonbiocompatible membranes have been utilized [37, 44, 50]. Yet, even in these latter cases a minute ventilation decrease was present [44, 50], which demonstrates how little the importance of this phenomenon is as a cause of dialysis hypoxemia. Another observation which testifies to the functional integrity of the lungs during dialysis is that $PaO_2$ increases significantly when the patients assume a sitting from supine posture: this suggests a reduced driving force for ventilation. In fact, we have found that during dialysis $PaO_2$ increased from $80 \pm 16$ mmHg to $87 \pm 12$ mmHg, and pH from $7.409 \pm 0.04$ to $7.43 \pm 0.51$ while $PaCO_2$ decreased from $35.5 \pm 4.2$ to $33.6 \pm 4.4$ mmHg, when the patients changed from the supine to the sitting position (m $\pm$ sd; D.F. 37; $p < 0.001$). This interpretation is also supported by a reduced VT/TI (tidal volume/inspiratory time = mean inspiratory flow) taken as an index of ventilatory driving force [50]. However, since complement activation, leucocyte, and platelet aggregation are clearly demonstrated phenomena of early dialysis [37, 49–53], a further hypothesis might be suggested, that the substances released from leucocyte aggregation depresses the activity of respiratory centers and/or respiratory chemoreceptors in the lungs [47, 48], adding this type of inhibitory effect to that of dissolved $CO_2$ depletion. In particular, the early hypoventilation during the first 15–30 minutes of dialysis would be better justified [54]. In support of a depression tendency for the respiratory and vasomotory centers, particularly in old patients, are the data of a recent and interesting investigation in a group of old dialyzed people, who demonstrated that they were particularly prone to symptomatic hypotension during standard ASPD, using cuprophan dialyzers [55]. These patients were characterized by predialytic $PaO_2$ significantly lower than that found in an age-matched group of patients, who did not suffer intradialytic symptomatic hypotension ($PaO_2$ $79.3 \pm 2.1 < 98.3 \pm 2.4$ mmHg, as predialytic values in the hypotensive and normal group; $p < 0.001$). During dialysis $PaO_2$ decreased in both groups with the same fractional rate constant, so that at the end of dialysis the $PaO_2$ values were not statistically different ($72.9 \pm 3.8 \simeq 82.6 \pm 3.3$; m $\pm$ s.e.) in the two groups. No difference was found in predialysis and postdialysis $PaCO_2$ levels, as if less $CO_2$ were given off in the hypoxemic group. When 100% $O_2$ was administered to the hypotensive group so as to correct hypoxemia, no improvement was found in the frequency of hypotensive attacks. As noted above, these data may suggest an inertness status for the respiratory and vasomotory centers, worsened by the metabolic deprivation of dissolved $CO_2$ and maybe $O_2$ administration, and one asks what would happen if high concentrations of exogenous $CO_2$ were administered in the dialysate to such patients, not so much as ventilatory activity is concerned but rather vasomotory stability. To conclude the topic, it is worth noting that the well-known antihypotensive effect of low temperature [56, 57] appears as effective in improving dialysis associated hypoxemia [58], perhaps by enhancing both the vasomotory and respiratory center activity.

*Interdialytic Variations of A–B status: the problem of extrarenal bicarbonate set-point*

It has been shown that the $H^+$ ions, given off by metabolic processes, are not completely eliminated by standard acetate single pass dialysis (ASPD) in most cases, so that a more or less positive $H^+$ ion balance takes place (table 8–3). On the contrary, even if with dialysis bicarbonate concentrations as low as 27–32 mmol/l, a constantly negative balance is shown (table 8–3). In spite of that, the patients present themselves for the following dialysis in conditions, that may be of strong, mild, or no acidosis (figure 8–5). Moreover, no correlation can be found between acid generation, postdialysis plasma bicarbonate concentration, and the level of predialysis acidosis, provided that the patients are not treated with high bicarbonate concentrations in the dialysate (figure 8–5) (predialysis plasma bicarbonate concentration versus PCR × 0.77; r = 0.177; patients n° 14; determinations n° 40; p = n.s.). It is also worth noting that wide variations in the predialytic plasma bicarbonate values can be frequently observed with time in the same patient [17] without any important dietary or dialysis schedule modification. The conclusion is that the different degrees of predialysis acidosis cannot be simply attributed to fluctuations in endogenous acid production as well as in the amount of buffer delivered [17]. In other words, it appears as if the urnemic well-compensated dialysis patients were able to maintain their own A-B status, opposing any exogenous either alkalinizing or acidifying factor. Such behavior is consistent with the presence of an equilibrium concentration (set-point) for bicarbonate in the extracellular fluid compartment, that is under nonrenal, nondialysis control factors [15]. As previously stated and generally speaking, A-B set-point can be interpreted as an amount of titratable acid and conversely, of titratable (basic) buffers per unit of volume at which the rates of $H^+$ generation and disposition balance each other [15, 59, 60]. Set-point can be considered genetically determined and controlled by a network of hormonal and metabolic agents that operate at the level of the kidney, intestine, bone, etc [61–63]. The same concept is valid for plasma and bony fluid Ca concentration and for its homeostatic system [65]. The less efficient this apparatus as a whole, the more $H^+$ ion bulk must expand in order for the $H^+$ ion excess to be irreversibly eliminated. While uremia causes the pool to expand, dialysis reduces it, not so much by loading the patients with buffers as by curing the metabolic derangement of uraemic intoxication. Since the daily $H^+$ generation can be considered small in comparison with its titratable pool [16, 17, 34, 64], the buffers delivered by dialysis are able to neutralize only a very small fraction of it and for only a very short time. This fact can be recognized by a slope for predialysis increase of plasma bicarbonate concentration 3 times slower than that for postdialysis bicarbonate increase (figure 8–4). All recognize that a second line of A-B defense is represented by bone [62, 65–68]. It should be for this reason that the bone of uremic dialyzed patients contains a reduced buffer concentration in its internal fluids (bone minicirculation) [67–69] as if it were an inert reservoir of buffer, for $H^+$ ion neutralyzation. On the contrary, the lining cells of bone make a living barrier between the minicirculation of bone and extracellular fluid, so that their electrolyte distribution and concentration are quite different, with bicarbonate and pH being far higher inside the bone (bicarbonate ~800 versus 24 mmol/l and pH 8.8 versus 7.40) [65, 69, 70]. A prerequisite of bone turnover is that of renewing bone phosphate and carbonate by eliminating from the inside of it $H^+$ ions in exchange for extracellular $Ca^{++}$, $Mg^{++}$, $Na^+$, $K^+$, etc., so as to obtain bicarbonate and carbonate, dibasic and neutral phosphate from carbonic and phosphoric acids [65, 70]. The discarded $H^+$ will be thereafter eliminated from the extracellular space by the kidney, which is why in growing children the urinary net acid excretion can attain 3 mmol/kg per day instead of 1 mmol/kg as in adult populations [71]. It is this activity that couples bone accretion and A-B regulation, that is under the control of the calciotropic hormones, such as active vitamin D metabolites and PTH [62, 65]. It as been demonstrated that $H^+$ ions enter the internal space of bone in exchange for calcium in order that extracellular buffer can be regenerated under the control of vitamin D and PTH, too [69, 72–74]. In fact, nephrectomized animals are killed by acid loads, only if previously para-thyroidectomized or treated with vitamin D poisons [73, 74]. Also in uremic patients, the buffering capacity of bone is probably inadequate since, besides the deranging effect of uremia by itself, active vitamin D availability is reduced or absent in its dihydroxilated form, causing secondary PTH hypersecretion [75]. In this condition the calcemic and alkalemic vitamin D and PTH-mediated effects appear inversely related to the entity of the osteomalacic component of uremic osteodystrophy [15, 70, 76]. Since osteomalacic-bone-cell activity is blunted as far as both bone mineral accretion and A-B regulation are concerned, the reduced buffer reservoir of bone in uremic dialyzed patients might be interpreted as if the set-point for bone fluid bicarbonate concentration were put at a lower value. In conditions of serious vitamin D depletion, PTH hypersecretion seems to cause the paradoxic effect of worsening metabolic acidosis as can be demostrated by the rapid improvement of acidosis after the hyperplastic PTH secreting glands have been removed in both uremic and nonuremic renal-patients [77, 78]. Since 1976 we have had the opportunity to observe the prompt and significant increase in predialytic plasma $HCO_3$ concentration even without or before any variation of serum calcium, induced by vitamin D administration [60, 70, 79, 80]. The types and amounts of vitamin D subsequently used were: vitamin $D_2$, $4 \times 10^5$ U/day per 3–4 days, followed by $4 \times 10^5$ U every 2–4 weeks; 25-OH-$D_3$, 50–100 $\mu$g/day; AT 10, 0.16–0.5 $\mu$g/day; 1–25 $OH_2D_3$, 0.25–0.50 $\mu$g/day. There was no difference as to the effects obtained with the various kinds of vitamin D. Moreover, the effect lasted as long as vitamin D was administered (table 8–4 and figure 8–6) [79, 80]. With time also serum Ca increased, while PTH decreased (table 8–4). The lower the serum Ca and bicarbonate were found to be before dialysis, the greater the increment of both after vitamin D, particularly when situations of osteomalacic bone disease were apparent [79, 80]. In some cases predialytic bicarbonate was as high as 26–28 mmol/l, starting from about 15 mmol/l, and was kept constant in spite of the depleting effect of dialysis (figure 8–6). This behavior was also shared by some of the most serious hyperparathyroid patients who, after

216

*Table 8–4.* At 10 effects (0.5–0.16 mg/day for 6 months) on predialysis values of CA and S-(HCO₃) PL.

|  | Before | After |
| --- | --- | --- |
| S-(Ca)mg/dl | $8.74 \pm 0.88$ | $9.72 \pm 0.62$*** |
| S-(PO4)mg/dl | $4.03 \pm 0.64$ | $3.86 \pm 0.63$* |
| S-(PTH)ng/ml | $3.27 \pm 2.31$ | $1.92 \pm 2.70$** |
| S-(HCO)mEq/l | $17.25 \pm 1.34$ | $21.20 \pm 2.37$*** |

t test for paired data *** $p < 0.001$, ** $p < 0.01$, * $p < 0.05$.
From reference [80]. With permission of the publisher.

parathyroid glands ablation, entered the following dialysis with plasma bicarbonate far higher than those observed at 1 hour after the end of the preceeding dialysis (unpublished data). Of course, neither the dialysis schedule nor dietary composition nor urea-generation rate were modified. That a dialysis-independent set-point for extracellular bicarbonate concentration does exist in uremic patients is also proved by the significant decrease in serum Ca and $HCO_3$ concentration that acetazolamide can induce together with an increment in PTH secretion [81, 82]. The effect is promtly reversed, within days, by drug withdrawal [82]. This demonstrates that the calcemic and

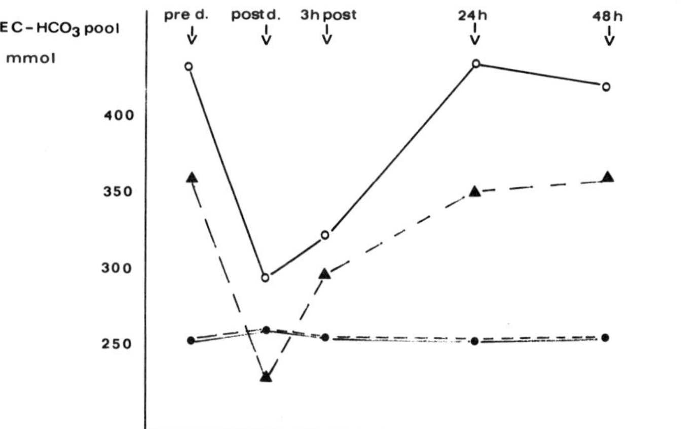


*Figure 8–6.* The vitamin D effects on the extrarenal setpoint of plasma bicarbonate concentration. In a patient who started dialysis with serum bicarbonate of 14 mmol/l and a pool of 250 mmol (*lower line*), the administration of vitamin D₂ at 60x ×10³ u/day made the predialysis serum bicarbonate rise to 21 mmol/l and the extracellular pool to 350 mmol (mid line). Subsequently, the administration of 250H, 100 μg/day, increased the predialytic plasma bicarbonate concentration to 26 mmol/l (*upper line*). In spite of the depletive effect of dialysis (ASPD), the generation system sensitized by the hormone rapidly reconstituted the extracellular bicarbonate to the predialysis values, proving that a setpoint for extracellular bicarbonate was operating independently of any renal or dialysis influence. (From reference [15]; with permission of the publisher.

217

alkalemic effect of PTH is operating in the uremic patients, at least when they have normal or near normal values of predialysis serum bicarbonate concentrations. The concomitant increase of serum Ca and $HCO_3$ concentration and the improvement of osteoid mineralization, secondary to carbonate and neutral phosphate generation and accumulation, clearly indicate that a common mechanism of $H^+$ ion disposition underlies, that is activated by vitamin D even in the absence of any kidney function [15, 65, 80]. This means that plasma bicarbonate does not increase at the expense of bony buffer, nor does the latter at the expense of plasma bicarbonate since both of them increase. What fate may await the excess of $H^+$ ions that must be disposed is not known, but it is clearly apparent that an irreversible elimination of them does exist, independent of any kidney function or dialysis buffering efficiency.

## References


1. Hoenich, N., Frost, T.H., Kerr, D.N.S. (1978) Dialysers. In *Replacement of Renal Function of Dialysis*, William Drukker, Frank Parsons and Johan Maher (eds.) The Hague-Boston-London: Martinus Nijhoff Medical Division, pp. 80–124.
2. Parsons, F.M. and Davison, A.M. (1978) The composition of dialysis fluid. In *Replacement of Renal Function by Dialysis*; William Drukker. Frank Parsons and Johan Maher (eds.). The Hague Boston-London: Martinus Nijhoff Medical Division, pp. 162–171.
3. Drukker, W., Jungerius, N. and Albert, C. (1967) Report on regular dialysis treatment in Europe. III Proc. Eur. Dial. Transplant. Ass. 4: 3–9.
4. Tolchin, N., Roberts, J.L., Hayashi, J. and Lewis, E.J. (1977) Metabolic consequences of high mass. transfer hemodialysis. Kidney Internat. 2: 366–378.
5. Graefe, U., Milutinovich, J., Follette, W.C., Vizzo, E.J., Babb, A.L. and Scribner, B.H. (1978). Less-dialysis-induced morbidity and vascular instability with bicarbonate in dialysate. Ann. Intern. Med. 88: 332–336.
6. Locatelli, E., Pedrini, L., Costanzo, R., Di Filippo, S., Marai, P., Pozzi, C. and Bonacina, G. (1981) Longterm hemodialysis treatment with sodium removal by convection. Proc. Eur. Dial. Transplant. Ass. 18: 146–151.
7. Locatelli, F., Pedrini, L., Ponti, R., Costanzo, R., Di Filippo, S., Marai, P., Pozzi, C. and Bonacina, G. (1982). "Physiological" and "pharmacological" dialysate sodium concentrations. Int. J. Artif. Organs 5: 17–24.
8. Mioni, G., Mombelloni, S., Cristinelli, L. and Panzetta, G. (1977) Kinetics of Bicarbonate from acetate generation during dialysis: metabolic aspects and energy balance. Kidney Internat. Abstract Italian Soc. Nephrol. Ancona 13: 4, 333.
9. Vreman, H.J., Assomul, U.M., Kaiser, B.A., Blaschke, T.F. and Weiner, M.W. (1980) Acetate metabolism and acid-base homeostasis during hemodialysis: influence of dialyser efficiency and rate of acetate metabolism. Kidney Internat. 18: S.62–S.64.
10. Lewis, E.J., Tolchin, N. and Roberts, J. (1980) Estimation of the metabolic conversion of acetate to bicarbonate during hemodialysis. Kidney Internat. 18: S.51–S.55.
11. Kaiser, B.A., Potter, D.E., Bryant, R.E., Vreman, H.J. and Weiner, M.W. (1981) Acidbase changes and acetate metabolism during routine and high efficiency hemodialysis in children. Kidney Internat. 19: 70–79.
12. Mioni, G., Gropuzzo, M., Favazza, A., Messa, P., Montanaro, D., Adorati, M., Paviotti, G., Messa, M. and Lo Greco, P. (1982) La reazione di ativazione dell'acetato nel trattamento emodialitico. Minerva Nefrol. 29: 137–150.
13. Mioni, G., Gropuzzo, M., Messa, P. and Montanaro, D. (1981) La regolazione dell'equilibrio acido-base nel paziente in uremia terminale. *Attualità Nefrologiche e*


218

*Dialitiche*. Milan, Italy: Wichtig Editore srl, pp. 195–207.

14. Wingert, K.J., Weiner, M.W. (1979) Acetate transfer across membranes of artificial kidneys in vitro. Kidney Internat. 15: 593–600.

15. Mioni, G., Gropuzzo, M., Favazza, A., Mesa, P., Montanaro, D., Adorati, M., Paviotti, G., Antonucci, F., Lo Greco, P., (1983) Pathophysiology of acid-base balance. In *Chronic Renal Failure, Uraemic Acidosis and Extracorporeal Treatment. Proceedings of the Milan Workshop 1981*. Milan, Italy: Wichtig Editore srl, pp. 19–39.

16. Ward, A.R., Wathen, R.L. (1982) Utilization of bicarbonate for base repletion in hemodialysis. Artif. Organs 6: 396–403.

17. Gennari, F.J. (1985) Acid-base balance in dialysis patients. Kidney Internat. 28: 678–688.

18. Drukker, W., Parsons, F.M., Gordon, A. (1978) Practical application of dialysate regeneration the Redy system. In *Replacement of Renal Function by Dialysis*, William Drukker, Frank M. Parsons, and John, F. Maher (eds.) The Hague-Boston-London: Martinus Nijhoff Medical Division, pp. 244–258.

19. Cambi, V., Hampl, H., Savazzi, G., Arisi, L., Bignardi, L., Garini, G., Rossi, E., Paeprer, H., Kessel, M., Migone, L. (1978) Principles and clinical application of ultrashort dialysis. Trans. Am. Soc. Artif. Int. Organs 24: 443–449.

20. Orlandini, G.C. (1981) Technical aspect of bicarbonate hemodialysis. In *Uremic Acidosis, Proc. Workshop on Uremic Acidosis*. Milano: Wichtig Editore, pp. 125–134.

21. Siliprandi, N. *Chimica biologica*, 2nd ed., Vol. 1, pp. 233–316; Vol. 2, pp. 66–148. Padova: Piccin Editore.

22. Sargent, J.A., Gotch, F.A. (1980) Mathematical modeling of dialysis the raphy. Kidney Internat. 18: S-2–S-10.

23. Aurigemma, N.M., Feldman, N.T., Gottlieb, M., Igram, R.H., Lazarus, J.M., Lowrie, E.G. (1977) Arterial oxygenation during hemodialysis. N. Engl. J. Med. 207: 871–873.

24. Sargent, J.A., Gotch, F.A. (1979) Bicarbonate and carbon dioxide/transport during hemodialysis. Asajo J. 2: 61–71.

25. Dolan, M.J., Whipp, B.J., Davidson, W.D., Weitzman, R.E., Wassermann, K. (1981) Hypopnea associated with acetate hemodialysis: carbon dioxide-flow-dependent ventilation. N. Engl. J. Med. 305: 72–75.

26. Alloatti, S., Nebiolo, P.E., Garneri, G., Gaiter, A., Giacchino, F., (1985) Bicarbonate transport during acetate and bicarbonate dialysis. G. Ital. Nefrol. 2: 103–108.

27. Skutches, C.L., Sigler, M.H., Teehan, B.P., Cooper, J.H., Reichard, G.H. (1983) Contribution of dialysate acetate energy metabolism: metabolic implications. Kidney Internat. 23: 57–63.

28. Sigler, M.H., Skutches, C.L., Teehan, B.P., Cooper, J.H., Reichard, G.H. (1983) Acetate and energy metabolism during hemodialysis. Kidney Internat. 24: S-97–S-101.

29. Tolchin, N., Roberts, I.L., Lewis, E.J. (1978) Respiratory gas exchange by high efficiency hemodialyzers. Nephron 21: 137–145.

30. Nissenson, A.R. (1980) Prevention of dialysis-induced hypoxemia by bicarbonate dialysis. Trans. Am. Soc. Artif. Intern. Organs 26: 339–342.

31. Rohmer, D., Nassry, M., Sherlock, J., Letteri, J., Ledwith, J. (1981) A comparison of the respiratory dynamics during hemodialysis using acetate and bicarbonate dialysate in a sorbent regenerative system. Trans. Am. Soc. Artif. Intern. Organs 27: 167–179.

32. Beckman, Astra (TM). Automated stat/routine analyzer system. Carbon dioxide chemistry measurement module, p. 2-1–10-1. Operating instructions 015-55559.

33. Ahmad, S., Pagel, M., Vizzo, J., Scribner, B.H. (1980) Effect of the normalization of acid-basa balance on postdialysis plasma bicarbonate. Trans. Am. Soc. Artif. Intern. Organs 26: 318–321.

34. Gotch, F.A., Sargent, J.A., Keen, M.L. (1982) Hydrogen ion balance in dialysis therapy. Artificial Organs 6: 388–395.

35. Man, N.K., Fournier, G., Thirean, P., Gaillard, J.L., Funck-Brentano, J.L. (1982) Effect of bicarbonate-containing dialysate on chronic hemodialysis patients: a comparative study. Artificial Organs 6: 421–425.

36. Hunt, J.M., Chappel, T.R., Henrich, W.L., Rubin, L.W. (1984) Gas exchange during dialysis. Amer. J. Med. 77: 255–260.

37. Burns, C.B., Scheinhorn, D.J. (1982) Hypoxemia during dialysis. Arch. Intern. Med. 12: 1350–1353.

38. Vaziri, N.D., Wilson, A., Mukai, D., Darwish, R., Rutz, A., Hyatt, J., Moreno, C. (1984) Dialysis hypoxemia. Amer. J. Med. 77: 828–833.

39. Romaldini, H., Stabile-Neto, C., Faro, S., Santos, M.L., Ramos, O.L., Ratto, O.R. (1982) Pulmonary ventilation during hemodialysis. Nephron 32: 131–134.

40. Faro, S., Stabile, C., Santos, M.L., Romaldini, H., Ratto, O.R. (1985) Central venous blood composition and the pulmonary ventilation during hemodialysis. Nephron 41: 45–49.

41. Raja, R.M., Kramer, M.S., Rosembaun, J.L., Bolisay, C.G., Krug, M.J. (1981) Hemodialysis associated hypoxemia. Role of acetate and pH in etiology. Trans. Am. Soc. Artif. Intern. Organs 27: 180–183.

42. Heineman, H.O., Goldring, R.M. (1974) Bicarbonate and the regulation of ventilation. Amer. J. Med. 57: 361–370.

43. Patterson, R.W., Nissenson, A.R., Miller, J., Smith, R.T., Narins, R.G., Sullivan, S.F. (1981) Hypoxemia and pulmonary gas exchange during hemodialysis. J. Appl. Physiol. 50: 259–264.

44. Igarashi, H., Kioi, S., Gejyo, F., Arakawa, M., (1985) Physiologic approach to dialysis-induced hypoxemia. Nephron 41: 62–69.

45. Eiser, A.R., Jayamanne, D., Kokosong, C., Che, H., Slifking, R.F., Neff, M.S. (1980) Contrasting alteration in oxigen consumption and R.Q. during acetate and bicarbonate hemodialysis (abstract). Am. Soc. Nephrology 13: 38A.

46. Nissenson, A.R., Patterson, R.W., Narins, R.G., Miller, J., Smith, R.T., Sullivan, S.F. (1978) Dialysis induced hypoxemia is due to increased $O_2$ consumption and $CO_2$ dialysance with normal lungs (abstract). Am. Soc. Nephrol. 11: 47A.

47. Stremel, R.W., Huntsman, D.J., Casaburi, R., Whipp, B.J., Wasserman, K. (1978) Control of ventilation during intravenous $CO_2$ loading in awake dog. J. Appl. Physiol. 44(2): 311–316.

48. Phillipson, E.A., Duffin, J., Cooper, J.D. (1981) Critical dependence of respiratory rhythmicity on metabolic $CO_2$ load. J. Appl. Physiol. 50(1): 45–54.

49. Craddock, P.R., Fehr, J., Brigham, K.L., Kronemberg, R.S., Jacob, H.S. (1977) Complement and leucocyte-mediated pulomonary dysfunction in hemodialysis. N. Engl. J. Med. 296: 769–774.

50. De Backer, W.A., Verpooten, G.A., Borgonjou D.J., Vermeire, P.A., Lius, R.R., De Broe, M.E. (1983) Hypoxemia during dialysis effects of different membranes and dialysate compositions. Kidney Intern. 23: 738–743.

51. Jones, R.H., Broadfield, J.B., Parsons, V. (1980) Arterial hypoxemia during hemodialysis for acute renal failure in mechanically ventilated patients: observations and mechanisms. Clin. Nephrol. 14: 18–22.

52. Broutbar, N., Shinaberger, J.H., Miller, J.H., Nachman, M. (1980) Hemodialysis hypoxemia: evaluation of mechanisms utilizing sequential ultrafiltration-dialysis. Nephron 26: 96–99.

53. Jacob, A.J., Gavellas, G., Zarco, R., Perez, G., Bourgoignie, J.J. (1980) Leucopenia, hypoxia and complement function with different hemodialysis membranes. Kidney Intern. 18: 505–509.

54. Hachim, R.M., Lowrie, E.G. (1982) Hemodialysis associated neutropenia and hypoxemia: the effect of dialyzer membrane materials. Nephron 32: 32–39.

55. Fujiwara, Y., Hagihara, B., Yamauchi, A., Shirai, D. (1985) Hypoxemia and hemodialysis-induced symptomatic hypotension. Clin. Nephrol. 24: 9–14.

56. Maggiore, Q., Pizzarelli, F., Zoccali, C., Sisca, S., Nicolò, F., Parlongo, S. (1981) Effect of extracorporeal blood coaling on dialytic arterial hypotension. Proc. Eur. Dial. Transplant. Assoc. 18: 597–599.

57. Maggiore, Q., Pizzarelli, F., Sisca, S., Zoccali, C., Parlongo, S., Nicolò, F., Creazzo, G.

(1982) Blood temperature and vascular stability during hemodialysis and hemofiltration. Trans. Am. Soc. Artif. Intern. Organs 28: 523–525.

58. Raja, R., Kramer, M., Alvis, R., Goldstein, S., De Los Angeles, A. (1984) Effect of varying dialysate temperature on hemodialysis hypoxemia. Trans. Amer. Soc. Artif. Intern. Organs 30: 15–17.

59. Mioni, G., Castellani, A., Cecchettin, M., Maiorca, R., Heynen, G., Franchimont, P., (1975a) A-B status and parathyroid hormone in dialyzed patients. Lancet i: 605.

60. Mioni, G., Castellani, A., Cecchettin, M., Maiorca, R., Heynen, G., Franchimont, P. (1976a) Acid-base status and parathyroid hormone in dialyzed patients. Lancet i: 812.

61. Engel, K., Kildeberg, P. (1977) Physiological view point on clinical acid-base diagnostics. Scand. J. Clin. Lab. Invest. 37: 21–26.

62. Hulter, H.N. (1985) Effects and interrelationships of PTH, Ca, vit D and Pi in acid-base homeostasis. Amer. J. Physiol. 284: F739–F752.

63. Hulter, H.N., Sigala, J.F., Sebastian, A. (1981) Effects of dexamethasone on renal and systemic acid-base metabolism. Kidney Internat. 20: 43–49.

64. Ward, R.A., Wathen, R.L., Williams, T.E. (1982) Effects of long-term bicarbonate hemodialysis (BHD) on acid-base status. Trans. Am. Soc. Artif. Intern. Organs 28: 295–298.

65. Parfitt, A.M., Kleerekoper, M. The divalent ion homeostatic system-physiology and metabolism of calcium-phosphorus, magnesium and bone. In *Clinical Disorders of Fluid and Electrolyte Metabolism*, 3rd ed., Morton H. Maxwell and Charles R. Kleeman (eds.) New York: McGraw-Hill Book Company, pp. 269–398.

66. Goodman, A.B., Leman, J.JR., Lennon, E.J., Relman, A.S. (1965) Production, excretion and net balance of fixed acid in patients with renal acidosis. J. Clin. Invest. 44: 495–506.

67. Bettice, J.A. (1984) Skeletal carbon dioxide stores during metabolic acidosis. Amer. J. Physiol. 247: F326–F330.

68. Pellegrino, E.D., Biltz, R.M. (1965) The composition of human bone in uremia. Medicine 44: 397–418.

69. Biltz, R., Pellegrino, E.D., Letteri, J.M. (1981) Skeletal carbonates and acid-base regulation. Mineral Electrolyte Metab. 5: 1–7.

70. Mioni, G. (1984) Aspetti della regolazione extrarenale dell'equilibrio acido-base. In *Progressi Clinici: Medicina*, Vol. 1, n°3. Padova: Piccin Editore, p. 23–36.

71. Sebastian, A., McSherry, E., Morris, R.C. (1976) Metabolic acidosis with special references to renal acidoses. In *The Kidney*, Barry M. Brennen and Floyd C. Rector (eds.) Philadelphia: W.B. Saunders Company, pp. 615–649.

72. Businsky, D.A., Krieger, N.S., Geisser, D.I., Grossman, E.B., Coe, F.L. (1983) Effects of pH on bone calcium and proton fluxes in vitro. Amer. J. Physiol. 245: F204–F209.

73. Fraley, D.S., Adler, S. (1979) An extrarenal role for parathyroid hormone in the disposal of acute acid loads in rats and dogs. J. Clin. Invest. 63: 985–997.

74. Arruda, J.A.L., Alla, V., Rubinstain, H., Cruz-Soto, M., Sabatini, S., Battle, D.C., Kurtzman, N.A. (1982) Metabolic and hormonal factors influencing extrarenal buffering of an acute acid load. Mineral Electrolyte Metab. 8: 36–43.

75. Avioli, L., Teitelbaum, S.L. (1976) Renal osteodistrophy. In *Disease of the Kidney*, Barry M. Brenner and Floyd R. Rector (eds.) Philadelphia: W.B. Saunders Company, pp. 1542.

76. Cochran, M., Nordin, B.E.C. (1969) Role of acidosis in renal osteomalacia. Brit. Med. J. 2: 276–279.

77. Muldowney, F.P., Carroll, D.V., Donohoe, J.F. and Freaney, R.F. (1971) Correction of bicarbonate wastage by parathyroidectomy. Q.J. Med. 40: 487–498.

78. Muldowney, F., Donohoe, J., Carroll, D., Powell, D., Freaney, R.F. (1972) Parathyroid acidosis in uraemia. Q.J. Med. 41: 321–342.

79. Casati, S., Graziani, G., Bellazzi, R., De Vincenzi, A., Araldi, A., Citterio, A., Mioni, G. (1983) Correzione dell'acidosi metabolica nell'uremico cronico in emodialisi periodica con I-25(OH)₂. Abstract XXIV Congress of Italian Society of Nephrology. Chieti 9–11 june.

80. Mioni, G., Messa, P., Favazza, A., Montanaro, D., Adorati, M., Paviotti, G., Antonucci, F.

(1983) Bone tissue metabolism and acid-base status in uraemic patients. In *Mineral Metab. Res. in Italy*, 4. Milano: Wichtig Editore, pp. 69–72.

81. Gomez-Fernarder, P., Sauz, A., Conesa, J., Torre, A., Ortega, O., Sachez-Sichilia, R. (1982) Effect of acetazolamide on hypoxemia during regular hemodialysis (RH). EDTA: 132.

82. De Marchi, S., Cecchin, E. (1986) The influence of Acetazolamide on the extrarenal buffer mechanism in uremia communication the 7th congress of the Italian Society of Mineral metabolism research. Parma. November 1985. In *Mineral Metabolism Research in Italy*, Vol. 6. Milano: Wichtig Editore.

# 9. Modeling dialysis therapy

Peter C. Farrell

It is now well accepted in the dialysis community that properly delivered dialysis therapy is consistent with and can provide long-term patient survival. In actuality, patient survivals of greater than 80% have been obtained during more than a decade of treatment [1]. Similar experiences over 5 or more years are common in dialysis units which have had active hemodialysis programs during the past 15 to 20 years. However, most of these data have been obtained on patients with dialysis times which were a minimum of 4 hours per treatment and extending up to 10 hours [1]. Indeed, there is considerable scepticism when one talks about long-term survival in the context of short-time dialysis [2]. It is important, however, to keep the issue in perspective if we are to have a rational debate about the efficacy of short-time dialysis. First of all we must recognize that we are dealing with a moving target, and in this context the following points are relevant.

1. Demographics are changing drastically; the dialysis population is getting older year by year.

2. Not only older but more fragile patients are being added to dialysis programs, e.g., the proportion of diabetic nephropathy patients is increasing inexorably, particularly in the United States.

3. Technology is changing; within the past 5 years dialyzers have become cheaper, easier to use, and significantly more efficient. They are also less likely to cause problems of any sort, whether due to intradialytic leaks or complement activation (For regenerated cellulose higher clearances are now obtained with smaller surface areas.)

4. There is now a better appreciation of patient nutritional requirements and how this relates to well-being. The connection between net urea generation and dietary protein intake is not only more widely appreciated but it is actually being applied, primarily, as a result of National Dialysis Cooperative Study findings.

5. The importance of improved dialysate composition has also become a topic of widespread interest with changes having occurred in the past few years in sodium concentration (from low to 'high' [~140 mmole/]), there has also been a swing away from acetate to bicarbonate as buffer base in certain instances, and the usefulness of adding dextrose to dialysate is now widely appreciated.

*Vincenzo Cambi (editor) Professor of Nephrology*

© *1987 Martinus Nijhoff Publishing, Boston. ISBN 0-89838-858-9. Printed in The United States.*

6. Since the work of Gotch and associates [3] there has been a growing interest in the application of urea kinetic modeling to aid in the selection of individualized dialysis times. At the same time, kinetic modeling has also been applied to heparin [4] and other extracorporeal procedures [5]. Although the use of kinetics cannot yet be considered widespread, it is gradually becoming accepted, and this has certainly resulted in better treatment. The reason is simple; what gets measured gets done, and patients benefit from closer attention to the delivery of therapy.

In short, with older and more fragile patients being added to dialysis programs, and with continuing changes occurring in the technology of therapy delivery, we are faced with great difficulties in interpreting the impact of shortening dialysis times on either morbidity or mortality. The two known boundary conditions are however, fixed: first, patients with inadequately functioning kidneys can be kept alive for many years on dialysis, and second, if these patients are not dialyzed, they will die within 1 to 2 weeks. Having said this, for the patient on dialysis, it is clearly the level of morbidity that matters on a day-to-day basis, and to be able to quantify the optimal dose of dialysis is of considerable importance. On this basis we should be talking less about short-time dialysis and more about individualization of dialysis therapy. Experience suggests that this approach, if based on a rational application of kinetic modeling, will result in reduced time on dialysis, as initially demonstrated by Gotch and associates in 1976 [3]. However, the important fact for this approach to work is that assumptions in kinetic modeling must be rational and supportable, and the results of the approach in terms of patient well-being must be both realizable and defendable. However, there is one important caveat that must temper expectations: patient mortality is much more likely to be controlled by the disease process itself rather than by the quality of the treatment.


**Modeling concepts**

Whereas thermodynamics refers to a study of equilibrium states, kinetics refers to the rates at which these states are reached. And it can be presumed that unless one understands how rapidly a system changes, one's understanding of the system is quite limited. By analogy to dialysis therapy, the thermodynamic portion is roughly comparable to predialysis chemistries whereas kinetics refers to the rates of change of solute concentrations during treatment, both intracellularly and extracellularly.

During hemodialysis therapy rapid concentration changes take place within the body, particularly for urea and (to a lesser extent) creatinine; the same also applies to electrolytes where both additions and subtractions to the blood occur during the dialysis procedure.

The key question that dialysis therapy poses is to estimate how much removal and replacement of various solutes is necessary for each patient on maintenance dialysis. In the past these decisions have been based upon empiricism, and the patient has actually been made to adjust to the dialysis therapy rather than the therapy being adjusted to patient needs.

Kinetic modeling offers one the opportunity to regulate the dose of therapy by analysis of the kinetics of treatment. Clearly, the use of modeling to select dialysis times requires assumptions. However, the latter can and should be thoroughly tested in an appropriately circumspect manner. In this way model hypotheses can be suitably altered as and when clinical data suggest the need. The main point is that modeling offers a more structured means of assessing health care delivery as well as providing the opportunity for greater elucidation of the disease. Some years ago Gotch [6] suggested a useful analogy between drug pharmacokinetics and dialysis therapy with the major difference being that for dialysis, instead of giving something on a regular or intermittent basis, one was actually taking away.

The dose of dialysis therapy could theoretically be based upon pharmacokinetic principles. However, the major difference between drugs and renal disease is that with the former one is dealing with a single substance, whereas with renal disease there are a myriad of substances; the obvious question concerns which substance(s) should form the basis of the model. This is a critical issue, since different doses of therapy may be derived from different model bases. How does one choose the correct metabolite or electrolyte upon which to base the model? There is no absolutely right answer to this question. However, logic, such as our current knowledge permits, can be applied to this choice.

In essence, modeling involves the mathematical representation of a system so that it becomes more understandable [4]. The major aims are to provide elucidation, as well as a clinical information base upon which to make decisions. It is important, however, not to overmodel the system by requiring knowledge of parameters that cannot be measured but have to be estimated. In other words, the model should reflect the known reality and not the way things might be.


**Which model**

Modeling of the patient-hemodialyzer system is certainly not a new concept, but is was not until the mid-1970s that kinetic modeling was applied directly to patient care and the selection of treatment schedules. However, the concept of basing dialysis therapy on marker molecules was proposed more than a decade ago when it was suggested that one should dialyze to remove intermediate metabolites between 300 and 2,000 daltons [7, 8].

Work from Scribner's group in Seattle induced many clinical investigators to adopt various dialysis strategies to elucidate the potential importance of so-called 'middle molecules.' These strategies involved crossover studies of (1) lowered dialysate flow rates, (2) large-area dialyzers for shorter times, and (3) studies on more permeable dialyzers. Unfortunately, none of the approaches to the programming or altering of dialysis schedules resulted in any significant elucidation of uremic toxicity. Nevertheless, important modeling concepts such as metabolic production rates and residual renal functions were highlighted and formed a basis for a more logical application of modeling to dialysis therapy, including urea kinetic modeling (UKM). This latter concept was pioneered by Gotch in the mid-1970s [3] on the premise that although urea was not a toxin per se, it certainly could be used as a marker of protein catabolism and, therefore, as a general indicator of patient metabolic activity [9].

Of necessity, the major premise behind the modeling of dialysis therapy is that some of the signs and symptoms of the uremic syndrome are linked to solute concentration-time profiles. Because of urea's obvious connection to catabolism in general, it is reasonable to assume that measured urea production will reflect increased production of other moieties such as potassium (through either cellular breakdown or ingestion) and hydrogen ions, as well as a family of protein catabolites. Urea kinetics has been applied with considerable success to both select dialysis regimens and to assess nutritional requirements of dialysis patients, both adult [10] and pediatric [11]. Mathematically, a number of different approaches can be taken to kinetic modeling whether of urea or other solutes. The model used also depends upon the type of extracorporeal treatment; whether closed-loop, single-pass, or hemofiltration, the principle is the same and, in the case of urea, straightforward.

Urea distributes rapidly over body water and, unlike drugs and other body constituents (such as tryptophan), it is unbound to plasma proteins. A single-pool first-order model is applicable and, taking into account intradialytic changes in distribution volume, the model can be easily solved and used for therapeutic purposes [5].

Creatinine has also been proposed as a useful marker of dialysis therapy. It follows 2-pool distribution and can be relatively easily modeled [12]. Although it is not completely dietary-independent, the net production of creatinine reflects skeletal muscle mass activity and it is certainly an adequate marker of renal function. Furthermore, creatinine index is a useful metabolic parameter. However, changes in skeletal muscle mass are likely to occur over several months and, for this reason, creatinine is not as good an indicator as urea of the metabolic changes occurring during and as a result of the dialysis process.

Another important waste metabolite, primarily because of its influence on parathyroid hormone levels, is inorganic phosphate. It is not, however, an easy solute to model. First, it is an intracellular anion and therefore follows at least a 2-pool distribution. Second, most dialysis patients are on aluminum hydroxide binders and therefore have a substantial and variable gut clearance of phosphate. It is possible, however, to model sorbent-mediated gut removal mechanism, but validation of this model would require a substantial amount of clinical and laboratory experimentation [12].

A further critical area to which modeling can be usefully applied is to study the dialysis patient's acid-base status. In the early clinical use of dialysis,

226

bicarbonate was used, but problems with calcium and magnesium salt precipitation saw the introduction of acetate ]13].

However, the advent of more efficient dialyzers raised concerns that since acetate influx can exceed the acetate metabolic rate, acute, adverse effects such as hypotension (due to the vasodilatory effects of acetate) may result. There was also concern about chronic acidosis with acetate dialysis, and some renal units moved to bicarbonate [14]. Nevertheless there are now nearly 2 decades of experience with the use of acetate as buffer base. It is also probable that some of the reported hypotensive episodes with acetate dialysis have less to do with acetate and more to do with too low a sodium level in the dialysate and no dextrose. Also, despite initial concerns about 'acetate intolerance' there now seems to be considerable doubt about its importance [15]. The modeling of acetate and acid-base balance in general is certainly of considerable academic interest but it is not a suitable reference base for selecting dialysis dose.

In short, urea is the most useful moiety on which to base kinetic assessment of adequacy of dialysis. Although not a toxin per se, it is indicative of toxin buildup, and it is directly related to dietary protein intake [16] which in turn, correlates with acid production, and both phosphate and potassium buildup. It is also easy to model and measure. In contrast, the next best candidates(2) for modeling are middle molecules. However, this modeling approach is associated with a number of major problems. The biggest limitations are that: (1) they are not correlated definitively with any set of uremic lesions: (2) their molecular weight keeps changing — they are now believed to be in the range of 500 to 700 daltons [17]; and (3) they do not represent a discrete entity.

The most ambitious attempt to quantify the needed dialysis prescription for an individual patient was the National Cooperative Dialysis Study (NCDS) [18]. This was a large undertaking supported by the U.S. National Institute of Arthritis, Diabetes Digestive and Kidney Diseases and conducted by Harvard University [19]. After much debate, the NCDS panel of advisors chose to use urea kinetic modeling as the yardstick to monitor the dose of dialysis therapy [17]. In addition, the NCDS data were recently subjected to intensive mechanistic analysis, as opposed to conventional statistical analysis, by Gotch and Sargent [20] who concluded that not only are the original conclusions of the study debatable but that dose of dialysis can be readily derived from total body clearances normalized to total body water.


**Urea kinetic modeling**

It is well known that urea distributes rapidly over body water and that a single-pool model of the body suffices for modeling purposes [5]. For a variable volume model with solute generation, the following equation applies:

$$\frac{d(VC)}{dt} = -KC + G \qquad (9.1)$$

where $V$ is urea distribution volume in relation to blood urea concentration $(C)$, $K$ is total clearance (dialyzer plus residual renal function), and $G$ is net urea generation rate.

The rate of change of blood volume with time is given by:

$$\frac{dV}{dt} = -Q_f \tag{9.2}$$

Where $Q_f$ represents the constant rate of fluid removal from the body. Blood-side dialyzer clearance is given by:

$$K_B = (Q_{Bi}C_{Bi} - Q_{Bo}C_{Bo})/C_{Bi} \tag{9.3}$$

Also

$$C_{Bi} = HC_{RBCi} + (1-H)C_{pi}$$

Where $C_{RBC}/C_{pi}$ are red cells/plasma concentrations and $H$ is hematocrit fraction.

In addition, the equilibrium partition coefficient between red cells and plasma $(k)$ is written as:

$$k = C_{RBC}/C_p \tag{9.4}$$

Hence

$$C_{Bi} = (1 - H + kH)\, C_{pi} \tag{9.5}$$

and

$$K_B = Q_{BO}\,(C_{Pi} - C_{Po})/C_{Pi} + Q_f \tag{9.6}$$

Note that $C_{Pi}$ and $C_{Po}$ are for equilibrated plasma samples [21]. Furthermore, it could be argued that since hematocrit changes between inlet and outlet of the dialyzer, this should be accounted for. However, even for large $Q_f$ the effect on the magnitude of clearance is only of the order of 1%; it can certainly be neglected. Dialysate-side clearance $(K_D)$ is inherently more accurate than $K_B$ [21] and is given by:

$$K_D = Q_{Do}C_{Do}/C_{Bi}$$

or

$$K_D = Q_{Do}C_{Do}/(1 - H + kH)\, C_{Pi} \tag{9.7}$$

Equations (9.6) and (9.7) should give identical values; with careful clinical studies we have found this to be so [21].

Since solute concentration is normally measured in plasma, it is more convenient to use urea distribution volume based on plasma concentration. Hence equation (9.1) becomes:

$$\frac{d(V_pC_p)}{dt} = KC_p\,(1 - H + kH) + G \tag{9.8}$$

228

where $K$ represents total blood clearance, that is, dialyzer plus residual clearance ($K_R$). When equation (9.7) is combined with the above, equation (9.8) becomes:

$$\frac{d(V_p C_p)}{dt} = -K_p C_p + G \tag{9.9}$$

where

$$K_p = Q_{Do} C_{Do}/C_{pi} + K_R$$

(Note that if blood-side clearance ($K_B$) were used. It would have to be multiplied by the factor $(1 - H + kH.)$)

With these points in mind, equation (9.9) can be easily integrated, with respect to initial/final plasma ($C_{Po}/C_{Pf}$) urea concentrations to yield:

$$C_{pf} = C_{po}\left(1 - \frac{Q_f}{V_o}t\right)^{\frac{K}{Q_f}-1} +$$
$$\frac{G}{K - Q_f}\left[1 - \left(1 - \frac{Q_f}{V_o}t\right)^{\frac{K}{Q_f}-1}\right] \tag{9.10}$$

where $V_o$ is predialysis urea distribution volume based on urea plasma measurement; this relationship can also be used in modified form in the off-dialysis period.

## Use of the model

The two most relevant items to be obtained from the solution of equation (9.10) are urea distribution volume (with reference to plasma concentration) and net urea generation rate. Of the two, the latter is the most important since it is related to protein catabolic rate and in turn to dietary protein intake (DPI) [3, 16].

Borah and associates [22] showed that $G$ is linearly related to protein catabolic rate ($PCR$) and that, under conditions of nitrogen balance, $PCR$ equals $DPI$. Furthermore, Borah and associates [22] showed that nitrogen balance was negative on dialysis days, even for patients on a high $DPI$ (1.4g/kg/day); on the off-dialysis days, $PCR$ became positive and more than made up for the catabolism occurring on the dialysis days.

The correlation derived by Borah and associates [22] is:

$$PCR = 4.37\,[G + 2.52] \tag{9.11}$$

where $PCR$ is in g/day and $G$ is net urea production (mg/min). For large swings in patients weight, such as for pediatric patients or very large patients, the following modification has been suggested by Sargent [23]:

$$PCR = 4.37\,[G + 0.39W] \tag{9.12}$$

where $W$ is patient weight in kg. (The original Borah paper was based on adult patients who averaged 64 kg in weight.)

Under these conditions (minimal volume change and small $G$) equation (9.9) reduces to:

$$\frac{V_p dC_p}{dt} = -K_p C_p$$

Integration from the start $(C_{po})$ to the finish of dialysis yields:

$$C_p/C_{po} = \exp(-K_p t/V_p) \tag{9.13}$$

(Of note, this is the limiting case of equation (9.10) as both $G$ and $Q_f$ approach 0.)

The rate at which solute concentration falls is exponential and clearly governed by the normalized clearance-time product ($Kt/V$). This parameter determines solute removal efficiency in relation to body solute distribution volume. It has been deduced by Gotch and Sargent [20], on the basis of the National Cooperative Dialysis Study (NCDS), that this product should be $\geq 1.0$ to minimize the probability of clinical failure. In fact, Gotch and Sargent [20] have shown that the NCDS probability of failure (PF) of the dialysis therapy for thrice weekly dialysis becomes almost flat and un-influenced by the value of $Kt/V$ between the values of 0.9 to 1.5. In contrast, below a $Kt/V$ of 0.8, PF increases dramatically; from these data it can be argued that dialysis therapy should aim for a $Kt/V$ of greater than or equal to 1.0 on the basis of a weekly therapy frequency of 3. (This issue is taken further in the text to follow.)


**Applying urea kinetic modeling (UKM)**

As has been suggested, perhaps one of the most beneficial aspects of modeling for patients is that the technical aspects of the treatment are at least being measured and monitored. In this way some degree of quality control is being exercised over the delivery of therapy. However, the potential advantages of UKM to the dialysis unit and the patient extend far beyond this undeniably important yet rather simplistic benefit. For example, experience by various dialysis units in the use of UKM over periods from 2 years and up to 10 years have indicated the following UKM benefits [5]: (1) it is cost-effective; (2) it permits nutritional counseling and monitoring; (3) it guards against over-vigorous or prolonged treatments while maintaining adequacy of dialysis; (4) it provides excellent quality control on the dialysis procedure allowing for more technically efficacious delivery of treatment; and (5) It is an effective method of prescribing the correct amount of dialysis therapy.

The latter statement becomes clearer upon consideration of Gotch and Sargent's recent discussion and analysis of the NCDS data [20]. It has been nicely demonstrated from their data analysis that UKM can be used to deduce an effective dialysis schedule based on whole body urea clearance normalized to total body water ($Kt/V$).


## The national cooperative dialysis study revisited

Statistical analysis of the NCDS data were based upon the probabilities of clinical failure [24]. The latter were defined as PF1: the probability of failure for any patient who died of withdraw for medical reasons at any time during the experimental phase; and PF2: the probability of failure for any patient who died, withdraw for medical reasons, or was hospitalized prior to 24 weeks in the experimental phase. (The date of failure was the date of death, withdrawal or first hospitalization, whichever occurred first.)

The statistical analysis showed PF1 and PF2 were continuously decreasing functions of normalized protein catabolic rates ($PCR$) in the range 0.6 to 1.6 g/day/kg of body weight. Probability of failure was also apparently correlated inversely with dialysis time. In short, long hours of dialysis were better statistically than short hours, at any given average blood urea nitrogen (BUN) concentration, and even though there was little apparent difference between short dialysis and low average BUN and long dialysis high average BUN, it was abundantly clear that short dialysis with a high BUN was very poor therapy and associated with a high morbidity.

One could be forgiven therefore in interpreting these conclusions to mean that long dialysis ($t_d$ of 4.5 hours $\times$ 3 times per week) and a low predialysis BUN ($\sim$90 mg/dL) as well as a high $PCR$ of $\geq$ 1.2 g/day/kg would represent good dialysis. However, there are other ways of looking at the NCDS data, and Gotch and Sargent undertook a more careful look at the data, in terms of what they called a mechanistic approach, by cross-correlation of data on dietary intake, BUN, and whole body urea clearances; their conclusions were quite different [20].

In essence they found that, contrary to the statistical analyses, probability of failure was not a continuous function of protein intake and the level of dialysis treatment, as prescribed in the study. Indeed when they analyzed the outcome data as a function of $Kt/V$, it was found that the data were discontinuous with a cluster of points, independent of $Kt/V$, with a high probability of clinical failure (PF1, 0.42; PF2, 0.57) for $Kt/V$ less than 0.8 and much lower PF1(0.08) and PF2(0.13) values, also independent of $Kt/V$, for $Kt/V$ greater than 0.9 but less than 1.5.

Additionally Gotch and Sargent [20] point out that the NCDS study failed to address the relative importance of dialysis and nutrition in low $PCR$ pateints since $Kt/V$ was <0.70 in all cases where $PCR$ was <0.8. In essence, the so-called mechanistic analysis indicated that the probability of therapy failure did not decrease as Kt/V increased from 0.9 to 1.5 in proportion to $PCR$ increasing from 0.8 to 1.4 g/day/kg. It was therefore concluded that a fully adequate dialysis prescription is provided if $PCR$ is $\geq$1.0 and $Kt/V$ is

$\geq 1.0$. Furthermore, increasing the amount of dialysis and protein intake beyond these values would not provide any apparent clinical benefit with conventional cellulosic dialyzers in current use on a thrice weekly treatment schedule [20]. If this analysis is accepted, one further question remains, and this concerns the relative value of clearance to time in the $Kt$ product. In other words, how high can clearance be increased to reduce time on dialysis? There are differing views on this point [2,25], but most feel that it is not realistic to reduce $t_d$ to much less than 3 hours due to fluid balance and both electrolyte and acid-base balance control.

## Future trends: dialysis technology of modeling applications

Economics and patient desires will continue to put pressure on dialysis units to reduce dialysis times still further. And the process will most likely be determined not so much by modeling as by applying the results of the modeling process, or Gotch's so-called mechanistic approach [26], based on the maintenance of a $Kt/V$ value of 1.0 for thrice weekly treatments. The main question concerns the lower limit of the value of $t$ which will be consistent with efficacious delivery of therapy; I will return to this point in a moment.

There is little doubt in my mind that modeling concepts have had a significant yet too limited impact on dialysis procedures. And the impact of UKM has been the most significant for the reasons which have already been outlined. There is little doubt that, in those units which have adopted modeling procedures, both patients and the unit themselves have benefited. In short, the units have been run more efficiently, mostly as the result of time reductions, and patients have benefited considerably from the measuring and monitoring process. In addition, as a result of the NCDS, there has been a much better appreciation of the benefits of kinetic modeling. Of more importance the circumspect analysis of the NCDS data by Gotch and Sargent [20] has provided a very useful benchmark for assessing adequacy of treatment, namely a normalized total body urea clearance, $Kt/V$ of unity.

The achievement of $Kt/V$ for urea of 1.0 is not of course a necessary and sufficient condition for adequacy of dialysis. On the dietary side, the ingestion of about 1.2 g/kg/day of reasonable quality biologic protein is also desirable, and UKM provides a means of monitoring $DPI$ over time [3, 5].

Clearly beyond these quantifiable dialytic parameters it is vital that patient morbidity is reduced to the lowest possible level. In this regard, however, it has to be recognized the renal replacement therapy by dialysis can only do so much because of the inherent limitations of the process itself.

If one accepts the concept of a $Kt/V$ of unit for thrice weekly dialysis then, for a given patient distribution volume (estimated as 0.58 times dry body weight) the question becomes the limit of dialysis time.

There are now dialyzers available which have mass transfer area ($K_oA$) properties which will provide clearances in excess of 180 ml/min. at blood dialysate flow rates of 200/500 ml/min. In fact, newly available polysulphone and cellulose acetate dialysers have $K_oA$ values of 750 to 1,000 ml/min which provide excellent clearance values as well as good biocompatability. At these kinds of $K_oA$ values dialysis times of 2 hours, at increased blood ($\sim$400 ml/min)/dialysate ($\sim$700 ml/min) flow rates, are readily achievable even in larger patients, e.g., 80 kg. This being the case, can other critical aspects of dialysis therapy such as electrolyte, acid-base balance, and fluid balances be adequately catered for?

Recently Gotch [26] predicted inter alia that by 1990, conventional dialysis treatment times will approach 2 hours. In his discussions about future trends in dialysis therapy he also addressed the aforementioned issues of acid-base and fluid balances as well as removal of electrolytes and other waste metabolites. Based on published data for urea, creatinine, and phosphate cell mass transfer coefficients, it was shown that the removal of these moieties would hardly be compromised in comparing 2-hour with 4-hour dialyses.

In fact, total body removal rates for these metabolites would be reduced by about 2% for urea and 5–6% for phosphate and creatinine, modest reductions indeed.

It appears, according to Gotch's modeling predictions, that a switch to bicarbonate as buffer base will be required. Estimates suggest that acetate metabolism to generate bicarbonate will be insufficient on 2-hour dialysis without significant transient acidosis. However, fluid balance should be controllable with precise volumetric control of ultrafiltration and the use of appropriate levels of sodium in the dialysate bath. Hence, despite scepticism about reduced dialysis times [25] and 2-hour dialysis in particular [2], it certainly seems achievable with acceptable clinical results.

With gradual recognition of the relevance of $Kt/V$, it is possible that UKM and dialysis modeling in general will become less important. I think that this would be a pity, particularly regarding areas such as dietary counseling and the monitoring of the treatment process; however, in principle with a good knowledge of patient dietary habits, based on a renal dietician's assessments, plus a handle on $Kt/V$, it should be adequate for all but the most difficult patients.

There is one final caveat that needs to be clearly understood. The dialyzer is capable of removing only relatively small, unbound moieties, and there are many endocrine and metabolic derangements which cannot be influenced by even the most careful and well-delivered dietary therapy. This must always temper our expectations in planning dialysis treatment schedules.


## References


1. Charra, B., Calemard, E., Cuche, M. and Laurent, G. (1983) Control of hypertension and prolonged survival on maintenance hemodialysis. Nephron 33: 96–99.
2. Cambi, V., Arisi, L., David, S., Bono, F. and Gardini, G. (1985) 2-h dialysis: A realistic goal? Contr. Nephrol. 44: 40–48.

3. Gotch, F.A., Sargent, J.A., Keen, M.L., Lam, M.A., Prowitt, M. and Grady, M. (1976) Clinical results of intermittent dialysis therapy guided by ongoing kinetic analysis of urea metabolism. *Trans. Am. Soc.* Artif. Intern. Organs; 22: 175.

4. Farrell, P.C., Ward, R.A., Schindhelm, K. and Gotch, F.A. (1978) Precise anticoagulation for routine hemodialysis. J. Lab. Clin. Med. 92: 164–172.

5. Farrell, P.C. (1983) Kinetic modeling: application in renal and related diseases. Kidney Int. 24: 487.

6. Gotch, F.A. (1975) Recommendation for quantification of dialysis therapy in research protocols. Kidney Int. 7: S246.

7. Babb, A.L., Popovich, R.P., Christopher, T.G. and Scribner, B.H. (1971) The genesis of the square-meter hour hypothesis. Trans. Am. Soc. *Artif. Intern. Organs* 17: 81.

8. Babb, A.L., Farrell, P.C., Milutinovic, J. and Scribner, B.H. (1972) Residual renal function: potential importance to hemodialysis therapy. Proc. Clin. Dial. Transplant. Forum 2: 48.

9. Sargent, J., Gotch, F., Borah, M., Piercy, L., Spinozzi, N., Schoenfeld, P. and Humphreys, M. (1978) Urea kinetics: a guide to nutritional management of renal failure. Am. J. Clin. Nutr. 31: 1696.

10. Sargent, J.A. and Gotch, F.A. (1981) Nutrition and treatment of the acutely ill patient using area kinetics. Dial. Transplant. 10: 314.

11. Harmon, W.E., Spinozzi, N. and Meyer, A. (1981) The use of protein catabolic rate to monitor pediatric hemodialysis. Dial Transplant. 10: 324.

12. Farrell, P.C. (1979) Hemodialysis. Am. Inst. Chem. Eng. Symp. Series 187: 10.

13. Mion, C., Hegstrom, R., Boen, S. and Scribner, B.H. (1964) Substitution of sodium acetate for sodium bicarbonate in the bath fluid during hemodialysis. Trans. Am. Soc. Artif. Intern. Organs 10: 110.

14. Graefe, U., Milutinovic, J., Folette, W., Vizzo, J., Babb, A.L. and Scribner, G.H. (1977) Less dialysis induced morbidity and vascular instability with bicarbonate in the dialysate. Ann. Intern. Med. 88: 332.

15. Maher, J.F., Bosch, J.P., Gotch, F.A., Kjellstrand, C.M. and Scribner, B.H. (1981) Acetate versus bicarbonate in dialysis. Trans. Am. Soc. Artif. Intern. Organs 26: 655.

16. Cottini, E.P., Gallina, D.L. and Dominguez, J.M. (1973) Urea excretion in adult humans with varying degrees of kidney malfunction fed milk, egg or amino acid mixture. Assessment of nitrogen balance. J. Nutr. 103: 11.

17. Chapman, G.V., and Farrell, P.C. (1981) Uremic middle molecules: separation and quantitation. Artif. Organs 4: 160–165.

18. Wineman, R.J. (1983) Rationale of the National Co-Operative Dialysis Study. Kidney Int. 23(13): S8–S10.

19. Lowrie, E.G., Laird, N.M. and Henry, R.R. (1983) Protocol for the National Co-Operative Dialysis Study. Kidney Int. 23(13): S11–S18.

20. Gotch, F.A. and Sargent, J.A. (1985) A mechanistic analysis of the National Co-Operative Dialysis Study (NCDS). Kidney Int. 28: 526–534.

21. Skalsky, M., Schindhelm, K. and Farrell, P.C. (1978) Accurate determination of in vivo dialyzer clearances. Dial. Transplant. 7: 217.

22. Bcrah, M.F., Schoenfeld, P.V., Gotch, F.A., Sargent, J.H., Wolfson, M. and Humphreys, M.H. Nitrogen balance during intermittent dialysis therapy of uremia. Kidney Int. 14: 491.

23. Sargent, J.A. (1981) Urea kinetics: a quantitative guide to nutrition and treatment in renal disease. Dial. Transplant. 10: 275.

24. Laird, N.M., Berkey, C.S. and Lowrie, E.G. (1983) Modeling success or failure of dialysis therapy. Kidney Int. 23: S101–S106.

25. Kjellstrand, D.M. (1985) Short dialysis increases morbidity and mortality. Contr. Nerphrol. 44: 65–77.

26. Gotch, F.A. (in press) Dialysis of the future.


234

# 10. Aluminum intoxication

Alex M. Davison

In 1972 Alfrey and his colleagues [1] described a new syndrome of unknown etiology that consisted of dementia, speech disturbances, seizures, and myoclonus. Following this initial description there were further reports indicating that this syndrome was being encountered in many dialysis units both in America and Europe [2–4]. The cause for this unusual progressive syndrome was not apparent, and many suggestions were put forward such as an infection with a slow virus, depletion of essential substances by dialysis, or the accumulation of some toxic substance during the dialysis procedure. Intensive investigations were undertaken to determine an etiological factor, but the most important finding was of the unusual geographical distribution of the patients [4–6] to areas where the water supply aluminum concentration was high due to the addition of alum as a clarifying agent at water treatment works. Some units had no patients with dialysis encephalopathy while in others it was a major cause of mortality. In addition, some patients seemed to develop the syndrome over a short period of time whereas others only became symptomatic after many years of treatment. It is now recognized that there is a close exponential relationship between the mean aluminum concentration in the water supply used to prepare dialysate and the time taken to develop dementia [6]. It is now widely accepted that aluminum is the major toxic factor in the etiology of dialysis encephalopathy and that the aluminum arises from both the dialysate and the oral ingestion of aluminum-containing, phosphate-binding drugs. It is interesting that although aluminum is the third most common element and most common metal in the environment, no metabolic role has yet been determined.

Although there is now a general awareness of the toxicity of aluminum in dialysis patients, there are a number of factors which make it necessary to keep in mind this potential hazard. There is an increasing trend toward a reduction in dialysis times, and this has been achieved by an alteration in the physical characteristics of dialyzers and also in the structure and nature of membranes. The increasing use of high flux membranes allows for more rapid ultrafiltration, but it will also allow for the transfer of potentially toxic contaminants from the dialysate to the patient. This is particularly so with

Vincenzo Cambi (editor) Professor of Nephrology
© 1987 Martinus Nijhoff Publishing, Boston. ISBN 0-89838-858-9. Printed in The United States.

respect to aluminum, and there may be a need to revise the accepted standards of water purity to accommodate these changes in membrane features. Although the increased efficiency of dialyzers may well be associated with increased phosphate removal, this may well be offset by the decreased dialysis duration. There may, therefore, be an increased use of phosphate-binding drugs and, therefore, an increased risk of aluminum toxicity. Consequently, in our desire to achieve shorter dialysis times, we must be aware of the increased membrane porosity and the possibility of the need for an increase in the use of intestinal phosphate-binding drugs. It should also be remembered that by unnecessarily prolonging the dialysis sessions, when using the more modern high flux membranes, there will be an increased possibility of toxic accumulation of dialysate contaminants. As with all significant advances in management, care must be taken to ensure that there are no adverse medical effects to the patient.

Initial reports concentrated on the neurological manifestations of the syndrome probably because they appear so obvious and unusual. In time, however, it was realized that these were frequently associated with a fracturing osteodystrophy [7] and also with a microcytic anemia [5] and that this latter feature may occur prior to any clinical manifestation of encephalopathy or bone disease [8]. In some reports the clinical manifestations became apparent after transplantation. There are thus wide clinical features but the classical signs are a progressive encephalopathy, a fracturing osteodystrophy, and a microcytic anemia.


**Encephalopathy**

The presenting clinical feature of dialysis encephalopathy is speech disorders (50%), behavioral disturbances (20%), dementia (20%), and neuromuscular disorders (10%) [9]. The speech abnormality appears to follow a fairly typical pattern in most patients. Initially the complaint is of stuttering or difficulty with speech toward the end of dialysis. With time, however, the stuttering becomes more prolonged and intermittent speech arrest may occur toward the end of a dialysis session. These symptoms increase until the patient may be rendered totally mute. Usually there is recovery of speech occurring several hours after dialysis, but as the syndrome progresses the speech disorder becomes more manifest.

The behavioral disorders encountered are nonspecific but can be the cause of much distress. The patient frequently develops an acute anxiety state toward the end of dialysis and may become extremely demanding on those assisting with his/her treatment. The acute anxiety state may last for several hours after dialysis, and frequently thereafter the patient is unable to explain why he/she felt so tense and anxious. During such time the patient requires considerable reassurance and the presence of other people including relatives and nursing staff. A particularly distressing feature is that often the patient is well aware of his/her surroundings but the inability to communicate makes him/her feel as a prisoner trapped within his/her own body. As with the speech disorders, the behavioral disturbances become more marked with time. The patient experiences intense frustration with the difficulty in communication, and a feeling of despair may well become apparent. In the late stages of the illness delusions, hallucinations, and paranoid behavior may become obvious, and later apathy and a loss of self-respect become major features. It is not uncommon for patients to contemplate and even attempt suicide.

A number of patients present with dementia which initially relates to disturbances of cognitive function and the inability to perceive and react appropriately to external influences. This creates a number of problems, particularly in patients who are being managed by home dialysis. They will soon find themselves unable to undertake simple dialysis procedures with which they were previously familiar, and this may become manifest by a totally inappropriate response when dealing with simple maneuvers relating to their dialysis. Recent memory may become impaired, and some patients become totally disorientated with respect to their surroundings and other people. A progressive intellectual deterioration gradually overtakes the patient resulting in a loss of reasoning power and understanding, with the patient eventually becoming totally demented.

The neuromuscular disorders associated with dialysis encephalopathy consist of myoclonus, drop attacks, incoordination, dysphasia, convulsions, and coma. In some patients the initial manifestation of the disease may be with myoclonus. There is frequently a symmetrical twitching of the limbs, and in some instances sudden flexion of both legs will result in the patient falling to the ground in a drop attack. The myoclonus may be provoked by some external auditory or visual stimulus, and although this is not a common feature it usually develops at some time during the illness in most patients. Other features within this category of disorders include the inability to coordinate limb movements, lower facial immobility, and dysphasia. Simple activities such as reaching for objects, feeding, and eating create enormous problems, and eventually these patients become totally dependent on others for their physical needs. Late in the illness the dysphasia is sometimes associated with an inhalation pneumonitis and consequent bronchopneu-monia. This is a relatively frequent cause of death in such patients. Convul-sive attacks vary in their degree of severity from localized or Jacksonian type fits to grand mal seizures. Most occur toward the end of dialysis or shortly thereafter.

The diagnosis of dialysis encephalopathy may be difficult, and other causes for dementia must be carefully considered. The plasma aluminum is elevated, frequently greater than 100 $\mu$g/l, and there is often an accompanying fracturing osteodystrophy (vide infra), and a microcytic anemia (vide infra). The EEG may show generalized slowing with runs of delta and spike wave activity, with the most severe changes being evident in recordings obtained immediately postdialysis. However, the EEG abnormality has not been demonstrated in all patients and is not specific for dialysis encephalopathy. The presence of bilateral synchronous spike and wave activity is suggestive of an excitatory discharge in the diencephalon and may explain the propensity toward myoclonus and other seizures. Computerised axial tomography of the brain shows little abnormality apart from some patients in which mild atrophy may be present. Brain biopsy has been performed as a diagnostic procedure but is unhelpful. The diagnosis, therefore, will be made by the presence of typical clinical symptoms associated with osteodystrophy and a microcytic anemia and confirmed by the finding of an elevated plasma aluminum.

There is no satisfactory treatment for dialysis encephalopathy, and prevention is clearly the best strategy. Aluminum exposure should be kept to a minimum and frequent monitoring of plasma and dialysate aluminum undertaken.

In the early stages of the disease, intravenous Diazepam may have a dramatic effect in improving the speech disorder, particularly when patients have a major problem with communication. In addition, the myoclonus frequently responds to Clonazepam, and considerable symptomatic relief may be obtained. The most important action that can be undertaken is avoidance of further exposure to aluminum and removal of accumulated aluminum by the use of chelating agents (vide infra).

Although there is no satisfactory cure for this syndrome, considerable benefit can be obtained from good patient management. For the patient who has a loss of coherent speech the inability to communicate frequently results in a great degree of frustration and an understanding of this frightening predicament can be particularly helpful. Sometimes patients are able to continue communicating their needs by writing or by identifying their thoughts and needs from a list of chosen pretyped words and sentences. The use of mechanical devices such as word printers may be of help in a number of cases. Considerable patient support is needed, particularly in the later stages of the illness when patients are unable to look after their physical needs and move about in a coordinated way. Frequently the families of such patients also require sympathetic and understanding support.

Encephalopathy is a most distressing condition for the patient, the family, and the staff responsible for treatment. Anxiety may occur in unaffected patients, and staff must be trained to manage the patients with encephalopathy, but just as important they must be capable of supporting and reassuring all patients under their care [10]. Aluminum intoxication must be prevented, and an awareness of the clinical features will hopefully allow diagnosis to be suspected at a time prior to permanent brain damage. The monitoring of plasma aluminum at regular intervals is essential and appropriate action must be taken if the concentration rises and particularly if it exceeds 100 $\mu$g/l.

238

## Osteodystrophy

Renal osteodystrophy frequently complicates end-stage renal failure and may worsen after starting hemodialysis. The bone changes consist of osteomalacia, hyperparathyroidism, osteopenia, and less commonly areas of osteosclerosis. It is now recognized that the osteomalacia may be induced by a deficiency of 1,25 dihydroxycholecalciferol, hypophosphataemia, or aluminum intoxication.

In 1971 Parsons and associates [11] reported an increased content of aluminum in bones of patients with end-stage renal failure. The greatest amount of aluminum was detected in those who had been on hemodialysis for the longest periods of time. The association between dialysis encephalopathy and spontaneous fractures was reported in 1977 by Platts and associates [4]. In this report there was a clear geographical distribution of affected patients, and it was suggested that some contaminant in the water used for dialysis was very probably responsible for the development of the fractures. This was further supported by the finding of Ward and his coworkers who reported that osteomalacia occurred in only 15% of patients who were dialyzed with a dialysate prepared from deionized water compared with 70% of patients using softened nondeionized water [7]. Subsequent studies demonstrated a highly significant correlation between the aluminum content of water used to prepare dialysate and the incidence of osteomalacic dialysis osteodystrophy.

Clinically the osteomalacia associated with aluminum intoxication is usually progressive and is associated with bone pain, fractures, frequently of the ribs and pelvis, myopathy, and is usually unresponsive to vitamin D or its biologically active metabolites. The plasma calcium is usually normal or slightly elevated. Plasma phosphate is elevated, alkaline phosphatase is either normal or slightly elevated, and plasma parathyroid hormone concentrations are rarely significantly elevated. Aluminum diminishes the secretion of parathyroid hormone and reduces the response of the parathyroid glands to hypocalcemia. Radiologically there is little evidence of hyperparathyroidism, the major feature being fractures or pseudofractures (Looser's zones). Bone biopsy reveals a reduced volume of mineralized bone with an increased thickness of osteoid seams, reduced osteoblastic activity, and an inability to label with Tetracycline.

The mechanism whereby aluminum inhibits normal mineralization of bone is at present a matter for much intensive study. There would appear to be considerable differences between cortical and trabecular bone in that trabecular bone is more affected. On bone biopsy it can be demonstrated that aluminum is localized at the interface between osteoid and the calcified matrix. In addition, there is evidence of direct correlation between the degree of osteomalacia and the amount of aluminum present. In vitro, it has been shown that aluminum interacts with citrate to form a potent inhibitor of mineralization, growth of calcium phosphate crystals in vitro, and calcium uptake by collagen [12]. The inhibitory effect of aluminum citrate complexes could be due to selective adsorption onto the crystal surface, thereby inhibiting further growth. Aluminum has a significant physical chemical inhibition of hydroxyapatite proliferation by acting on early crystals after initial nucleation events have taken place. There is also in vitro work suggesting that aluminum affects bone acid and alkaline phosphatase modifying the response of these enzymes to both parathyroid hormone and 1.25 di-hydroxycholecalciferol [13]. In addition, aluminum could have a direct inhibitory effect on osteoblastic activity in that the number of active bone-forming sites is reduced and that the activity of these sites is also reduced. The majority of evidence seems to point to a direct effect on the calcification front inhibiting the formation of normal mineralized bone. The resultant effect is a progressive osteomalacia which is resistant to treatment by vitamin D.


**Anemia**

The majority of patients with chronic renal failure have a normochromic normocytic anemia which responds poorly if at all to hemodialysis. The etiology of this anemia is multifactorial. In 1978 Elliott and MacDougal [5] reported that anemia was associated with osteomalacic dialysis osteodystrophy and with dialysis encephalopathy. Frequently the anemia preceded the onset of neurological symptoms or bony complications, and it has been suggested that anemia may be a useful early indicator for aluminum toxicity. The aluminum associated anemia is microcytic and hypochromic, and responds to a change to a dialysate with a low aluminum concentration [8]. The mechanism whereby aluminum induces anemia is unknown, but it has been suggested that it may be due to a disturbance in haem synthesis specifically involving delta aminolevulinic acid dehydrogenase.


**Source of aluminum**

The two main sources of aluminum intoxication in patients with chronic renal failure are oral ingestion and transfer of aluminum across the membrane during dialysis. Oral ingestion can occur from aluminum contamination of domestic water supplies, from aluminum released from cooking utensils, or from the ingestion of aluminum-containing drugs such as phosphate binders. The normal daily ingestion is probably in the region of 3–5 mg. In dialysis the sources can be either the water used to prepare the dialysate solution, the dialysate concentrate, release from dialysis equipment such as the Redy cartridge, and also from contamination of CAPD fluids.

The major source of aluminum accumulation following oral ingestion is the use of phosphate-binding agents. Dietary restrictions and phosphate removal during dialysis are usually inadequate to ensure good control of plasma phosphate in the majority of dialysis patients. In patients with normal renal function, aluminum is excreted by the kidney and thus in renal functional impairment there is accumulation. Berylene and colleagues in 1970 [14] reported increases in serum aluminum concentration in patients with end-stage renal failure who were being treated with aluminum cycle resins and aluminum hydroxide. Once the association between aluminum toxicity and dialysis encephalopathy became apparent, interest in intestinal aluminum absorption increased. It became apparent that in areas where the dialysate aluminum was low, the major source of aluminum accumulation was from intestinal absorption from aluminum-containing, phosphate-binding agents [15]. There is a tendency to prescribe such agents without reference to the nature or amount of phosphate ingestion. Obtaining a careful dietary history will allow for proper prescribing of such drugs to times when there is an intestinal phosphate load. This usually allows for a considerable reduction in the amount of medication, while at the same time maintaining good control of the plasma phosphate [16]. In view of the amphoteric nature of aluminum, ingestion of aluminum hydroxide into the acid environment of an empty stomach will result in increased intestinal absorption and therefore a greater chance of toxicity. It is likely that the majority is absorbed in the stomach and proximal duodenum. Aluminum can form complexes with fluoride, and thus the fluoride content of the diet may significantly affect absorption.

Transfer of aluminum from dialysate to plasma is now well recognized. Although there is a variable small amount of naturally occuring aluminum, the majority derives from the addition of alum as a clarifying agent in water treatment works, and aluminum is likely to spill over into the distribution system in variable amounts. Therefore, in any area where alum is used as a clarifying agent there is serious risk of aluminum intoxication.

Transfer during dialysis can occur from an apparently low concentration to a high concentration [17] due to the fact that the majority of aluminum in plasma is strongly bound to protein, possibly transferrin, and lower molecular weight substances. Even with a dialysate concentration as low as 10 $\mu$g/l there may be transfer to plasma with subsequent accumulation. Aluminum is amphoteric, and the insoluble form predominates at neutral pH. Small changes in pH can greatly increase the dialyzable form of aluminum, thereby increasing the potential of transfer to plasma. The aluminum concentration of the dialysate should be maintained below 10 $\mu$g/l. During dialysis aluminum may also arise from the Redy sorbent cartridge [18], although now that this has been recognized, modifications to its use have been made thereby eliminating this problem. There are also reports of aluminum accumulation from contamination of CAPD fluids [19]; therefore, it would seem wise to monitor at frequent intervals both dialysate fluid and plasma from all patients undergoing either hemodialysis or continuous ambulatory peritoneal dialysis.


**Management**

The management of aluminum intoxication falls into two parts: the first is to avoid aluminum accumulation, while the second is to treat those patients already exposed and with, or at risk of developing, symptoms. It is to be hoped now that the association of this progressive syndrome to aluminum toxicity has been established, patients coming to dialysis treatment will be regularly monitored and changes will have been made in the management to avoid toxicity. The population of patients on dialysis treatment is increasing due to both an increased rate of acceptance of patients and also the fact that patient survival is improving. There is thus a significant number of patients who were treated for variable lengths of time prior to the widespread recognition that aluminum was so toxic. Such patients require careful examination and investigation to detect aluminum overload.

*Prevention*

In the initial reports of encephalopathy it was considered that the major source of aluminum was from transfer from the dialysate across the membrane with subsequent tissue accumulation. Aluminum can occur naturally in low concentrations, but the major source arises from the addition of alum, as a clarifying agent, at water treatment installations. Alum causes suspended particulate matter to flocculate and sediment, leaving the supernatant water clear. Unfortunately the mechanics of this process are imprecise, and frequently alum will be added in excessive quantities and result in aluminum appearing in the main distribution system. This explains the very wide day-to-day variation in domestic water aluminum concentration, and emphasizes the need for frequent monitoring of water supplies especially where alum is added in the course of water treatment.

The aluminum concentration of the water used to prepare dialysate should be less than 5 $\mu$g/l (0.2 $\mu$M/l), and should this value be exceeded, then appropriate water treatment is required. In view of the haphazard method of using alum as a clarifying agent I would recommend that in any area where alum is employed then water purification prior to the preparation of dialysate is essential. It is therefore vital that information be obtained from water authorities as to their modes of treatment. The most satisfactory method of removing aluminum is by reverse osmosis; deionization and softening are not adequate. The most appropriate method of water purification will depend to a large extent on the nature of contaminants in the local water supply but will consist of some form of filtration followed by softening and subsequent reverse osmosis. The membranes of reverse osmosis plants are expensive, and pre-treatment by softening will greatly prolong their use and therefore be very cost-effective. The treated water supply and the final dialysate should be monitored at least monthly, and the aluminum concentration kept below 5 $\mu$g/l for treated water and less than 10 $\mu$g/l for dialysate. Values in excess of these require careful examination of the water treatment facilities and/or the dialysate concentrate.

Now that the problem of water aluminum has been recognized and that water treatment has been generally introduced, it is becoming increasingly obvious that aluminum accumulation can occur from oral ingestion. Although

242

aluminum is a widespread element occurring naturally in food and water as well as being commonly used for cooking utensils, the major source for patients is undoubtedly from the use of phosphate-binding agents used to control hyperphosphataemia. The most widely used agent is aluminum hydroxide which is usually prescribed without reference to the phosphate content of the ingested food. Frequently excessive doses are prescribed but fortunately patients find these preparations unpalatable and so the amount ingested is usually less than that prescribed. Aluminum is amphoteric and most insoluble at neutral pH. The ingestion of aluminum hydroxide on an empty stomach will therefore result in the aluminum being in a more acid environment, thereby increasing its solubility and absorption. In addition, the quantity and type of food taken by patients varies greatly, and so it is important to obtain a good dietary history and then to prescribe the phosphate-binding agent appropriately. I usually find that aluminum hydroxide 0.5–1.0 g is sufficient for light meals and snacks, and that 1.0–2.0 g are sufficient for cooked meals. Obviously this will vary from country to country and for different patients, but if the medications are related to meals then the amount taken can usually be significantly reduced and the amount absorbed greatly diminished. In addition the patients should be advised of the phosphate content of food so that they can restrict excessive phosphate ingestion, thereby reducing further the need for phosphate-binding drugs. In this respect the help and advice of a dietitian is essential.

To further limit the ingestion of aluminum, alternative phosphate binders have been sought. Magnesium hydroxide, calcium carbonate, and ferric hydroxide have been suggested, but only calcium carbonate has achieved widespread use. Magnesium hydroxide combined with a magnesium free dialysate has been reported to result in a significant reduction in predialysis aluminum and control of plasma phosphate without an increase in plasma magnesium [20]. Although some promising new agents have been developed [21], none has yet become available for widespread use. In view of the disastrous consequences of aluminum toxicity, this is an area of research that merits urgent development. In the meantime, aluminum-containing, phosphate-binding drugs should be given in the lowest possible dose for adequate phosphate control and where possible should be combined with calcium carbonate.

The introduction of effective water purification and reduction in oral ingestion should prevent aluminum intoxication. However, there is a need for monitoring to ensure that the actions adopted are effective. I would recommend that the water supply to the dialysis facility, the treated water, and the final dialysate should be monitored monthly. In addition, red cell mean cell volume should be closely watched for any unexplained microcytosis. Bone radiology should be examined at yearly intervals and, where indicated, bone biopsy obtained and examined for aluminum accumulation at the calcification fronts. Plasma should be examined at least every three months, the plasma aluminum should be less than 80 $\mu$g/l but if greater than 100 $\mu$g/l then action should be taken, and if greater than 200 $\mu$g/l then symptoms are likely to develop. In uremia the majority of the excess aluminum is found in bone although increased concentrations are also found in other tissues such as cardiac muscle. Unfortunately there is not a good correlation between plasma aluminum and bone overload. Finally clinical examination, particularly of speech, should be regularly conducted and if any disorder detected, an EEG is indicated. Hopefully with good monitoring early action can be introduced, thereby preventing the appearance of any clinical manifestations.

*Treatment*

In spite of good management some patients may develop evidence of aluminum toxicity. In such a situation the source of the aluminum must be identified and eliminated. Secondly the accumulated aluminum must be removed.

Aluminum is not effectively removed by hemodialysis due to its high degree of protein and tissue binding. In 1980 Ackrill and his colleagues reported the successful removal of aluminum from a patient with dialysis encephalopathy by the use of desferrioxamine (DFO) [22], and since then there have been many reports confirming this procedure [23, 24]. Aluminum combines strongly to DFO in a 1:1 molar ratio, and this chelate is then subsequently removed by hemodialysis or hemofiltration. Following DFO infusion there is a substantial increase in plasma aluminum indicating mobilization from tissues. This increase, however, appears to cause little toxicity [22] presumably as it is so strongly bound to the DFO. There have, however, been reports that some batches of DFO contain significant amounts of aluminum and that some of the postinfusion increase could be due to aluminum contained in the DFO [25]. Many protocols have been suggested, but in the adult patient 2 g DFO infused intravenously in the 30 minutes immediately after a dialysis session is adequate for aluminum mobilization, and at this dose there does not seem to be significant iron chelation [26]. The mobilized and chelated aluminum is then most effectively removed by dialysis 48 hours later. Some patients may react to DFO, and so the first infusion should be given more slowly and under medical supervision. The infusions should be given at the end of each dialysis, but the duration of the course of treatment can only be determined by the response of the clinical manifestations and laboratory parameters. It is likely to take a minimum of 3 months; so far there do not appear to be any reports of adverse effects from the long-term use of DFO. There are reports of the beneficial effects of DFO treatment on the encephalopathy [22, 23], osteodystrophy [24], and microcytic anemia [27]. DFO treatment, by the mobilization of aluminum from bone, may be followed by evidence of increased bone activity indicated by an increase in alkaline phosphatase and the development of hyperparathyroidism [28]. Care must therefore be taken with the long-term followup of these patients.

244

In patients on continuous ambulatory peritoneal dialysis, aluminum can be removed following intravenous or intramuscular [29] desferrioxamine. In such patients vascular access may prove difficult and repeated intramuscular injections painful. Recently, there have been reports of successful treatment using intraperitoneal desferrioxamine (500 mg to each bag), and this route offers a safe and effective alternative mode of administration [30].

As with other conditions that appear to arise as a complication of hemodialysis, there is always a feeling that successful transplantation will resolve the problem. In dialysis encephalopathy this has not been our experience [31], although other authors have reported resolution of the syndrome after successful transplantation [32]. It is interesting to note that some patients develop their first symptoms after transplantation [32]. In our center only 2 of 7 patients have shown any improvement following transplantation with the rest showing fairly rapid deterioration to death. It is possible that the hospitalization and steroid therapy employed after transplantation results in the liberation of accumulated aluminum from bones, thereby significantly aggrevating the cerebral effects of aluminum intoxication. In our experience these patients have had little problems with rejection which raises the interesting possibility that aluminum may have a depressant effect on the immune system. This is supported by the experience of Hanson [33] who reported that the grafts did well but the patients did not. In patients who have been exposed to high aluminum concentrations in the past it is difficult to know when it will be safe to undertake transplantation without the risk of producing an encephalopathy-like syndrome.


**Conclusion**

Aluminum intoxication in hemodialysis patients arises due to the loss of the normal excretory pathway and accumulation from dialysate and ingestion of aluminum-containing, phosphate-binding drugs. It produces multisystem effects with the cardinal features being a progressive encephalopathy, a fracturing osteodystrophy, and a microcytic anemia. Effective measures now available for water purification and knowledge of intestinal absorption have resulted in a reduction in exposure to an acceptable and manageable amount. Action to keep the dialysate aluminum less than 10 $\mu$g/l and the plasma aluminum less than 80 $\mu$g/l should avoid the development of any toxicity. For patients with clincial or laboratory evidence of accumulation, successful depletion can be achieved with DFO.


**References**

1. Alfrey, A.C., Mishell, J.M., Burks, J., Contiguglia, S.R., Rudolph, H., Lewin, E. and Holmes, J.H. (1972) Syndrome of dyspraxia and multifocal seizures associated with chronic

hemodialysis. Trans. ASAIO. 18: 257–261.

2. Barratt, L.J. and Lawrence, J.R. (1975) Dialysis associated dementia. Aust. N.Z.J. Med. 5: 62–65.

3. Flendrig, J.A., Kruis, H. and Das, H.A. (1976) Aluminum and dialysis dementia. Lancet i: 1,235.

4. Platts, M.M., Goode, G.C. and Hislop, J.S. (1977) Composition of the domestic water supply and the incidence of fractures and encephalopathy in patients on home dialysis. Brit. Med. J. ii: 657–660.

5. Elliott, H.L. and MacDougall, A.L. (1978) Aluminium studies in dialysis encephalopathy. Proc. EDTA 15: 157–163.

6. Davison, A.M., Walker, G., Oli, H. and Lewins, A.M. (1982) Water supply aluminium concentration, dialysis dementia, and effect of reverse osmosis water treatment. Lancet ii: 785–787.

7. Ward, M.K., Feest, T.G., Ellis, H.A., Parkinson, I.S., Kerr, D.N.S., Herrington, J. and Good, G.L. (1978) Osteomalacia dialysis osteodystrophy: evidence for a water-borne aetiological agent, probably aluminium. Lancet i: 841–845.

8. Short, A.I.K., Winney, R.J. and Robson, J.S. (1980) Reversible microcytic hypochromic anaemia in dialysis patients due to aluminium intoxication. Proc. EDTA., 17: 226–233.

9. Bone, I. (1978) Progressive dialysis encephalopathy, 'Dialysis Dementia.' In *Dialysis Review*, A.M. Davison (ed.) Tumbridge Wells: Pitman Medical, pp. 216–229.

10. Lewins, A.M. (1982) Aluminium intoxication. Proc. EDTNA 11: 210–220.

11. Parsons, V., Davis, C., Goode, C., Ogg, C. and Siddiqui, J. (1971) Aluminium in bone from patients with renal failure. Brit. Med. J. iv: 273–275.

12. Thomas, W.C. (1982) Trace metal-citric acid complexes as inhibitiors of calcification and crystal formation. Proc. Soc. Exp. Biol. Med. 170: 321–327.

13. Lieberherr, M., Grosse, B., Cournot-Witmer, G., Thiel, C.L. and Balsan, S. (1982) In vitro effect of aluminium on bone phosphatases: a possible interaction with PTH and vitamin $D_3$ metabolites. Calcif. Tissue. Int. 34: 280–284.

14. Berlyne, G.M., Ben-Ari, J., Pest, D., Weinberger, J., Stern, M., Gilmore, G.R. and Livine, R. (1970) Hyperaluminaemia from aluminium resins in chronic renal failure. Lancet ii: 494–496.

15. Fleming, L.W., Stewart, W.K., Fell, G.S. and Halls, D.J. (1982) The effect of oral aluminium therapy on plasma aluminium levels in patients with chronic renal failure in an area with low water aluminium. Clin. Nephrol. 17: 222–227.

16. Cannata, J.B., Alegria, P.R., Cuesta, M.V., Herrera, J. and Peral, V. (1983) Influence of aluminium hydroxide intake on haemoglobin concentrations and blood transfusion requirements in haemodialysis patients. Proc. EDTA-ERA. 20: 719–724.

17. Kaehny, W.D., Alfrey, A.C., Holman, R.E. and Shorr, W.J. (1977) Aluminium transfer during haemodialysis. Kidney Int. 12: 361–365.

18. Shapiro, W.B., Schilb, T.P., Waltrous, C.L., Levy, S.R. and Porush, J.G. (1983) Aluminium leakage from Redy sorbent cartridge. Kidney Int. 23: 536–539.

19. Wolf, A., Graf, H., Pinggera, W.F., Sturmvoll, H.K. and Meisinger, V. (1980) Serum aluminium and continuous ambulatory peritoneal dialysis. Ann. Intern. Med. 92: 130–131.

20. O'Donovan, R., Monitz, C., Baldwin, D., Brewer, J., Hammer, M., Rogerson, M. and Parsons, V. (1985) Control of hyperphosphataemia by oral magnesium carbonate and zero magnesium dialysate without aluminium binders. Proc. EDTA-ERA 22: 1,229–1,232.

21. Schneider, H., Kulbe, K.D., Weber, H. and Streicher, E. High-effective aluminium free phosphate binder in vitro and in vivo studies. Proc. EDTA-ERA 20: 725–730.

22. Ackrill, P., Ralston, A.J., Day, J.P. and Hodge, K.C. (1980) Successful removal of aluminium from a patient with dialysis encephalopathy. Lancet ii: 692–693.

23. Arze, R.S., Parkinson, I.S., Cartlidge, N.E., Britton, P. and Ward, M.K. (1981) Reversal of dialysis encephalopathy after desferrioxamine treatment. Lancet ii: 1,116.

24. Brown, D., Dawbor, J.K., Ham, K.N. and Xipell, J.M. (1982) Treatment of dialysis osteomalacia with desferrioxamine. Lancet ii: 343–345.

246

25. Wagner, K., Lenz, T., Keller, F., Neumayer, H.H., Fitzner, R., Pipenhagen, V., Dulce, H.J., Distler, A. and Molzahn, M. (1985) Does desferrioxamine induce aluminium load in patients on chronic haemodialysis? Proc. EDTA-ERA 22: 388–391.
26. Ciancioni, C., Poignet, J.L., Mauras, K., Panthier, G., Delous, S., Allain, P. and Mau, N.K. (1984) Plasma aluminium and iron kinetics in haemodialyzed patients after iv infusion of desferrioxamine. Trans. ASAIO 30: 479–482.
27. Simon, P., Ang, K.S. and Cam, G. (1985) Impaired transport of the iron-transferrin complex and microcytic anaemia in haemodialysis patients with aluminium intoxication. Proc. EDTA-ERA 22: 374–381.
28. Ihle, B.V., Buchanan, M.R.C., Stevens, B., Becker, B. and Kincaid-Smith, P. (1982) The efficacy of various treatment modalities on aluminium associated bone disease. Proc. EDTA 19: 195–202.
29. Kingswood, C., Banks, R.A., Bunker, T., Harrison, P. and Mackenzie, C. (1982) Fracture osteomalacia, CAPD, and aluminium. Lancet i: 70–71.
30. Payton, C.D., Junor, B.J.R. and Fell, G.S. (1984) Successful treatment of aluminium encephalopathy by intraperitoneal desferrioxamine (abstracts). Scottish Renal Association.
31. Davison, A.M. and Giles, G.R. (1981) The effect of transplantation on dialysis dementia. Proc. EDTA 16: 407–412.
32. Sullivan, P.A., Murnaghan, D.J. and Callaghan N. (1977) Dialysis dementia: recovery after transplantation. Brit. Med. J. ii: 740.
33. Hanson (1976) In discussion during Congress EDTA, Hamburg. Proc. EDTA 13: 362.

# 11. Water treatment for the preparation of dialysate

Alex M. Davison

In the early days of regular hemodialysis treatment, little attention was given to the quality of the water used to prepare dialysate. It was some time before it became recognized that variations in the quality of the water used to prepare dialysate could be associated with adverse reactions in the dialysis patient. In those patients treated with a dialysate prepared from excessively hard water, a syndrome developed in which there was a marked rise in blood pressure 3 to 6 hours after commencing hemodialysis, and this was associated with sweating, an abnormal sensation of warmth, nausea, profound lethargy, and weakness. This hard water syndrome [1] was recognized as being due to acute hypercalcemia and hypermagnesemia from the high concentration of these substances in the dialysate due to abnormally high concentrations being present in the water used to prepare the dialysate. Thereafter it did not take very long to understand that the quality of water for drinking purposes was clearly different from that required for dialysate preparation.

Even after 30 years of hemodialysis experience the full importance of adequate water treatment is only being recognized; although acute syndromes can be readily detected, it is only with increasing longevity of the dialysis patient that the full extent of chronic exposure to low concentrations of toxic substances is being fully appreciated. Unlike the gastrointestinal mucosal barrier, the dialysate membrane is not selective, and substances will pass across depending upon their size, charge, and molecular shape. In addition to this is the fact that certain substances which are present in dialysate in lower concentrations than in plasma may still cross the dialysis membrane and lead to toxic accumulation. This is because a number of substances in plasma are protein bound and therefore their free diffusable concentration is low, and if this is less than the concentration in the dialysate, then net transfer will take place, thereby increasing the total body burden.

There have been considerable changes in dialysis techniques and also dialysis equipment in the past 20 years. There has been a general shortening of dialysis hours due to structural changes in dialyzers, and changes in the thickness and nature of the dialysis membrane. The changes in membranes were stimulated by the 'middle molecule hypothesis,' which suggested that the persisting uremia of dialysis patients was due to the retention of

*Vincenzo Cambi (editor) Professor of Nephrology*
© *1987 Martinus Nijhoff Publishing, Boston. ISBN 0-89838-858-9. Printed in The United States.*

substances of a molecular weight greater than that removed by conventional membranes. In addition, there was a desire to produce a more 'biocompatible' membrane which would result in less cellular and humoral interaction. The older membranes, such as cuprophan, rely on diffusion of substances, while the more modern high flux membranes with larger pore radii provide for increased convection. While this may well satisfy the desire for more rapid ultrafiltration, shortened dialysis times, and improved biocompatibility, there will be increased possibility for transfer of contaminants from the dialysate and therefore the need for an increased standard of purity of the water used to prepare dialysate.

The quality of water varies throughout the year due to variations in rainfall, water treatment, and flow changes in the distribution system. In addition there is increasing use of a grid system for national water distribution, and therefore an individual house may be supplied with water from differing reservoirs at different times of the year. This makes it essential not only to adequately treat water used for preparing dialysate but also to monitor the quality of water being provided to dialysis installations. It must be remembered that the hourly exposure of a patient to dialysate is approximately 30 litres and in a year, approximately 19,000 litres; therefore, even substances which are present in only trace amounts may have the potential for producing toxicity in long-term treatment patients.

Contamination of water can occur in a variety of ways. It may occur anywhere between the area of rainfall, through the water treatment works, within the water distribution systems, or within the dialysis unit. There are a number of methods for the removal of contaminants from water, but there is no system that will universally remove all materials. The choice of water treatment plant will therefore depend on a knowledge of the type and amount of contamination in the water supplying the particular dialysis installation. If the correct systems of water treatment are chosen, then it should be possible to provide the patient with a water supply pure enough to ensure freedom from toxicity even with long-term treatment.


**Sources of Contaminants**

The water supply may be contaminated anywhere from the rainfall area to the final delivery system to the patient (table 11–1). In the provision of adequate dialysis care it is important to know details of the local collection, treatment, and distribution of water used to prepare dialysate.


*Water collection*

Water is usually collected from surface-fed reservoirs or from underground wells. Surface-fed reservoirs are likely to contain water with a variable amount of suspended particulate matter. The amount and type will vary

250

*Table 11–1.* Sources of water contamination

Water collection
  Fertilizers
  Herbicides
  Minerals
  Organic Material
  Pesticides
  Suspended particulate matter
Water treatment plants
  Aluminium
  Chloramines
  Chlorine
  Copper
  Fluoride
Water distribution system
  Bacteria
  Iron
  Lead
  Nitrates
  Pyrethrins
Dialysis equipment
  Bacteria
  Copper
  Zinc

depending upon the rainfall and the surrounding terrain. When rain falls after a prolonged dry period, it is likely readily to run from the surface and contain a considerable amount of suspended material such as clay, sand, or peat. Similarly the organic content of water will vary throughout the year, organic substances are formed from the decomposition of vegetation, and this process is at its greatest in autumn when grasses, ferns, and leaves start to decay. Where water is drawn from a well source it may contain a large amount of dissolved minerals depending upon the composition of the strata through which the water percolates. In addition, from both sources there is potential for contamination with agricultural products in the form of fertilizers, pesticides, herbicides, and detergents. Clearly the amount of these substances will vary from area to area, but there is increasing use of these substances; in many instances the toxicity for dialysis patients is unknown.

*Water treatment works*

Water authorities are charged with providing potable water, and to achieve this a number of substances are added in water treatment plants. In areas where the reservoir water contains a recognizable amount of suspended particulate matter, alum is added as a flocculating agent. Unfortunately there is no satisfactory control system available, and accordingly a variable amount of aluminum will be released into the distribution system. This has the effect of variably elevating the water supply is aluminum concentration, thereby producing a toxicity syndrome in dialysis patients consisting of dementia, myopathy, osteomalacia, and anemia. Ferrous sulphate can be used as an alternative to alum, but this affects a number of industrial processes and is not widely used. Chlorine is added to water as a widely accepted method of controlling bacterial contamination. In some areas chloramines, condensation products of chlorine and ammonia, are added. These are able to cross the dialysis membrane, and they subsequently denature hemoglobin by a direct oxidation and inhibition of the hexose monophosphate shunt, thereby producing a hemolytic anemia characterized by the presence of Heinz bodies [2]. In many areas fluoride is added to the water for the prevention of dental caries. If the dialysate fluoride concentration is in excess of 0.1 mg/l it is likely that significant quantities will cross the dialysis membrane with the potential of producing adverse effects on bone metabolism [3]. In some areas where the water supply is obtained from shallow surface reservoirs, copper sulphate is added to kill algae. In amounts exceeding 0.5 mgs/l it is likely to produce a number of dialysis-related effects such as nausea, headache, hepatic damage, and hemolysis [4].

*Water distribution systems*

The water distribution system may well be a source of contamination. The pipes used for distribution may be composed of either lead or iron, and these substances may leach into the water, producing unacceptably high concentrations. In addition, bacteria may grow particularly if there are any stagnant or dead spaces. The bacteria may produce pyrogens and toxins giving rise to adverse reactions during dialysis, and they may also produce nitrates which can give rise to methemoglobulinemia, hypotension, and nausea [5]. A fresh water louse Asellus aquaticus breeds in water mains and may give rise to an unpleasant odor and taste. For this reason water supplies are frequently treated with pyrethrins the toxicity of which is unknown. It is unlikely, however, that the amount used in water treatment has any adverse effects for dialysis patients.

*Dialysis equipment*

There are now a number of well-documented reports in which the source of the contaminant has been traced to the dialysis equipment. This is usually taken the form of metals leaching from the water distribution system, and to date there have been reports relating to copper [6], zinc [7], and aluminum [8]. In addition, the water distribution system from the water treatment plant may have stagnant areas and blind loops. These are ideally suited for bacterial growth, and adverse reactions may result from pyrogens and toxins. The bacterial counts in the dialysate water supply should not exceed 100 per ml, and careful planning is required to ensure that distribution systems do not

252

have any stagnant areas. Chlorine added to the municipal water supply to prevent bacterial growth will be removed by certain water purification apparatus, carbon filters, and so water 'down-stream' from such devices are liable to bacterial contamination.


**Water Treatment Methods**

A number of methods are available for the treatment of water used to prepare dialysate for hemodialysis. These include sediment filtration, water softeners, carbon filters, reverse osmosis, and deionization. It is important in the design of a water treatment facility that appropriate methods are used in the correct sequence in order to obtain water of the best possible quality as well as ensuring the maximum life from the installed equipment. Obviously the equipment chosen will be determined to a considerable extent by the quality of the local water supply, but will in general contain a sediment filter to remove particulate matter, water softening to remove calcium and magnesium, activated carbon filtration to remove chlorine, chloramines, organic materials, and pyrogens, reverse osmosis to remove dissolved minerals and organic materials and/or deionization to remove dissolved ions (table 11–2).


*Sediment filtration*

Sediment filters are used to remove particulate matter to protect other water treatment equipment from clogging. A number of types are available, and

*Table 11–2.* Equipment for effective removal of contaminants

| | |
|---|---|
| Aluminium | Reverse osmosis |
| Bacteria | Reverse osmosis, disinfection |
| Calcium | Softener, reverse osmosis, deioniser |
| Chloramine | Carbon filter |
| Chlorine | Carbon filter |
| Copper | Reverse osmosis, deioniser |
| Fertilizers | Reverse osmosis |
| Fluoride | Deioniser, reverse osmosis |
| Herbicides | Reverse osmosis |
| Iron | Oxidative filter, softener, Reverse osmosis |
| Lead | Reverse osmosis |
| Magnesium | Softener, deioniser |
| Nitrate | Reverse osmosis |
| Organic material | Organic scavenger, resins, Carbon filter |
| Particulate matter | Sediment filtration, ultrafiltration |
| Pesticides | Reverse osmosis |
| Sodium | Reverse osmosis, deioniser |
| Zinc | Reverse osmosis, deioniser |

they are described by the pore size which indicates the cut-off above which particles are retained by the filter: most commonly a 1 $\mu$ filter is used. The water pressure drop across the filter must be monitored as once the capacity of the filter is exceeded the pressure drop will increase, and there may be the breakthrough of particulates into the effluent from the filter. Once the pressure drop exceeds the value specified by the manufacturers the filter must be replaced.

The problems associated with sediment filtration are bacterial contamination and growth of algae. One consequence of excessive bacterial growth may be pyrogen reactions in the patient. For this reason regular disinfection and replacement are required.

*Water softeners*

Water softeners contain the sodium forms of strong cation exchanges, thereby removing calcium, magnesium, and other polyvalent cations such as iron and manganese in exchange for sodium ions. Once all the available sodium ions in the resin have been exchanged, it becomes exhausted and has to be regenerated. This is undertaken by using a solution of sodium chloride. The capacity of the water softener is dependent upon the amount of sodium available for exchange; therefore, in selecting appropriate equipment, it is essential to know the calcium and magnesium content of the local water supply as well as the volume of water that requires to be treated for each dialysis session.

The resins used in water softeners are capable of supporting bacterial growth, and this may give rise to pyrogen reactions in the patient. Back washing of the resin during regeneration will help to reduce this problem, but regular culturing is recommended and disinfection with hypochlorite undertaken as required.

If the water softener is regenerated on site it is important to ensure that this does not happen during a dialysis procedure, otherwise the dialysate sodium may rise to unacceptable values. The water softener should be provided with an automatic bypass valve which should be activated during regeneration.

*Carbon filtration*

Activated carbon filters remove chlorine, chloramines, and dissolved organic material, and are essential in the pretreatment of water prior to reverse osmosis. Carbon is particularly useful for the removal of organic materials in the molecular weight range of 60–300 daltons. Granular activated charcoal is best but, as it comes from a variety of sources, it is not of uniform quality and therefore care must be taken in equipment selection. This is particularly true with respect to chloramine which, if inadequately removed, may give rise to hemolysis. In addition, carbon filters which have become saturated with absorbed material may release chloramines into the effluent, thereby producing potential harm to the patient.

254

Carbon filters are liable to support bacterial growth because of their porosity and affinity for organic material. In addition, the removal of chlorine from the water may cause increase in microbial growth in the downstream water treatment apparatus, and therefore regular monitoring and appropriate disinfection are essential.

Carbon filters may release small particles of carbon, 'fines,' and this may cause clogging of other apparatus. It is important, therefore, to use a sediment filter downstream from the carbon filter.

Organic material can also be removed by organic scavengers using macroreticular resins which remove most organics present in mains water. These resins have the capacity for regeneration using a 10% brine solution with sometimes the addition of caustic soda.

*Reverse osmosis*

Reverse osmosis water treatment is the most effective method for removing dissolved inorganic substances, dissolved organic materials, bacteria, pyrogens, and particulate matter. Rejection of material is based on molecular sieving, and substances with a molecular weight greater than 200 daltons are rejected. Reverse osmosis membranes are capable of removing 90–95% of monovalent ions and 95–99% of divalent ions, and in the absence of any membrane leaks are able to exclude all bacteria, viruses, and pyrogens.

If two solutions of different ionic concentrations are separated by a semipermeable membrane, solvent flows from the less concentrated to the more concentrated. The pressure that must be applied to the concentrated solution to prevent such a flow is the osmotic pressure. If the pressure applied to the more concentrated side is greater than the osmotic pressure, then solvent will flow to the less concentrated side; this process is called reverse osmosis. In commercially available equipment several types of membranes have been used. Cellulose acetate has been extensively used, and more recently membranes of polyamide, polyimide, and polyfurane have been introduced. In addition, thin film composite membranes have also recently become available. The configuration of the membranes in the reverse osmosis apparatus varies, but the most commonly available are either spiral wound or hollow fibers. The spiral wound type are probably more satisfactory as the hollow fibers are susceptible to plugging and leaks.

Failure of the membrane can occur for a number of different reasons. If there is inadequate removal of calcium and magnesium by pretreatment with a water softener, then there is liable to be scale formation on the membranes with a subsequent loss of efficiency. Some membranes can be damaged by the presence of chlorine or chloramines, and cellulosic membranes are susceptible to bacterial degredation. Cellulose acetate membranes are sensitive to alkaline water. Care must be taken, therefore, to adequately pretreat the water entering the reverse osmosis device to ensure that the maximum life is obtained from the filter.

The efficacy of the reverse osmosis treatment can be monitored by determining the resistivity of the feed water and the product water, thereby calculating the percentage rejection. Once rejection falls below a critical value the membrane requires replacement.

Reverse osmosis membranes are susceptible to bacterial contamination, and this may well produce patient symptoms if there has been inaequate disinfection or membrane leaks which may be small enough not to be detected by any change in resistivity monitoring.

*Deionization*

Deionizers use an ion exchange principle, but they differ from water softeners in that they remove both cations and anions; cationic exchangers are made from a polysterene matrix which has been sulphonated with concentrated sulphuric acid. In this phase cations are exchanged for hydrogen ions. Anionic exchanges are made by chlormethalating and aminating the matrix and anions are exchanged for hydroxyl ions.

Deionizers may be of a mixed bed type where there is both cationic and anionic exchange resins, or a dual bed type in which there are two tanks one containing the cationic resin and the other the ionic resin. The mixed bed system is most efficient. The exchanged hydrogen ion and hydroxyl ion combine to form water. As with other ion exchange systems the deionizer has a finite capacity, and the duration of satisfactory performance will depend on the total quantity of dissolved ions in the feed water. The efficiency of the deionizer can be measured by monitoring the resistivity of the effluent, and regeneration can be undertaken as the deionizer nears exhaustion.

A problem may arise in that a deionizer nearing exhaustion may produce an effluent of an unacceptable degree of acidity. This occurs because in most deionizers there is an imbalance between cation and anion exchange capacity favoring cations. If the effluent becomes significantly acidic then two hazards may well arise. Firstly the acidic effluent may cause copper to leach from any of the piping of the delivery system [6] or from the dialysis equipment. The amount may reach toxic proportions, and patients may complain of anorexia, nausea, vomiting, diarrhea, and abdominal pains associated with hemolysis. This syndrome has now been well documented, and no copper should be present in either the water distribution system or the dialysis apparatus. Secondly heparin loses its anticoagulant activity once the pH falls below 7, and it is almost completely ineffective at a pH less than 6.7. Thus if the effluent water is acidic, there is a possibility of the inactivation of heparin and the subsequent clotting of the dialyser [9].

Once exhausted, the previously absorbed ions may be eluted to the effluent, those of lower affinity being most readily displaced; thus for cations this would cause the sequential elution of hydrogen, sodium, potassium, magnesium, and then calcium. For anions it would be fluoride, hyroxyl, bicarbonate, chloride, nitrite, sulphate, and subsequently nitrate.

Deionizers are liable to bacterial contamination which may cause pyrogenic reactions in the patients. They are also expensive particularly if they require frequent regeneration due to a high ionic concentration in the feed water. In addition, they do not remove chlorine or chloramines but can be particularly useful for improving the quality of postreverse osmosis treated water, especially in those situations where there is a high fluoride and nitrate content. Used in this situation the combination of reverse osmosis and deionization will produce an extremely high quality water, and the deionizer will have a particularly long life and therefore be cost-effective.

*Other Methods*

Ultrafiltration is a water treatment process similar to reverse osmosis, but the sieving coefficient is very much higher. Ultrafiltration is therefore effective for removing micro-organisms, pyrogens, colloids, and particulate matter. They can be particularly useful in areas where the supply water is contaminated with significant amounts of bacteria or in which there is a high concentration of suspended particulate matter. They can then be used as pretreatment prior to reverse osmosis treatment thereby protecting a reverse osmosis membrane from bacterial contamination and scaling from particulate matter.

Distillation is another method for water purification, but it is extremely expensive, particularly with respect to energy costs. Although distillation itself is very effective, certain volatile contaminants maybe carried over and cause untoward effects. In addition, the system design is such that it is prone to bacterial contamination.

**Treated Water Distribution**

In a dialysis unit the ultra-pure water produced by the water treatment plant must be conveyed to the dialysis station. If the storage tank and distribution system is made of inappropriate material, there is a danger that substances will be leached which may well be toxic to the patient. There are well-documented reports in the literature of copper water pipes being implicated as a source of copper contamination producing headache, chills, sweating, nausea, and exhaustion during dialysis. Similarly zinc has been implicated producing nausea, vomiting, and fever. A further report associated aluminum leaching from an anode in the water system as a cause of aluminum intoxication in hemodialysis patients [8].

The storage tanks and distribution system may also be a source of bacterial proliferation. The storage tank should be of a size adequate to enable dialysis within the unit to continue in the event of an unexpected failure of the water treatment plant. The size, therefore, will depend upon the number of treatment stations being served and the average length of dialysis being undertaken. The distribution system should not have any dead ends or lengths where there is only intermittent flow. In our experience the problem of bacterial proliferation within the distribution system has been solved by the installation of a ring main system whereby the water is continually circulating through the distribution system and then returned to the storage tank following exposure to ultraviolet light. In this way there are no parts of the system in which the water flow is stagnant and therefore liable to bacterial overgrowth.


## Conclusion

The correct design of a satisfactory water treatment system is dependent upon the quality of the mains water being supplied by the water authority. Ideally the installation should be duplicate so that in the event of a breakdown or the requirement for routine servicing, continuous ultra-pure water can be produced. I therefore recommend that the mains water should be initially treated by a sediment filter to remove suspended particulate matter. It should then pass through a water softener to remove divalent cations and then a carbon filter or organic scavenger to remove chlorine and chloramines. A further filtration is then required to remove any carbon 'fines.' The water should then pass through reverse osmosis treatment, and in those areas where there is very high fluoride or nitrate contamination this can then be followed by 'polishing' with deionization. The water can then be stored in a suitable storage tank and distributed to the dialysis stations through PVC piping arranged in a ring mains system with the return to the storage tank through an ultraviolet sterilizer. The quality of the water with respect to both bacterial and other contamination should be monitored at regular intervals, and the apparatus serviced according to manufacturers' recommendations. The installation of a parallel water treatment plant allows for the continuous provision of ultra-pure water while allowing for essential maintenance without disruption to the routine dialysis treatment.

The changes that have taken place in hemodialysis in the past few years have resulted in much improved patient management. Although many patients still become symptomatic during a dialysis session, changes in membranes have reduced both the incidence and severity of these reactions. The desire to reduce dialysis times by the introduction of high flux membranes has resulted in the increased possibility of contaminants, even if present in only trace amounts, being transferred from dialysate to patient. There is thus an increasing need to provide ultra-pure water for the preparation of dialysate. The move toward shortened dialysis times will not be reversed in view of widespread patient acceptance, and therefore we are beholden to ensure that there is no adverse medical effect from this trend. Apart from the dialysis membrane, the most important factor in achieving this aim is water of a high degree of purity. We must be prepared to provide the necessary equipment to achieve this standard, and thereafter institute regular monitoring of both patient and water to ensure that it is achieved.

# References

1. Freeman, R.M., Lawton, R.L. and Chamberlain, M.A. (1967) Hard water syndrome. New Eng. J. Med. 276: 1,113–1,118.
2. Kjellstrand, C.M., Eaton, J.W., Yawata, Y., Swofford, H., Kolpin, C. F., Buselmeir, T.J., von Hartitzsch, R. and Jacobs, H.S. (1974) Haemolysis in dialysed patients caused by chloramines. Nephron 13: 427–433.
3. Jowsey, J., Johnson, W.J., Taves, D.R. and Kelly, P.J. (1972) Effects of dialysate calcium and luoride on bone disease during regular hemodialysis. J. Lab. Clin. Med. 79: 204–214.
4. Manzler, A.D. and Schreinner, A.W. (1970) Copper induced acute hemolytic anaemia. A new complication of hemodialysis. Ann. Intern. Med. 73: 409–412.
5. Carlson, D.J. and Shapiro, F.L. (1970) Methemoglobulinemia from well water nitrates: a complication of home dialysis. Ann. Intern. Med. 73: 757–759.
6. Ivanovitch, P., Manzler, A. and Drake, R. (1969) Acute haemolysis following hemodialysis. Trans. ASAIO 15: 316–320.
7. Petrie, J.J.B. and Row, P.G. (1977) Dialysis anaemia caused by subacute zinc toxicity. Lancet i: 1,178–1,180.
8. Flendrig, J.A., Kruis, H. and Das, H.A. (1976) Aluminum intoxication: the cause of dialysis dementia. Proc. EDTA 13: 355–363.
9. Schwarzbeck, A., Wagner, L., Squarr, H.U. and Strauch, M. (1977) Clotting in dialysis due to low pH of dialysis fluid. Clin. Nephrol. 7: 125.

# 12. 'On-site' preparation of sterile apyrogenic electrolyte solutions for hemofiltration and hemodiafiltration

C.M. Mion and B. Canaud

Predilutional [1] and postdilutional hemofiltration (HF) [2] and hemodiafiltration (HDF) [3] have been proposed as alternatives to conventional hemodialysis (HD) for more than a decade, and yet by December 31, 1984, their utilization remained limited to less than 5% of end-stage renal disease (ESRD) patient population receiving some form of maintenance dialysis in Europe [4]. The restricted application of both HF and HDF contrasts with the claims insisting on marked improvement in dialysis tolerance obtained with convective solute removal, characterized by a reduction in the incidence of symptomatic hypotension and postdialytic fatigue [5–7]. This situation can, at least partly, be explained by the higher cost of HF/HDF induced by the use of commercially prepared sterile apyrogenic electrolyte solutions required to compensate for the large amounts of body fluids removed by convection` during each HF/HDF session.

Following the initial success of Henderson and his associates [8] in producing sterile pyrogen-free fluid by ultrafiltration through an Amicon XP50 polysulfone hollow fiber ultrafilter, the possibility to prepare safely on a routine basis sterile pyrogen-free infusate for HF/HDF has been further explored by several investigators [9–12]. These studies have confirmed the effectiveness and reliability of ultrafiltration to obtain on a very long-term sterile pyrogen-free substitution fluid prepared in the dialysis center.

In this chapter, the technical aspects of 'on-site' preparation of substitution fluid for HF/HDF are described. The hazards of bacterial contamination of the water and/or the equipment utilized for this purpose are thoroughly reviewed, and the appropriate measures that should be implemented to eliminate this risk are emphasized.

## Rationale

Many reasons may be advocated to justify the preparation of sterile pyrogen-free electrolyte solutions in the dialysis center for instantaneous use during HF and HDF.

First, considerable progress have been made in the technology of

*Vincenzo Cambi (editor) Professor of Nephrology*
© *1987 Martinus Nijhoff Publishing, Boston. ISBN 0-89838-858-9. Printed in The United States.*

membrane filtration and reverse osmosis (RO). Highly purified water is currently utilized in areas as diverse as analytical laboratories, the pharmaceutical and food industries, and in the manufacture of microprocessors. To meet this growing demand, a great variety of water treatment devices are presently available on the market; properly operated and adequately maintained and disinfected, these equipments can produce sterile apyrogenic water at a resonable cost [13].

Second, the large-scale evaluation of HF or HDF as alternative therapies of ESRD will be possible only if these techniques become cost-effective by comparison with conventional HD. The on-site production of substitution fluid at the bedside is a prerequisite for any attempt in reducing significantly the cost of HF/HDF, which can be estimated to be 50–200% higher than HD when 10 to 30 liters of commercially available substitution fluid are utilized [14]. Furthermore, by lowering the cost of replacement fluid by on-line production, the volume of exchange may be prescribed on an individual basis according to the patients' needs for adequate dialysis without increasing the treatment cost at an unacceptable level.

Third, sterile apyrogenic substitution fluid prepared by pharmaceutical companies is conditioned in 4.5-liter soft plastic bags. These bags, made of transparent polivinyl chloride, are protected by double packing with a stronger outer envelope attached under sterile vacuum conditions [15]. The sterility of the infusate is insured by autoclaving; contamination of the solution can occur, however, during handling and transport through accidental microperforation of the bag wall. In a survey of the West German experience with commercially prepared fluid for HF, a 0.2% incidence of pyrogenic reactions was observed: there was a high degree of morbidity, and 12 patients deaths were recorded. The death rate due to contaminated infusate was estimated at 1 death per 27,000 treatments [15]. Two preventive measures were recommended by the manufacturer to eliminate the risk of infusing contaminated fluid. The first was to check for the persistence of vacuum and the absence of fluid between the inner and outer bags, to confirm the integrity of the double packing. The second preventive measure was to control bags for cloudiness of fluid using a high-power light source. These two measures, however, are not absolutely foolproof: pyrogen reactions have been reported in patients infused with substitution fluid contained in intact bags with double packing [15], and electrolyte solutions may remain crystal clear even in the presence of heavy bacterial contamination with colony counts up to $10^6$ colonies forming unit/ml (CFU/ml) [16]. To increase the safety of commercially produced infusate, the interposition of a filter between bag and patient seems to be a more reliable preventive measure. This filter should allow for a volume flow up to 200 ml/min and reject bacteria, endotoxin, and their fragments. An ultrafilter with a cut-off point of $10^4$ daltons and an adequate surface area is therefore required, resulting in a significant cost increase, particularly if the filter is not reused [15]. In addition to accidental bacterial contamination, premixed prepackaged infusates have been shown to contain up to 9.2 pg/ml of endotoxins [17]. At this concentration, a 70 kg patient infused with 30 liters of substitution fluid during HF would receive 270 ng of endotoxin, a load largely in excess of the pyrogenic dose of 1 to 2 ng/kg body weight [18]. Whether plastic bags are the cause of the endotoxin content of the commercially prepared infusates is not proven, but it is interesting to note that water for injection and normal saline conditioned in conventioned glass bottles and prepared by the same pharmaceutical companies were commonly found to contain less than 1 pg/ml of endotoxin [17].

Finally, a growing clinical experience obtained by several groups of investigators [9–12, 14, 19–22] has confirmed over the years that on-site production of substitution fluid is a safe reproducible technique, not overly complicated, and easy to duplicate.


**Specifications concerning the preparation of 'water for injection'**

Substitution fluid for HF and HDF is directly infused in the patient's blood: it should therefore satisfy the sterility and apyrogenicity requirements for intravenous fluid. To meet this demand, the nephrologists interested in the preparation of sterile apyrogenic infusate should become familiar with the specifications of various pharmacopeiae about the quality of water that may be used in the preparation of intravenous solutions. These specifications are not universal, however, and some discrepancies exist between the United States Pharmacopeia (USP) and most European pharmacopeiae. It should be stressed, however, that these pharmacopeiae requirements are presented by national regulating agencies in the form of good manufacturing practices for solutions prepared by the pharmaceutical industry that are stored and transported. There is at present no specific recommendations made by health authorities concerning the preparation and quality control of substitution fluid (or other compounded solutions) made for extemporaneous intravenous infusion.

The main USP definitions concerning water used as a pharmaceutical solvent are presented in table 12–1. According to USP standards, 'Purified Water' and 'Water for Injection' may be obtained by reverse osmosis. Water for injection may be sterilized by appropriate membrane filtration [23]. These specifications can readily be implemented in on-site preparation of infusate, because this preparative technique rests exclusively on the effectiveness and reliability of reverse osmosis and submicron membrane filtration procedures. It is worth nothing, however, that water for injection should not contain any added substance.

Conversely, most European pharmacopeiae define water for injection as water purified by distillation. In fact, distillation necessitates complex equipments, that function with energy expenditure, require stringent main-tenance, and have elevated running costs. Even though distillation eliminates

*Table 12–1.* Definition of purified water for injection and sterile water for injection according to the United States Pharmacopeia [23]

---

A.   *Purified water:* water obtained by distillation, ion exchange treatment, reverse osmosis, or other suitable process. It is prepared from water complying with the regulations of the United States Public Health Service with respect to drinking water. Purified water contains no added substance.

    * *Caution:* Do not use purified water in preparation intended for parenteral administration. For such purposes use water for injection or sterile water for injection.

B.   *Water for injection:* water purified by distillation or reverse osmosis. It contains no added substance.

    * *Caution:* Water for injection is intended for use as a solvent for the preparation of parenteral solutions. For parenteral solutions that are prepared under aseptic conditions and are not sterilised by appropriate filtration or in the final container, first render the water for injection sterile and thereafter protect it from microbial contamination.

C.   *Sterile water for injection:* Water for injection sterilized and suitably packaged. It contains no antimicrobial agent or other added substance.

---

bacteria and pyrogens, the overall system may be prone to microbial proliferation because storage tanks are necessary with this form of water treatment. Early attempts to develop a home peritoneal dialysis system utilizing water distillation and water sterilization was abandoned after a few years in spite of successful clinical application because of the bulkiness of the equipment, long hours for preparing and sterilizing the dialysate fluid, and elevated costs [24]. Although stills with production capacities adapted to the on-site production of infusate are available on the market, it appears that distillation is not the method of choice for this purpose.

Whatever the procedures utilized to produce purified water and water for injection and to prepare sterile apyrogenic electrolyte solutions, the greatest awareness should be maintained among involved personnel concerning the permanent risk of microbial contamination of the finished product. The long-term success of on-site preparation techniques will rest upon enforcement of rigid adherence to tested protocols of sterilization, disinfection, and maintenance practices. A detailed description of the various aspects of bacterial contamination of aqueous media is presented in the following section to help setting up a surveillance and control program adequately designed for the elimination of this health hazard.

## Bacterial contaminants of water

The bacterial and pyrogen content of water varies greatly depending on its source. In most cases, however, dialysis centers are supplied with municipal water meeting the requirements for drinking water. In city water treatment plants, drinking water is sanitized by adding free chlorine, chloramines, or ozone. The bactericidal action of these agents maintain bacterial contamination at a low level, provided there are no leaks in the pipes of the city distribution system and the concentration of disinfecting agents remains adequate down to the point of utilization. When the water is pumped from a well, great care should be taken to protect the well from environmental contamination, particularly by organic substances that could potentiate bacterial growth. Furthermore, the water should be adequately chlorinated to prevent bacterial proliferation during storage in the holding tank [10]. Microorganisms and their breakdown products commonly found in drinking water and water treatment systems are presented in table 12–2. Gram positive and Gram negative bacteria are almost universally found in cultured samples, whereas mycobacteria are isolated only from 45–60% of tap water samples studied [25]. Fungi and yeasts are rarely found in municipal water. Viruses have been isolated from 6.7–43.5% of samples obtained by concentrating large volume of sanitized drinking water (studied volumes of water ranging from 20 to 1,890 liters) [26].

*Magnification of bacterial contamination in water treatment systems*

When adequately treated, tap water contains less than 100 CFU/ml: the colony counts averaged 38 CFU/ml in one study [27] and remained below 10 CFU/ml in another [11]. The best way to maintain such a low contamination would be to feed directly tap water into a reverse osmosis apparatus without pretreatment. In most cases, however, feed water of RO units is of poor quality and should be pretreated to eliminate colloids, particulates, calcium, magnesium, iron, and/or manganese that induce scale

*Table 12–2.* Contamination of water by microorganisms and their breakdown products (adapted from reference [45])

| | Microorganisms | Metabolic or Breakdown Products |
|---|---|---|
| I. Common contaminants | Gram neg bacteria | Endotoxins<br>Lipopolysaccharides<br>Lipid A<br>Peptidoglycans |
| | Gram pos bacteria | Peptidoglycans<br>Teichoic acids<br>Exotoxins<br>Proteins |
| | Mycobacteria | Peptidoglycans<br>Polysaccharides<br>Proteins |
| | Algae | Peptidoglycans |
| II. Unusual contaminants | Fungi and yeasts | Polysaccharides<br>Protein |
| | Viruses | Hemagglutinin |

formation on the RO membrane with loss of efficiency. Further, some types of RO membranes necessitate chlorine removal.

Three components of water pretreatment systems are the major cause of bacterial contamination: sediment filters, resins of water softeners and deionizers, and carbon filters. Sediment filters are made of felts, woven yarns, or packed fiberglass: these filter media behave like ideal ecological niches for the attachment and growth of bacterial organisms, which result in the contamination of downstream equipment. Continuous chlorination of the water treatment system and replacement of sediment filters at appropriate intervals will minimize this problem.

Water softener resins are susceptible to bacterial contamination. These resins have large microbiological entrapment capabilities and facilitate bacterial multiplication [28]. Although backwashing of the resins during regeneration tends to limit this phenomenon, the microorganisms are not readily dislodged because they are adsorbed to the resin and enmeshed with the resin matrix. Attempts to disinfect resins with formaldehyde have been disappointing [11, 29]. In a microbiologic study of water pre-treatment systems [11], the authors of this chapter observed that the weekly disinfection of the softener resins with 4% formaldehyde had no effect on bacterial growth: over a period of 4 weeks, the bacterial content of the water passing through the resins increased from $10^1$ CFU/ml on the first day up to $10^4$ on the 28th day of observation. However, when the sediment filters and the carbon filters were changed each week together with resin formalinization, the water bacterial content decreased and the number of bacteria oscillated during the week from $10^1$ to $4-7\times10^3$ CFU/ml.

Deionizers resins are also susceptible to bacterial contamination. When tap water contains high levels of fluoride or aluminum, the installation of a deionizer downstream from an RO unit may be necessary. This combined process yields a 'polished' water with a low inorganic content and high resistivity; such a procedure, however, results in the seeding of RO treated water by bacteria released from the deionizer resins [29].

When carbon filters are required for chlorine removal, as, for example, with the RO membranes made of polyamide, bacterial contamination of water is unavoidable. The microporous structure of granulated activated carbon and its affinity for organics facilitates the adsorption of bacteria, whereas the removal of chlorine promotes bacterial growth.

*Bacterial flora of tap water, water treatment, and hemodialysis systems*

As shown in table 12–3, Gram positive bacteria are isolated both from tap water and water treatment systems. In the experience of the authors of this chapter, Bacillus seems to be the predominant organism in tap water, where its persistence in spite of chlorination at the water treatment plant may be related to its spore-forming characteristics (11). However, other studies have shown that Gram negative bacteria, such as Pseudomonas aeruginosa and

266

*Table 12–3.* Bacteria isolated from tap water, water treatment systems, and hemodialysis systems

|  | Tap Water | Water Softener | Hemodialysis Systems |
|---|---|---|---|
| Gram pos bacteria | Bacillus sp | Bacillus sp<br>Corynebacterium sp<br>Micrococcus sp<br>Staphylococcus sp<br>Streptococcus sp | Bacillus sp |
| Gram neg bacteria | Pseudomonas sp<br>(P aeruginosa,<br>P maltophilia,<br>P cepacia)<br>Flavobacter sp | Escherichia coli<br>Pseudomonas sp<br>Flavobacterium sp<br>Serratia sp<br>Achromobacter sp<br>Aerobacter sp<br>Alcaligenes sp | Pseudomonas sp<br>Flavobacterium sp<br>Acinetobacter sp<br>Alcaligenes sp<br>Erwinia sp<br>Achromobacter sp<br>Aeromonas sp<br>Xanthomonas sp<br>Serratia sp<br>Moraxella sp<br>Klebsiella sp<br>Enterobact Cloacae |
| Anaerobes |  | Clostridium sp |  |
| Mycobacteria | M chelonei<br>M kansasii<br>M xenopi<br>M gordonae<br>M scrofulaceum | Mycobacterium sp | M chelonei<br>M chelonei-like<br>  organisms |

Flavobacterium species, may represent the main contaminants of municipal waters [27, 28].

In water treatment systems as in hemodialysis systems, it has been repeatedly shown that the type of microorganisms involved are primarily Gram negative water bacteria, among which Pseudomonas and Flavobacterium represent the two most frequently encountered genera. In a remarkable series of studies, the investigators from the Center for Disease Control (Public Health Service, U.S. Department of Health, Education and Welfare, Phoenix, Arizona, U.S.A.) have demonstrated that Gram negative bacteria can multiply relatively fast in a variety of hospital-associated fluids ranging from distilled, deionized, RO, and softened water, which are normally considered devoid of nutrients [30]. 'Naturally occurring' strains of Pseudomonas aeruginosa, grown in distilled water, were shown to have a generation time (i.e., time required for a population to double) of 4.8 hours [31]. Furthermore, 'naturally occurring' Ps aeruginosa demonstrated a higher resistance of a variety of disinfectants than subcultured cells of the same strain [32]. These observations suggested the potential for the development of formaldehyde resistant Pseudomonas strains, a possibility that has been confirmed for Ps mesophilica [33].

Mycobacteria are frequently isolated from tap water [24] and have been identified as the cause of infection in uremic patients, occurring either in isolated cases [34, 35] or in outbreaks among ESRD patients receiving peritoneal dialysis with reverse osmosis peritoneal dialysis systems [36] or treated with hemodialysis and using processed dialysers [37]. Mycobacterium chelonei and M chelonei like organisms (MCLO) were isolated during the investigation of a peritoneal dialysis outbreak by the Center for Disease Control: the growth characterics in water of these atypical mycobacteria and their resistance to disinfectants were studied [38]. M chelonei was shown to be able to multiply in commercial distilled water attaining population levels of $10^5$ to $10^6$ cells per ml, with generation times from 8 to 15 hours at 25°C. Results of disinfectant studies demonstrated that isolates of M chelonei and M fortuitum were markedly resistant to chlorine and to formaldehyde. Isolates of M chelonei obtained from peritoneal dialysis machines [38] and isolates of MCLO from hemodialysis systems [37] survived in 2% aqueous formaldehyde solutions up to 24 hours although they did not survive exposure to 4% formaldehyde for the same duration. For comparison, it is worth noting that cultures of P aeruginosa, P Cepacia, Klebsiella, and E coli ranging from $1.4 \times 10^4$ to $2.4 \times 10^6$ CFU/ml showed no survivors in 2% formaldehyde at 10 minutes of exposure [38].

Yeasts and fungi are seldom encountered in tap water and have not been identified as a health hazard arising from hemodialysis systems. However, yeasts (Candida sp., Rhodotorula sp) and fungi (Aspergillus sp, Cryptococcus sp, Geotrichum sp, Paecilomyces sp, Penicillium sp, and Streptomyces sp) represented 21.5% of the isolates obtained from cultures of backflushed samples from exhausted softener tank resins [28].

*Recommended procedures to reduce bacterial contamination*

Water pretreatment systems behave as culture media and their utilization, which is almost always necessary, results in a marked increase in bacterial content of water. This trend will be further exaggerated if strict procedures for maintenance and disinfection of pretreatment equipment are not established. Several approaches can be used to maintain the system at an acceptable level of bacterial contamination. First, the configuration of the hydraulic flow path should be linear and should exclude dead ends, by-passes, and three-way faucets that may create zones of water stagnation into the system [39]. Second, continuous disinfection can be efficiently obtained from the head of the pretreatment chain down to the carbon filters by adequate chlorination implemented by a proportioning pump; an automatic chlorine titration device should monitor the pump to guarantee water free chlorine concentrations ranging from 0.35 to 1 mg/l. At these chlorine levels, most Gram negative bacteria fail to survive after 1 minute contact time [38]. Third, sediment filters should be changed at frequent intervals (at least monthly) both to avoid the release of collected particles that could occur should the exclusion capacity of the filter be exceeded, and to prevent excessive bacterial growth. Likewise, the regeneration cycles of water softeners should be scheduled at short intervals (i.e., daily or every other day). Fourth, whenever possible, storage tanks for softened water should be avoided, and pretreated water should be fed directly in the reverse osmosis unit. Finally, the bacterial content of softened water can be reduced drastically by placing an ultrafilter or a microbiological filter (0.22 $\mu$m pore size filter membrane) downstream from the water pretreatment chain: however, strict disinfection procedures should be prescribed to protect these membrane filtration devices from becoming heavily contaminated and losing their efficiency (vide infra).

*Endotoxins and other water contaminants from bacterial origin*

Bacterial endotoxins are constant constituents of the outer part of the Gram negative bacterial cell wall, and are the most significant pyrogen for the preparation of intravenous solutions. Constantly shed into the environment of the living bacterium and entirely released from the cells when the bacterium undergoes autolysis, endotoxins are characterized by their ubiquitous nature. Extreme care should be taken to eliminate even minute quantities of these substances when preparing substitution fluid for HF/HDF. Besides its well-known pyrogenicity, endotoxin has been shown to have profound effect on a broad spectrum of biological activities. Among an array of pathophysiological disturbances, endotoxin has the capacity to activate the mononuclear phagocytes, as well as the complement and the coagulation system, release vasoactive amines and modify hemodynamics, induce platelet aggregation and initiate intravascular disseminated coagulation, produce shock and ultimately death [40].

Endotoxins are heat-stable compounds that are not inactivated by usual disinfectants such as formaldehyde and chlorine. Their inactivation can be obtained by extended dry heat cycles, alkaline or acidic conditions, and also by polymyxin B.

Chemically, endotoxins are members of a class of phospholipids called lipopolysaccharides (LPS). LPS are highly purified endotoxins that do not contain protein, whereas unpurified endotoxins contain lipid, carbohydrate, and protein. The term endotoxin seems therefore preferable when referring to the unpurified endotoxin that contaminate water and chemicals used for the preparation of substitution fluid. As shown in figure 12–1, LPS consist of three distinct regions that are biochemically linked to each other. The inner region is a hydrophobic lipid called lipid A. The central region, called the core, is an acidic oligo saccharide that is similar for large groups of bacteria. The outer region is hydrophilic; it is composed of long, whisker-like projections, the O-antigenic side chains, that contain repeating oligosaccharide units. These side chains determine the serological specificity of the organisms by their primary structure and spatial configuration [40]. Typical endotoxins usually have a minimal particle weight on the order of $10^6$ daltons.

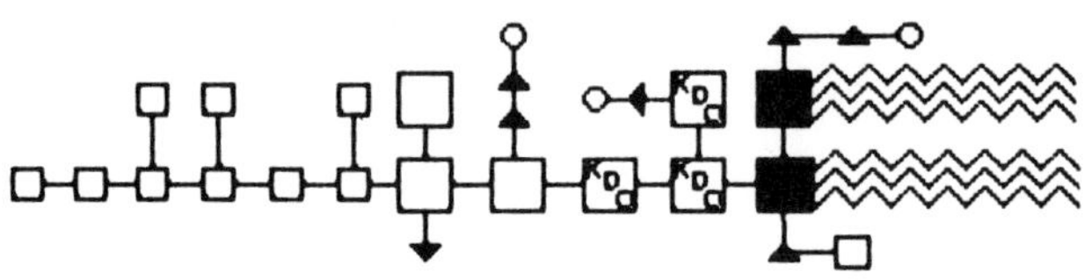

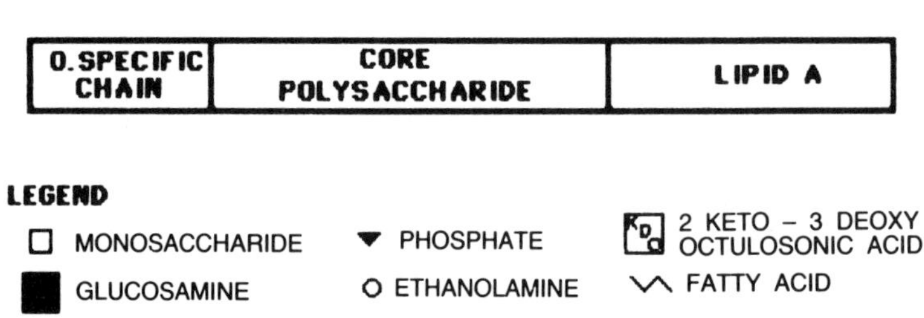


*Figure 12–1.* Schematic representation of the structure of lipopolysaccharides and their major constituents. In most cases, the core is terminated by a 2-keto-3-deoxyoctulosonic acid (KDO) placed at the junction between the core and lipid A (from reference [49]).

These molecules are polymers made by association of subunits having molecular weights of 120,000 to 10,000 daltons. Depending on environmental factors, endotoxins may form large aggregates or dissociate in smaller subunits. In the presence of magnesium and calcium, LPS form bilayer sheets of vesicles with a diameter of the order of 0.1 $\mu$m. Conversely, when endotoxin preparations are treated with a surfactant or detergent, a disaggregation process results in the production of subunits which have a molecular weight of approximately 10,000 to 25,000 daltons, a diameter of 8 to 12 angströms, and a length of 200 to 700 angströms [41–43]. Studies using molecular filters have shown that the vesicles and bilayer sheets will pass through a 0.22 $\mu$m membrane filter, but will be retained by a 0.025 $\mu$m pore size. Small micellar forms will pass through 0.025 $\mu$m membrane filter, but will be retained by $10^6$ normal molecular weight limit (mmwl) molecular filter. Finally, when LPS dissociates in its smallest subunit due to the action of sodium deoxycholate, a surface active agent, it will pass through a $10^6$ nmwl molecular filter, but will be retained by a $10^4$ nmwl molecular filter [44]. Lipid A can be as small as 2,000 daltons and could be expected to pass through molecular filters of lower nmwl pore size. Free lipid A, however, is a water-insoluble material prepared from LPS by mild acid hydrolysis, and there is no evidence that such a degradation takes place in aqueous media. It is important to note that lipid A retains all the biological activities of intact endotoxin molecules [40].

Other microbial products that contaminate water, are also potential pyrogens. Among them, peptidoglycan is one the major candidates [45]. Peptidoglycan is a rigid macromolecule that forms the basal layer of the bacterial cell wall and surrounds the cytoplasmic membrane of cell bacteria. It

270

is made of polymerized disaccharide tetrapeptide subunits. Small fragments of peptidoglycan are shed from the cell wall of the bacterium into the environment [46]. The enzymatic hydrolysis of peptidoglycan by bacterial enzymes divides the molecule into dipeptides, tetra, and pentapetpides and also in larger fragments (E. Lederer, personal communication). The N-acetyl muramic dipeptide structure, which is a major constituent of intact peptido-glycan, is the most representative among these breakdown products. With a molecular weight of 492 daltons, this dipeptide can readily pass through cellulosic dialysis membranes. N-acetyl muramic dipeptide has been shown to be pyrogenic for humans, but relatively large doses (i.e., several $\mu$g per kg body weight) are required to obtain a febrile response. In rabbits, the minimal pyrogenic dose is about 10,000-fold higher than that for bacterial lipopolysaccharides [47, 48]. Peptidoglycan derivatives have also been shown to induce alterations in the activity of mononuclear phagocytes [49].

*Microbiology of electrolyte concentrates*

Although substitution fluid could be prepared by dissolving dry reagent grade chemicals in RO-treated water (i.e., water for injection), it is more practical to use commercially prepared premixed electrolyte concentrates conditioned in plastic containers. Electrolyte concentrates and RO-treated water can easily be mixed using a proportioning pump [19–22] or a gravimetric method [9, 11].

Acetate-containing concentrate is most commonly used in the preparation of substitution fluid [8–12, 19, 20]. One liter of this solution contains the ade-quate amount of a balanced electrolyte mixture necessary for the preparation of 35 liters of diluted infusate. The molarity of this highly concentrated solution is not compatible with bacterial growth and survival. Acetate concentrate is, therefore, considered as an autosterilizing solution. On rare occasions, acetate concentrate was found to be contaminated with Penicillium sp, an environmental fungus (C. Mion, unpublished observation).

The use of bicarbonate substitution fluid has also been recommended particularly in HDF [22]. Two concentrates of different composition are required to prepare bicarbonate infusate [50]. The first solution contains sodium chloride, divalent cations, and acetic acid: it is concentrated 35 times and is considered as bacteriostatic. The second solution contains adequate amounts of sodium bicarbonate and sodium chloride and is provided in a concentration of 20:1 because of the poor solubility of bicarbonate. It has been suggested that bacteriostasis should be also insured by the molarity of this bicarbonate concentrate [50]. In fact, isolates from cultures of this concentrate have been found positive for Staphylococcus epidermidis with less than 100 CFU/ml [50], and also for a variety of bacteria including Pseudomonas putida, Staphylococcus saprophyticus, St hominis, Corynebac-terium sp, and Micrococcus sp, with colony counts ranging form $10^2$ to $10^3$ CFU/ml (unpublished observations from the authors of this chapter).

## Cold sterilization and depyrogenation of substitution fluid prepared for instantaneous use

Sterilization is defined as the use of a physical or chemical procedure to destroy all microbial life, including highly resistant bacterial endospores [51]. Steam autoclaving is the conventional technique used by the pharmaceutical industry to sterilize electrolyte solutions following adequate depyrogenation and suitable packaging. Heat sterilization ensures an 'overkill' that increases the margin of safety necessary to sterilize fluids that will be transported and later used after a storage period of unpredictable duration. Heat sterilization is obviously not applicable to on-site production of substitution fluid in a dialysis center. In such a setting, reverse osmosis, ultrafiltration (sometimes called molecular filtration), and submicron membrane filtration should be considered together as complementary procedures necessary to accomplish cold sterilization and depyrogenation of infusate. For the sake of brevity, the

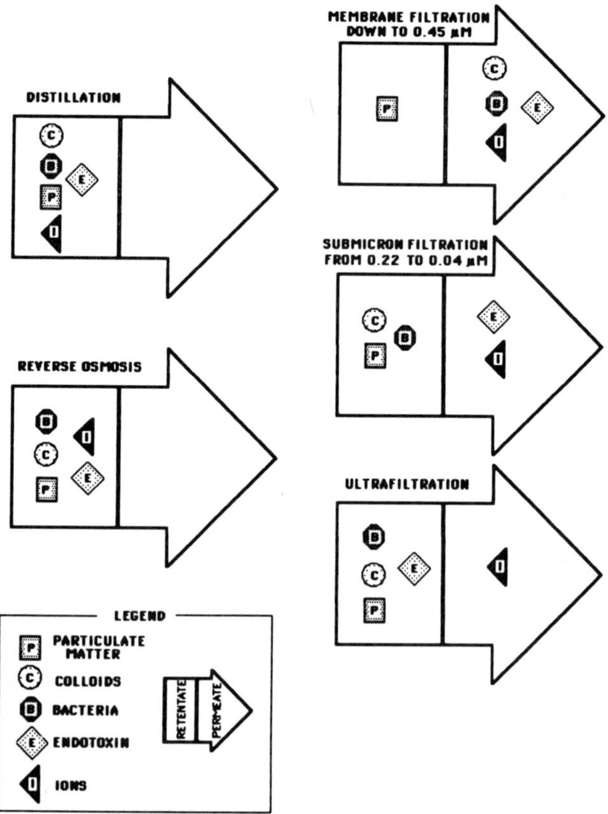


*Figure 12–2.* Compared effectiveness of various methods of water purification. Particulate matter corresponds in this figure to particles 1 $\mu$m or larger.

272

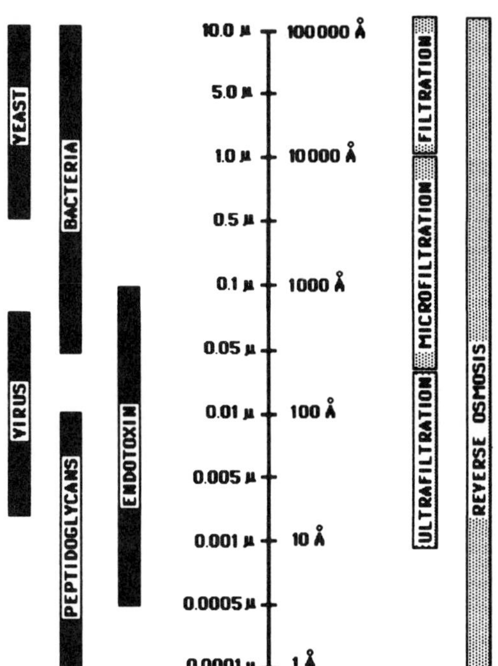


*Figure 12–3.* Approximate molecular or particle sizes of major water microbial contaminants and removal efficiency of common types of membrane filtration processes.

term 'cold sterilization' will be used in the following sections of this chapter to define in general terms procedures in which these practices are utilized singly or in combination. Figure 12–2 compares schematically the various processes that are available for water purification and their relative effectiveness regarding the removal of particulate matter, colloids, bacteria, endotoxins, and ions. In figure 12–3, the size range of endotoxins and microorganisms are compared to the cut-off point of the membranes utilized for cold sterilization of water and solutions. In practices, the safest approach will be to utilize these three processes in combination: sterile apyrogenic water will be produced by reverse osmosis; the sterility and apyrogenicity of electrolyte solutions will be ensured without alteration in their composition by ultrafiltration; a supplemental barrier for bacteria removal will be provided by submicron membrane filtration, a process that can also be used for quality monitoring of sterility [52].

*Some problems encountered with cold sterilization procedures*

When implementing on-site preparation of infusate for HF/HDF in a dialysis center, the nephrologist, the nursing team, and the technicians should be aware of the limitations of cold sterilization procedures. Some of the

273

problems encountered with liquid-filtrating sterilization may be summarized as follows:

1. Absolute sterility is difficult to prove. As a result, sterility is commonly defined in terms of the probability that a contaminating microorganism will survive treatment [51]. Steam and ethylene oxide sterilization are usually challenged and verified with $10^6$ to $10^9$ dried bacterial endospores, and sterilization is defined as the state in which the probability of any one spore surviving is less than $10^6$ or lower [51]. These criteria do not apply to cold sterilization. The efficiency with which the filter membranes remove incident bacteria or other particles is expressed as titer reduction ($T_R$), a term used in filtration operations when the purpose is to achieve microbially sterile filtrates. $T_R$ is the ratio of influent to effluent particle counts and is also the reciprocal of fractional penetration [53]. The production of sterile effluent by filtration will depend both upon membrane characteristics (i.e., pore size rating for submicron filters; sieving coefficients for ultrafiltration membranes) and on the physical integrity of the membrane. It will also depend on the level of microbial contaminants present in the influent fluid.

2. Membranes used in RO modules or filtration devices can be damaged when brisk changes in hydrostatic pressure occur into the system.

3. No technique is presently available to continuously monitor an effluent for its content in bacteria and endotoxins.

4. The sterility and apyrogenicity of fluids sterilized by filtration will depend not only on the membrane integrity but also on the tightness of the package components and on the seals of the assembled permeators or filters. Microbial contamination of the downstream portion of a filtration device can occur from retrograde contamination. If this occurs, the sterility of the filtered fluid will be compromised even if the membrane filter is intact.

5. When not in use, cold sterilization systems are prone to bacterial colonization with water-borne bacteria [54].

6. Sterile infusate produced by cold sterilization procedures should be used in the shortest possible delay after passing through the last sterilizing filter of the system. With on-line production, the fluid is extemporaneously infused in the patient's blood stream, and the risk of contamination is extremely low [19–22]. With batch preparation procedures, however, the sterile fluid is stored in a container for the duration of the treatment and is exposed to bacterial proliferation.

To overcome these shortcomings, several precautions are therefore required. The cold sterilization system should be run smoothly in the range of hydrostatic pressures recommended by the manufacturer. The system should include several levels of membrane filtration to minimize the possibility of a defective membrane compromizing its sterilizing effectiveness. A last stage filter should be placed as close as possible to the infusion site. The system should also be protected against the risk of accidental retrograde contamination. It should be filled with disinfectant solution immediately after use with no exception.

274

*Reverse osmosis, ultrafiltration, and submicron membrane filtration as methods for preparing sterile apyrogenic fluids*

Reverse osmosis, ultrafiltration, and submicron membrane filtration have been shown to remove bacteria effectively from liquid media, but endotoxin removal can be only be effected by the two first procedures.

Reverse osmosis is a membrane process which is based both on ionic exclusion (90–98% rejection for monovalent ions, 95–99% for divalent ions) and molecular sieving (removal of molecules over 200 daltons molecular weight). The first demonstration that RO-treated water is sterile and apyrogenic was made by Madsen and associates [55]. This advantage was utilized by Tenckhoff and associates [56] who developed a peritoneal dialysis system utilizing reverse osmosis to produce sterile apyrogenic dialysate at a low cost for home peritoneal dialysis. There are two main types of membranes assembled in two major configurations: cellulosic and spiral wound modules, and polyamide and hollow fiber modules. Cellulose acetate membranes are sensitive to pH greater than 8 and may be degraded by bacteria. Polyamide membranes are sensitive to free chlorine and chloramines. Pretreatment is, therefore, essential to appropriate performance of the RO device [14]. There is no available study comparing prospectively the relative efficiency in removing bacteria from supply water of cellulosic spiral wound versus polyamide hollow fiber membranes. Experimental [57, 58] and clinical data [11, 58], however, suggest that the former is more efficient than the latter, but neither is an absolute barrier to bacteria [54]. Figure 12–4 illustrates the remarkable efficiency of polyamide hollow fiber modules in removing pyrogen from contaminated water effluent from a pretreatment chain [59]. Several outbreaks of infectious peritonitis have been attributed to microbial infestation of peritoneal dialysis machines [36, 60, 61]. The cause of these outbreaks was found to be the lack of appropriate disinfection schedules. Microbial colonization of the reverse osmosis module can occur with microorganisms penetrating small defects in the membrane of leaky seals, and from retrograde contamination. This hazard can be reduced by placing ultrafilters at the water inlet and at the two outlets (i.e., reject and product water) of the RO module [11]. Disinfection of the RO module with 2% formaldehyde for 12 hours' exposure time after each use remains the only reliable approach to prevent bacterial colonization.

Ultrafiltration is a membrane process utilizing polymeric membranes made of polysulfone, polyamide, polyacrylonitrile, and polymethylmetacrylate. These membranes are effective for removing microorganisms and also endotoxins in spite of elevated sieving coefficients for molecular species in the range of 10 kD to 20 kD [62, 63]. The hydraulic permeability of these membranes is 20 to 30 times that of cellulosic dialysis membranes; ultrafiltration devices utilizing these membranes can be operated at low transmembrane pressure to ultrafiltrate water and aqueous media with low viscosity. Except in one study utilizing a polysulfone membrane [64],

275

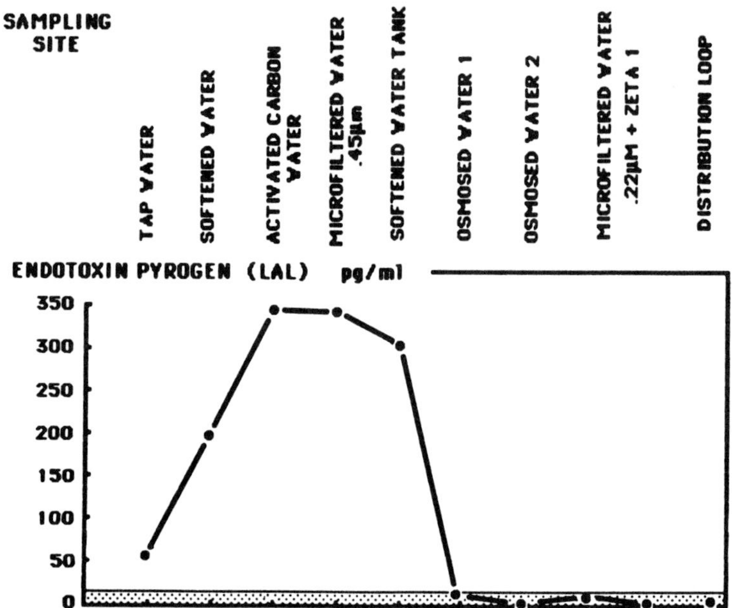


*Figure 12–4.* Water pyrogen content in the water pretreatment and treatment system of the dialysis unit at Montpellier University Hospital. The peak value of 350 pg/ml is observed in the carbon filter. Note the striking reduction of endotoxin level at less than 10 pg/ml after passage of the water through the first reverse osmosis unit (hollow fiber membrane).

ultrafiltration has been confirmed as a very effective process for depyrogenating pure water as well as various parenteral solutions [44, 65–67]. It has been determined that using a 10,000 molecular weight cut-off ultrafiltration system, four log and two log reductions in the E coli endotoxin content of water, and a parenteral solution, respectively, can be achieved in a single pass system [67]. The amount of endotoxin removed depends upon the quality of the membrane, the design of the system, and the load of endotoxin in electrolyte solutions. Further, polyamide ultrafilters have been shown to reject human interleukin 1-inducing substances (i.e., bacterial filtrates of E coli and Pseudomonas sp) even with grossly damaged ultrafilters, an observation suggesting that these molecules are rejecting not only by size but also by adsorption [68]. These results indicated a considerable margin of safety with depyrogenating ultrafiltration. For reasons of convenience, hollow fiber hemofilters are commonly used as ultrafilters, as the fittings on the polycarbonate housing permit their easy connection into the cold sterilization system [8]. Most of the hemofilters available on the market will produce readily ultrafiltratin rates of 500 ml/min of water per hemofilter, for a transmembrane pressure of 100 mmHg [62–64]. Ultrafilters should be placed at several levels in the system: (1) at the water inlet of the RO unit to protect the more expensive RO membranes from bacterial contamination and

276

fouling by colloids and particulates [9, 11, 14]; (2) at the product water outlet of the RO unit [11], while the electrolyte concentrate should be added upstream to this filter to facilitate the thorough mixing of RO-treated water and electrolytes and to eliminate bacteria and pyrogen possibly present in the concentrate; (3) at a short distance from the infusion site on the blood circuit as the last stage of treatment to control bacteria and pyrogens in the product infusate [10, 11]. Formaline utilized in the preparation of 2–4% formaldehyde solutions should also be depyrogenated by ultrafiltration.

To contain the cost of ultrafiltration in acceptable limits, the reuse of ultrafilters is mandatory. There are no available data about filter life, when hemofilters are used for sterilizing depyrogenating procedures. Filter life will depend upon the total filtered water volume and upon the amount of contaminants present in the filtered media. Empirically, hemofilters have been used for periods ranging from 2 weeks to 3 months without observing significant changes in transmembrane pressure or ultrafiltration rates (authors personal experience). Further, backflushing the filters will restore satisfactory ultrafiltration rates when flow rates slow. Finally, ultrafilter life may be further prolonged by adding a 0.2 $\mu$m filter proximal to the ultrafilter to trap bacteria and other particulates that may be present [8].

Submicron membrane filtration is a membrane process like reverse osmosis and ultrafiltration utilizing cellulose-ester or nylon membranes, that are rated at 0.2 $\mu$m, 0.1 $\mu$m, or 0.04 $\mu$m pore size by their manufacturers. These membranes are effective in removing bacteria, and 0.2 $\mu$m filter membranes have become a standard for cold sterilization of fluids. The ability to remove influent level of $10^7$ per cm$^2$ of the organism Pseudomonas diminuta, 0.3 $\mu$m diameter $\times$ 1 $\mu$m long, is a widely accepted definition of 0.2 $\mu$m rated sterilizing grade filter membranes [69]. These membranes have also the ability to remove particulates, but it should be noted that 0.2 $\mu$m rated membranes may pass particulates. Bacteria of smaller size have also been shown to pass 0.2 $\mu$m rated membranes, but this occurs only with prolonged continuous filtration over several days [70]. On the other hand, these membranes do not remove endotoxins [44] except if their surface is positively charged with zeta potential. In the latter case, the amount of adsorbed endotoxin from distilled water is difficult to predict; further, these membranes do not remove pyrogens effectively from electrolyte solutions [71]. Filter membranes are available at low cost in various dimensions. A convenient size is 47 mm diameter, that can be fitted in a special filter holder (Swinnex TM, Millipore Corp, Bedford, MA., U.S.A.) and steam sterilized before placing it on-line as part of the cold sterilization system. This filter accommodates flow rates of about 200–250 ml/min for a transmembrane pressure of about 200 mmHg. Forty to 60 liters of infusate may be filtered without clogging this filter membrane, provided the influent solution is prepared with ultrapure water. The membrane is disposable and should not be reused. The submicron filter membrane should be positioned in the last segment of the cold sterilization system, just before the last ultrafilter. There are two advantages in placing a 0.2 $\mu$m filter membrane at this site: (1) it forms an additional bacterial barrier using a disposable membrane recognized as a standard for the cold sterilization of fluids [69]; (2) at the end of the sessions, the filter membrane may be cultured on standard media for bacteriologic monitoring of on-site preparation of HF/HDF substitution fluid [52].

To summarize, an on-line sterilization system is schematically represented in figure 12–5. The system, which is depicted with a linear configuration, includes several levels of membrane filtration. A water pretreatment system is represented since it is commonly necessary. Drinking water entering the system has a relatively low bacterial content. Bacterial proliferation due to the presence of sediment filters, and softener resins will be contained by chlorination down to the carbon filter. As the latter removes chlorine, microbial contamination will reach a peak value in the carbon filter and the attached downstream sediment filter. It will be reduced in the following segments by several orders of magnitude by ultrafiltration and reverse osmosis. The product water effluent from the RO unit will be ultrapure, with very few (if any) bacteria and low levels of endotoxin as shown in figure 12–4. In the following segment, the infusate produced by the admixture of ultrapure water and concentrate in the proportioner will be sterilized and depyrogenated by passing through an ultrafilter and an 0.2 $\mu$m filter membrane. Finally, a last stage of ultrafiltration will provide the ultimate safety ensuring the infusion of sterile pyrogen-free substitution fluid to the patient.

**Practical approaches to on-site preparation of HF/HDF substitution fluid**

Clinical investigations on the feasibility and reliability of on-site production of HF/HDF substitution fluid were initiated in the late seventies. In the absence of standard equipment, it is no surprise that different practical approaches have been developed by each group of investigators. Recently, at least two systems, one for postdilutional HF and the other for HDF, have been specifically designed to produce on-line apyrogenic substitution fluid. The exhaustive description of the various systems developed for on-line or batch preparation of substitution fluid is beyond the scope of this chapter. The techniques described have been selected either because they have received large-scale clinical application [10, 72] or because they are presently available on the market in the form of standardized equipment [20, 22]. These systems may be classified in two groups: equipment designed for the individual patient and central systems for the dialysis center.

*On-line or batch preparation systems for the individual patient*

The semiautomated technique for batch preparation of the infusate was first developed for use with existing HF monitors based on gravimetric balancing

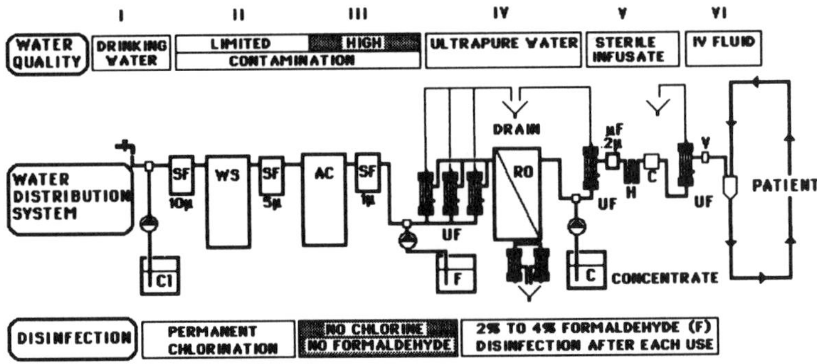



*Figure 12–5.* Schematic representation of a cold sterilization system for on-line preparation of substitution fluid. The highest degree of bacterial infestation is at the carbon filter and the downstream sediment filter because of the lack of chlorine in this segment. Abbreviations: SF = sediment filter; WS = water softener; AC = activated charcoal; CL = chlorine; F = formalin; UF: ultrafilters; $\mu$F: submicron filter membranes; H = heater; C = conductivimeter; V = anti reflux valve.

of ultrafiltrate and replacement flow rates [11]. This approach, used by the authors of this chapter with a Gambro HFM 10 equipment (Gambro AG, Lund, Sweden), can be applied to any other HF monitor. The configuration of the sterilizing system is depicted schematically in figure 12–6. A batch of infusate is prepared by adding the concentrate upstream from an ultrafilter to the RO product water (flow rate 1.2–2 liters/minute) by means of a manually adjusted pump while conductivity is monitored. The admixture is then stored in a clean polivinyle chloride bag lining a rigid container suspended on one of the scale arms of the machine, the ultrafiltrate tank being suspended on the other scale arm. Thirty-five liters of replacement fluid are prepared for each session. Before entering the patient's extracorporeal blood stream, the

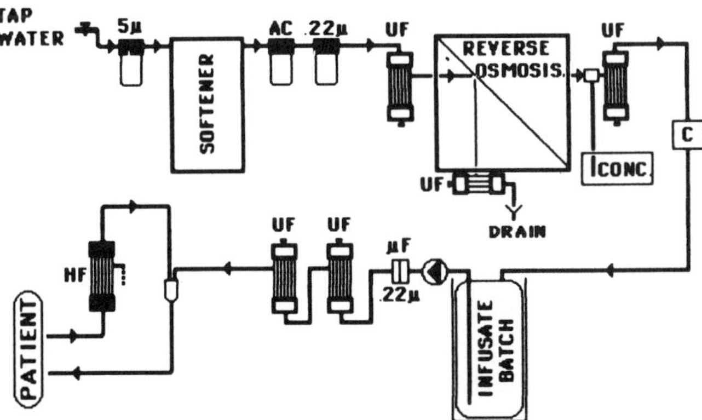



*Figure 12–6.* Individual equipment for the manual batch preparation of substitution fluid, utilizing a gravimetric balancing system.

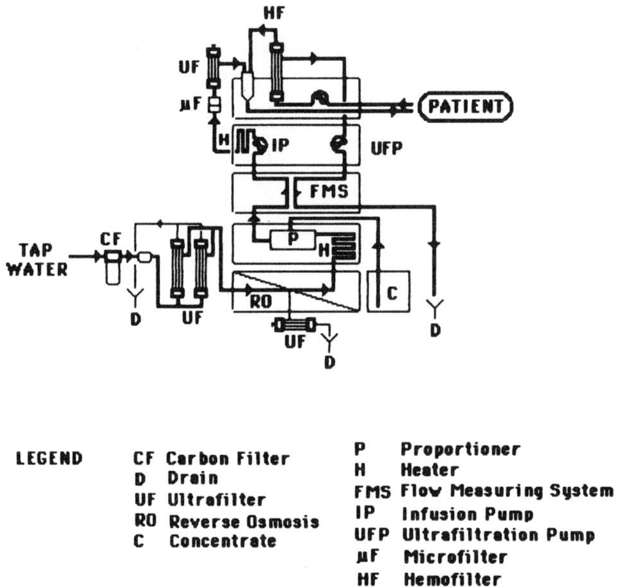


*Figure 12–7.* Automatic hemofiltration system with on-line production of substitution fluid (RO-HFS model, Gambro AG, Lund, Sweden).

infusate passes through a 0.2 $\mu$m filter membrane, two ultrafilters placed in series, and a heater. This system has been used in the center and at home [9, 11]. Its main drawbacks are the lengthy preparative procedures, necessitating the presence of competent personnel, and the storage of the infusate in the batch for the duration of the treatment. This approach, which is still valuable for centers equipped with gravimetric HF monitors, should be considered obsolete as on-line automated HF machines become available on the market.

The on-line HF system developed by Gambro represents a complete cold sterilization system and is shown in figure 12–7. This apparatus includes a RO module, two levels of ultrafiltration (one ultrafilter at the water inlet, one at the infusion site on the blood circuit), and 0.2 $\mu$m filter membrane [20]. This equipment, which is equally suitable for in-center or home HF, can be directly supplied with tap water. Disinfection and rinsing cycles are part of an automated program to ensure the safety of the system.

The on-line HDF system developed by Fresenius (model A 2008 C, Fresenius AG, Bad Homburg, FRG), is represented on figure 12–8. This equipment is derived from a conventional HD machine. The dialysate circuit is modified, allowing 100 ml/min of dialysis fluid to pass through a separate flow path including two ultrafilters and a 0.2 $\mu$m filter membrane. To guarantee the microbiologic quality of the infusate during treatment, it is preferable to supply the HDF system with product water effluent directly from an RO unit [22]. An automatic cycle ensures disinfection and rinsing of

280

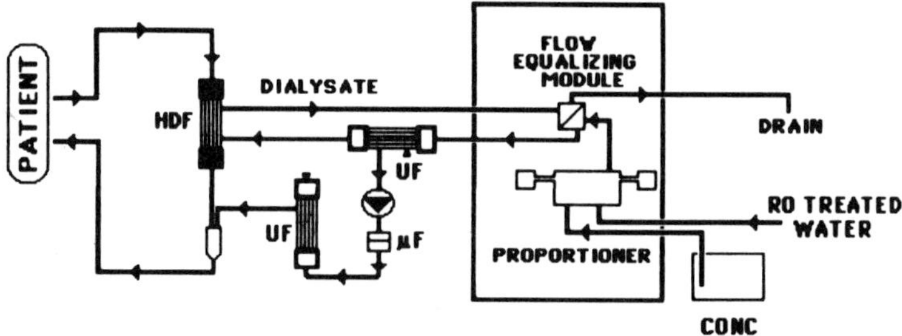



*Figure 12–8.* Automatic hemodiafiltration system with on-line production of substitution fluid (model A 2008 C, with modified dialysate circuit, Fresenius AG, Hamburg, FRG).

the dialysate and infusate circuit at the end of each treatment and before use.

These two automated systems with on-line production of infusate have been proved to be bacteriologically more acceptable for HF [20] and for HDF [72]. Furthermore, these equipments are as easy to operate than conventional HD systems: they facilitate the acceptance of HF and HDF by nursing personnel and open a new era for the routine prescription of these two alternative modes of blood purification.

*Central systems for batch production of infusate*

These systems, schematically represented in figure 12–9, have been developed to supply several gravimetric HF monitors with adequate amounts of infusate in periods of time short enough to satisfy the functioning requirement of a dialysis center, without jeopardizing the safety of the patient. Two groups of investigators have reported on the long-term use of central systems [10, 12]. In both cases, a high flux proportioning unit produces the substitution fluid under sterile conditions in a side room, and the

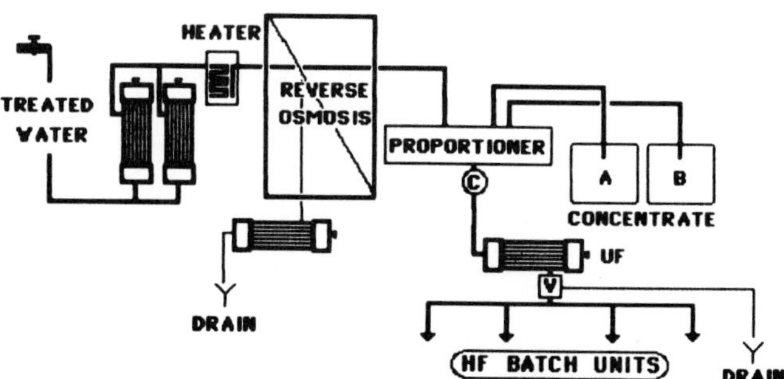



*Figure 12–9.* Schematic representation of a central proportioning system for batch production of substitution fluid. This system is convenient with any HF balancing system in a dialysis unit. The infusate distribution circuit is not represented in this figure and should be identical to that shown on figure 12–6.

sterile infusate stored in plastic bags is then distributed to the HF monitors in the dialysis room.

In one center, the proportioner was a Drake Willock proportioning pump [10], while a volumetric system (model Aachen, Fresenius AG, Bad Homburg, FRG) was utilized at another center [12]. Once centrally produced, each batch of fluid is distributed with a trolley cart to each HF station and placed on the corresponding scale arm of the HF monitor. The infusate is then pumped from the batch to the blood circuit through a heater and three membrane ultrafilters in series [10] or a 0.2 $\mu$m filter membrane [12].

*Disinfection procedures of HF/HDF equipments*

The microbiologic safety of on-site preparation of substitution fluid rests upon the rigorous enforcement of strict disinfection procedures of the equipment. Surprisingly, information concerning disinfection procedures of cold sterilization membrane systems for infusate preparation is quite scarce. In one study, daily formalinization of the RO unit and of the ultrafilters was performed with a 4% formaldehyde solution and a minimum exposure time of 8 hours [11]. In another study, an on-line HDF system was rinsed with peracetic acid after each treatment, and, in the evening, an 85°C pasteurization for 20 minutes was followed with 2.5% formaldehyde exposure overnight [22].

To obtain the effective disinfection of the systems described in the previous paragraph of this chapter, at least two major points should be carefully implemented: (1) the disinfectant should be in contact with all parts of the system, including the RO unit and the ultrafilters placed upstream [30]; (2) the concentration and the contact time of the disinfectant should be adequate to produce high level disinfection, that is, to eliminate all microorganisms except bacterial spores [73].

In spite of its toxicity [74, 75], formaldehyde still remains the most commonly used disinfectant. There are many reasons for preferring formaldehyde to other chemical germicides: it is stable in aqueous solutions; it is a highly effective disinfectant that is considered as sporicide and a cold sterilant at a concentration of 8% and a contact time of 12 hours at 20°C [73]; it ensures high level disinfection at a 4% concentration and an exposure time of 24 hours [73]; it is compatible with a wide spectrum of membranes and other materials; because of its excellent solubility in water, it is relatively easy to eliminate by adequate rinsing from dialysis systems [76, 77]; it can be detected in water or infusate in concentration below 1 mg/l [77]; finally, it costs less than any other disinfectant.

In view of their experience with on-site preparation of infusate [11, 72, 78] and also by extrapolation from accepted reuse standards for hemodialyzers [79, 80], the authors of this chapter believe that 4% formaldehyde solution should be routinely used to disinfect cold sterilization membrane systems.

The system should be filled with disinfectant solution at the end of each day in a center or after each treatment in home HF, with a minimum exposure time of 8 hours. To obtain the desired concentration of formaldehyde in the water and infusate circuit, appropriate amount of formaline (i.e., 37% formaldehyde solution) should be infused into the system both at the water inlet upstream of the ultrafilters protecting the RO unit and at the electrolyte concentrate inlet. This precaution is required, even when an acetate concentrate is used, because part of the formaldehyde infused upstream of the RO module is lost to the drain with the rejected water.

**Quality control**

Five parameters should be regularly monitored to control the quality of the substitution fluid prepared according to the techniques described in this chapter:

1. The electrolyte composition and osmolality of the solution should correspond to the prescribed formulae, which are presented in table 12–4. This will be easily obtained by continuous conductivity monitoring during infusate production. Trace elements should not exceed the maximum levels recommended for dialysate [81].

2. The solution should not contain any added substance. Particularly, the concentration of residual formaldehyde should be kept at levels below 1 mg/l as recommended for reused dialyzers [77, 82]. As shown in figure 12–10, rinsing formaldehyde out of the RO module to attain such low levels requires up to 3 hours (B. Canaud and C. Mion, unpublished observations). Sensitive color reagents based on Shiff or Hantzch reactions [77] can detect trace amounts of formaldehyde, but the Clinitest reaction should be abandoned because of its lack of sensitivity.

3. The sterility and apyrogenicity of the infusate should be monitored epidemiologically by means of a log of all febrile reactions occurring during or

*Table 12–4.* Composition of substitution fluids (in mmol/l) for hemofiltration and hemodiafiltration

|  | Buffer | |
|  | Acetate | Bicarbonate |
| --- | --- | --- |
| Sodium | 142.0 | 142.0 |
| Potassium | 1.5 | 1.5 |
| Calcium | 1.75 | 1.75 |
| Magnesium | 0.75 | 0.75 |
| Chloride | 111.0 | 107.0 |
| Acetate | 35.0 | 4.0 |
| Bicarbonate |  | 35.0 |
| Dextrose | 11.0 | 11.0 |
| Total osmolality | 301.5 | 301.5 |

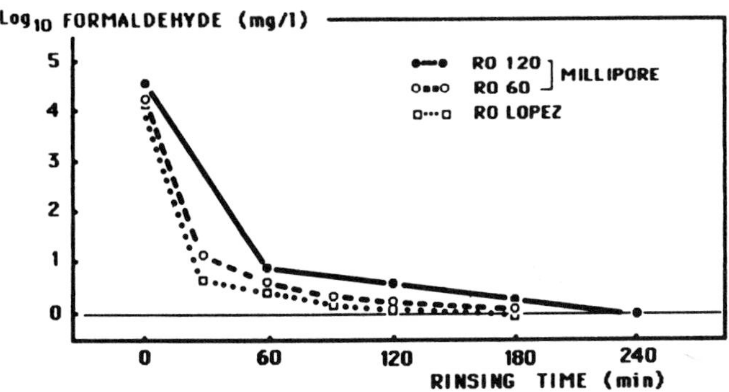


*Figure 12–10.* Formaldehyde concentration in product water of reverse osmosis modules as a function of rinsing time. In the RO 120 study, the RO module and the ultrafilters placed at the inlet and outlet of the RO unit were rinsed simultaneously.

in the hours following HF/HDF. According to published data [9–11, 78] it is reasonable to expect an incidence of febrile reactions below 0.5%. A febrile reaction rate of 0.5% or greater should therefore require careful reevaluation of all the procedures involved with on-site preparation of substitution fluid.

4. The sterility of the fluid should be regularly assessed. Microbiologic quality control can be implemented in the dialysis center by culturing the 0.2 $\mu$m filter membrane of the sterilizing system at the end of HF/HDF treatment [52]. The membrane removed from its filter holder should be carefully placed with aseptic procedures on to a Petri dish containing standard method solid culture media [83]. How often should membrane cultures be performed may be a matter of controversy as environmental microbiologic sampling often produces useless information and may also foster a sense of false security [84]. The sampling and culturing procedures developed by the authors of this chapter have been carefully assessed by simultaneously filtering the same contaminated solution with both 0.2 $\mu$m and 0.45 $\mu$m filter membranes mounted in parallel: both membranes yielded identical results in culture [52]. Cultures of 0.2 $\mu$m membranes utilized in the filtration of the total amount of infusate injected to the patient provides meaningful information and reflects accurately the total contamination of the product infusate. Although information gathered from membrane culture is by necessity obtained after a lag period of a few days, it was found useful in the early detection of a degradation in routine production and disinfection procedures before febrile reactions occurred in the patients (B. Canaud and C. Mion, unpublished data). The control of infusate sterility could be accomplished according to the following guidelines:

a. When initiating a program of on-site infusate production culture of 0.2 $\mu$m filter membranes could be done at the end of each treatment for a period of 2 to 3 months. On-site cultures procedures would be established in close cooperation with a microbiologist, while dialysis personnel would be trained and the reliability of the results would be assessed.

284

b. Once culture protocols and baseline control values would be established and found reproducible, membrane culture would be done less frequently. A reasonable culturing schedule could be once a day with on-line automated HF machines. The cultures should be done on the 0.2 $\mu$m filter membrane used during the last session of the day: at this time, the HF equipment would be rinsed of all disinfectant for several hours, and negative membrane cultures would therefore indicate the maintained sterilizing effectiveness of the HF system.

c. With batch prepared infusate, membrane cultures should be performed on certain number of batches (e.g., 10–15%) to provide statistically significant information for the long-term surveillance of preparation and disinfection procedures.

5. The apyrogenicity of the substitution fluid should also be monitored. The limulus amebocyte lysate (LAL) assay is the only specific test available for the on-site evaluation of infusate pyrogen content [85–87]. However, the simple clot test (PyrogentR Test, Mallinckrodt Inc, St Louis, Mo., U.S.A.) which can be easily performed in the dialysis unit, is a time-consuming procedure. After mixing 0.1 ml of test solution and 0.1 ml of LAL reagent, the sample should be incubated undisturbed for at least 1 hour at 37°C [85]. Further, the LAL clot test has a lower level of sensitivity of 0.06 ng/ml, which allows only for the detection of relatively heavy endotoxin contamination of the infusate. Therefore, it appears preferable to have the LAL test performed with a more sensitive spectrophotometric method using a chromogenic substrate: the lower sensitivity of this assay which is commonly of 0.010 ng/ml can be reduced to the 0.001 ng/ml [17]. In practice, infusate samples can be collected during each HF/HDF treatment, preferably at the end of the session. A certain number of these samples (e.g., 10%), will be routinely tested for quality control of apyrogenicity. Other collected samples should be preserved for the 24 hours following the HF/HDF sessions to be available for testing in case of a febrile reaction occurring during treatment or a few hours after it is completed.


**Problems of responsibility**

To date, on-site production of substitution fluid for HF/HDF is considered an experimental procedure and utilized only by a few groups of motivated investigators. In these circumstances, untoward consequences resulting from inadequate infusate quality is the exclusive responsibility of the clinical investigator. With the development of automated HF system specially designed for the continuous on-line production of sterile pyrogen-free substitution fluid, the responsibility will be shared to a certain extent by the manufacturers and by the dialysis practitioners.

Before installing an automated HF system, the manufacturer should obtain a certified analysis of the feed water from the dialysis center. This analysis should provide detailed information on the presence of inorganic and organic substances as well as on the degree of bacterial contamination (i.e., bacteria and endotoxins). The fouling index of the water should be measured to evaluate the particulate and colloid content of tap water. Based on these data, the manufacturer should recommend the type and capacity of the water pretreatment and/or treatment system needed to produce the water of high quality that will minimize the risk of particulate clogging of ultrafilter and RO membranes and the risk of bacterial proliferation. The recommendations should take into account the known or anticipated seasonal variations in water quality. A disclosure document should be prepared indicating expected contaminants at various parts of the treatment system [14]. Detailed information should also be provided according to accepted standards concerning the selection of water treatment equipment. Upon installation, the on-line HF system should be validated by the manufacturer for a duration of time sufficient to obtain reliable laboratory evidence that the cold sterilization membrane system effectively produces sterile apyrogenic solutions. Along with the usual maintenance guidelines and trouble-shooting procedures, the manufacturer should recommend the validated methods for disinfecting the system with precise indications concerning disinfectant concentration and minimum contact time at room temperature (20°C). Information concerning the duration of rinsing procedures to obtain an infusate free of disinfectant should also be available.

Beyond installation and validation of the system, everything else will be the responsibility of the dialysis practitioner. Effective measures should be implemented for the chemical and microbiologic monitoring of water quality. Disinfection schedules of proven efficiency should be strictly enforced. One of the most important requirements for the success of on-site preparation of substitution fluid is to give adequate information to all personnel involved with these procedures. Every member of the nursing team should have a clear understanding of the pursued goal, be fully aware of the potential hazards and existing pitfalls, and get an adequate training about the overall procedure, especially concerning its microbiologic aspects.

## Conclusion

The on-site preparation of substitution fluid meeting the requirements of intravenous solutions may appear as a difficult endeavor. In fact, the difficulty is more apparent than real. On the one hand, an important knowledge has accumulated during the seventies on the multifaceted aspects of the microbial contamination of water and hemodialysis systems. The epidemiologic and bacteriologic studies conducted by the investigators of the Center for Disease Control provide essential basic information which can readily be applied to the development of water treatment systems and HF/HDF equipments with a minimal risk of bacterial infestation. On the other hand, the evolving technology of membrane filtration, ultrafiltration, and reverse osmosis offers a variety of water filtration devices that are easy to interconnect and that permit the safe production of sterile apyrogenic water and electrolyte solutions. These membrane processes are utilized by the semiconductor industry to prepare highly purified water in large quantity. Their long-term effectiveness has been successfully implemented in the industrial environment. It would be a discouraging paradox if a similar result could not prevail in the field of long-term maintainance dialysis. The present evolution in water treatment systems suggests that the possibility to produce at low cost sterile apyrogenic water will be increasingly utilized in dialysis units not only for HF/HDF purposes but also as a standard of the future for conventional hemodialysis [59].

# References


1. Henderson, L.W., Besarab, A., Michaels, A. and Bluemle, L.W., Jr. (1967) Blood purification by ultrafiltration and fluid replacement (diafiltration). Trans. Am. Soc. Artif. Intern. Organs 13: 216–222.
2. Quellhorst, E., Rieger, J., Doht, B., Belkmann, H., Jacob, I., Kraft, B, Mietzsch, G. and Scheler, F. (1976) Treatment of chronic uremia by an ultrafiltration kidney — first clinical experience. Proc. EDTA 13: 314–321.
3. Leber, H.W., Wizemann, V., Goubeaud, G., Rawer, P. and Shütterle, G. (1978) Simultaneous hemofiltration/hemodialysis: an effective alternative to hemofiltration and conventional hemodialysis in the treatment of uremic patients. Clin. Nephrol. 9:115–121.
4. Brunner, F.P., Broyer, M., Brynger, H., Challah, S., Fassbinder, M., Oulès, R., Rizzoli, G., Selwood, N.H. and Wing, A.J. (1985) Combined report on regular dialysis and transplantation in Europe, XV, 1984. Proc. EDTA-ERA 22: 5–53.
5. Quellhorst, E., Schuenemann, B and Boryhardt, J. (1978) Clinical and technical aspects of hemofiltration. Artif. Organs 2: 334–338.
6. Baldamus, C.A., Schoeppe, W. and Koch, K.M. (1978) Comparison of hemodialysis and hemofiltration in an unselected dialysis population. Proc. EDTA 15: 228–234.
7. Shaldon, S., Deschodt, G., Beau, M.C., Claret, G., Mion, H. and Mion, C. (1979) Vascular stability during high flux hemofiltration. Proc. EDTA 16: 695–697.
8. Henderson, L.W. and Beans, E. (1978) Successful production of sterile pyrogen-free electrolyte solution by ultrafiltration. Kidney Int. 14: 522–525.
9. Ramperez, P., Beau, M.C. Deschodt, G., Flavier, J.L., Nilsson, L., Mion, C. and Shaldon, S. (1981) Economic preparation of sterile pyrogen free infusate for hemofiltration. Proc. EDTA 18: 293–296.
10. Luehman, D., Hirsch, D., Ebben, J., Collins, A., Shapiro, F. and Keshaviah, P. (1984) Central on-site preparation of substitution fluid for hemofiltration. Trans. Am. Soc. Artif. Intern. Organs 30: 195–198.
11. Mayr, H.U., Stec, F., Canaud, B., Mion, C. and Shaldon, S. (1984) Microbiological aspects of the batch preparation of replacement fluid for hemofiltration. Blood Purif. 2: 158–163.
12. Haas, T., Dongradi, G., Villeboeuf, F., de Viel, E., Verrier, J. and Hillion, D. (1985) Technical and clinical data on high performance hemofiltration: twelve patients during one year. Artif. Organs 9: 164–168.
13. Keshaviah, P. and Luehmann, D. (1984) The importance of water treatment in hemodialysis and hemofiltration. Proc. EDTA-ERA 21: 111–129.
14. Ramenofsky, J.A., Prestidge, H., Ford, C., Sanfelippo, M.L. and Henderson, L.W. (1981)

Novel applications for hemofiltration membranes. Trans. Am. Soc. Artif. Intern. Organs 27: 613–617.

15. Frei, U. and Koch, K.M. (1983) Fever and shock during hemofiltration. Contr. Nephrol. 36: 107–114.

16. Felts, S.K., Schaffner, W., Melly, M.A. and Koenig, M.O. (1972) Sepsis caused by contaminated intravenous fluids. Epidemiologic, clinical and laboratory investigation of an outbreak in one hospital. Ann. Int. Med. 77: 881–890.

17. Tominaga, H., Tanaka, S. and Tominaga, N. (1986) Endotoxin levels of sterile injection solutions or substitution fluid for hemofiltration in Japan and Australia. Nephron 42: 128–132.

18. Wolff, S.M. (1972) Biological effects of bacterial endotoxins in man. J. Infect. Dis. 128: 251–256.

19. Henderson, L.W., San Felippo, M.L. and Beans, E. (1978) 'On-line' preparation of sterile pyrogen-free electrolyte solutions. Trans. Am. Soc. Artif. Intern. Organs 24: 465–467.

20. Shaldon, S., Deschodt, G., Granolleras, C., Branger, B., Oulès, R., Gullberg, C.A. and Mayr, H. (1984) Experience with on-line hemofiltration. In *Progress in Artificial Organs*, K. Atsumi, M. Maekawa and K. Ota (eds.). Cleveland, OH: ISAO Press n° 204, pp. 586–588.

21. Shinzato, T., Sezaki, R., Usuda, M., Maeda, K., Ohbayashi, S. and Toyota, T. (1982) Infusion free hemodiafiltration and dialysis with no need for infusion fluid. Art. Organs 6: 453–456.

22. Canaud, B., N'Guyen, Q.V., Lagarde, C., Stec, F., Polaschegg, H.D. and Mion, C. (1985) Clinical evaluation of a multipurpose dialysis system adequate for hemodialysis or for post-dilution hemofiltration/hemodiafiltration with on-line preparation of substitution fluid from dialysate. Contr. Nephrol. 46: 184–186.

23. *The United States Pharmacopeia*, 20th Revision. (1980) Easton, PA: Mack Publishing Co.

24. Tenckhoff, H., Shilipetar, G., Van Paaschen, W.H. and Swanson, E. (1969) A home peritoneal dialysate delivery system. Trans. Am. Soc. Artif. Intern. Organs 15: 103–107.

25. Collins, C.H., Grange J.M. and Yates, M.D. (1984) A review: mycobacteria in water. J. Appl. Bacteriol. 57: 193–211.

26. Baron, D. (1985) Les virus humains dans l'environnement hydrique. In *Flammarion Medecine Sciences*, J. Maurin (ed.). Paris: Virologie médicale, pp. 825–836.

27. Lauer, J., Streifel, A., Kjellstrand, C.M. and Deroos, R. (1975) The bacteriological quality of hemodialysis solutions as related to several environmental factors. Nephron 15: 87–97.

28. Stamm, J.M. Engelhard, W.E. and Parsons, J.E. (1969) Microbiological study of water-softener resins. Appl. Microbiol. 18: 376–386.

29. Katz, D., Laney, H., Linquist, J.A. and Persike, E.C. (1976) Formaldehyde disinfection to eliminate bacterial contamination of deionizers. Dial. Transpl. 5 (5): 42–78.

30. Favero, M.S., Petersen, N.J., Carson, L.A., Bond, W.W. and Hindman, S.H. (1975) Gram-negative water bacteria in hemodialysis systems. Health Lab. Sci. 12: 321–334.

31. Favero, M.S., Carson, L.A., Bond, W.W. and Petersen, N.J. (1971) Pseudomonas aeruginosa: growth in distilled water from hospitals. Science 173: 836–838.

32. Carson, L.A., Favero, M.S., Bond, W.W. and Petersen, N.J. (1972) Factors affecting comparative resistance of naturally occurring and subcultured Pseudomonas aeruginosa to disinfections. Applied Microbiol. 23: 863–869.

33. Hakim, R.H., Friedrich, R. and Lowrie, E.G. (1985) Formaldehyde kinetics and bacteriology of dialyzers. Kidney Int. 28: 936–943.

34. Katz, M.A. and Hull, A.R. (1971) Probable mycobacterium septicemia: complication of home hemodialysis. Lancet 1: 499.

35. Azadian, B.S. Beck, A. Curtis, J.R., Cherrington, L.E., Gower, P.E., Phillips, M., Eastwood, J.B. and Nichols, J. (1981) Disseminated infection with Mycobacterium chelonei in a hemodialysis patient. Tubercle 62: 281–284.

36. Band, J.D. Ward, J.I., Fraser, D.W., Petersen, N.J., Silcox, V.A., Good, R.C. Ostroy, P.R. and Kennedy, J. (1982) Peritonitis due to Mycobacterium chelonei-like organism associated with intermittent chronic peritoneal dialysis. J. Infect. Dis. 145: 9–17.

37. Bolan, G., Reingold, A.L., Carson, L.A., Silcox, V.A., Woodley, C.L., Hayes, P.S., Hightower, A.W., McFarland, L., Brown, J.W., III, Petersen, N.J., Favero, M.S., Good, R.C. and Broom, C.V. (1985) Infections with Mycobacterium chelonei in patients receiving dialysis and using processed hemodialysers. J. Infect. Dis. 152: 1013–1019.

38. Carson, L.A., Petersen, N.J., Favero, M.S. and Aguero, S.M. (1978) Growth characteristics of atipycal mycobacteria in water and their comparative resistance to disinfectants. Appl. Environm. Microbiol. 36: 839–846.

39. Favero, M.S., Carson, L.A., Bond, W.W. and Petersen, N.J. (1974) Factors that influence microbial contamination of fluids associated with hemodialysis machines. Applied Microbiol. 28: 822–830.

40. Westphal, O., Jann, K. and Himmlpach, K. (1983) Chemistry and immunochemistry of bacterial lipopolysaccharides as cell wall antigens and endotoxins. Prog. Allergy 33: 9–37.

41. Ribi, E., Haskins, W.T., Milner, K.C., Anacker, R.L., Ritter, D.B., Goode, G., Trapani, R.J. and Landy, M. (1962) Physicochemical changes in endotoxin associated with loss of biological activity. J. Bacteriol. 84: 803–814.

42. Ribi, E., Anacker, R.C., Brown, R., Haskins, W.T., Malmgren, B., Milner, K.C. and Rudbach, J.A. (1966) Reaction of endotoxin and surfactants. I Physical and biological properties of endotoxin treated with sodium deoxycholate. J. Bacteriol. 92: 1493–1509.

43. Hannecart-Pokorni, E., Dekegel, D. and Dupuydt, F. (1973) Macromolecular structure of lipopolysaccharides from Gram negative bacteria. Eur. J. Biochem. 38: 6–13.

44. Sweadner, K.J., Forte, M. and Nelsen, L. (1977) Filtration removal of endotoxin (pyrogens) in solution in different state of aggregation. Appl. Environm. Microbiol. 34: 382–385.

45. Dinarello, C.A. (1983) Pathogenesis of fever during hemodialysis. Contr. Nephrol. 36: 90–99.

46. Ryter, A. (1982) Structure et anatomie fonctionnelle. In *Bacteriologie Médicale*. L. Le Minor and M. Veron (eds.). Paris: Flammarion Médecine Sciences, pp. 1–7.

47. Dinarello, C.A., Elin, R.J., Chedid, L. and Wolff, S.M. (1978) The pyrogenicity of the synthetic adjuvant muramyl dipeptide and two structural analogues. J. Infect. Dis. 138: 760–767.

48. Parant, M., Riveau, G., Parant, F., Dinarello, C.A., Wolff, S.M. and Chedid, L. (1980) Effect of indomethacin on increased resistance to bacterial infection and on febrile responses involved by muramyl dipeptide. J. Infect. Dis. 142: 708–715.

49. Lemaire, G., Tenu, J.P. Petit, J.F. and Lederer, E. (1985) Effects of microbially derived products on mononuclear phagocytes. In *The Reticuloendothelial System. A Comprehensive Treatise. 8: Pharmacology,* J.W. Hadden and A. Szentivanyi (eds.) New York, London: Plenum Press, pp. 181–245.

50. Sargent, J.A., Gotch, F.A. Lam, M. Prowitt, M. and Keen, M. (1977) Technical aspects of on-line proportioning of bicarbonate dialysate. Proc. Dial. Transpl. Forum 7: 109–115.

51. Favero, M.S. (1985) Seterilization, disinfection, and antisepsis in the hospital. In *Manual of Clinical Microbiology*, 4th ed. E.H. Lennette, A. Balows, W.J. Hausler, Jr. and H.J. Shadomy (eds.). Washington, D.C.: American Society for Microbiology, pp. 129–137.

52. Mayr, H.U., Stec, F. and Mion, C.M. (1984) Standard methods for the microbiologic assessment of electrolyte solution prepared on line for hemofiltration. Proc. EDTA-ERA 21: 454–460.

53. Pall, D.B., Kirnbauer, E.A. and Allen, B.T. (1980) Particulate retention by bacteria retentive membrane filters. Colloids & Surfaces 1: 235–256.

54. Petersen, N.J., Carson, L.A. and Favero, M.S. (1977) Microbiological quality of water in an automatic peritoneal dialysis system. Dial. Transpl. 6(2): 38–40.

55. Madsen, R.F., Nielsen, B., Olsen, O.J. and Raaschou, F. (1970) Reverse osmosis as a method of preparing dialysis water. Nephron 7: 550–558.

56. Tenckhoff, H., Meston, B. and Shilipetar, G. (1972) A simplified automatic peritoneal dialysis system. Trans. Am. Soc. Artif. Intern. Organs 18: 436–439.

57. Kabei, N., Kolff, W.J. and Foux, A. (1977) Evaluation of hollow-fiber reverse osmosis permeators for use in peritoneal dialysis. Dial. Transpl. 6(1): 59–88.

58. Blagg, C.R. and Tenckhoff, H. (1975) Microbial contamination of water used for hemodialysis. Nephron 15: 81–86.

59. Canaud, B., Peyronnet, P., Armynot, A.M., Nguyen, Q.V., Attisso, M. and Mion, C. (1986) Ultrapure water: a need for future dialysis. Abstracts: 23rd Congress of EDTA-ERA, p. 113.

60. Furman, K., Koornhof, H.J. Frizelle, K., Block, C. Van Wyk, H. and Allcock, E.R. (1979) Unsafe automatic peritoneal dialysis in Johannesburg (abstract). Kidney Int. 16: 86.

61. Berkelman, R.L. Godley, J, Weber, J.A., Anderson, R.L. Lerner, A.M., Petersen, N.J. and Allen, J.R. (1982) Pseudomonas cepacia peritonitis associated with contamination of automatic peritoneal dialysis machines. Ann. Int. Med. 96: 456–458.

62. Colton, L.K., Henderson, L.W., Ford, C.A. and Lysaght, M.J. (1975) Kinetics of hemodiafiltration. I. In vivo transport characteristics of a hollow fiber blood ultrafilter. J. Lab. Clin. Med. 85: 355–371.

63. Göhl, H. Konstantin, P. and Gullberg, C.A. (1982) Hemofiltration membranes. Contr. Nephrol. 32: 20–30.

64. Klinkman, H. Falkenhagen, D. and Smollich, B.P. (1985) Investigation of the permeability of highly permeable polysulfone membranes for pyrogens. Contr. Nephrol. 46: 174–183.

65. Nelsen, L.L. (1978) Removal of pyrogens from parenteral solutions by ultrafiltration. Pharm. Technology 2(5): 46–49.

66. Cradock, J.C., Guder, L.A., Francis, A.L., Morgan, S.L. (1978) Reduction of pyrogens: application of molecular filtration. J. Pharmaceut. Pharmacol. 30: 198–199.

67. Abramson, D., Butler, L.D. and Chrai, S. (1981) Depyrogenation of a parenteral solution by ultrafiltration. J. Parenteral Sc. Technol. 35: 3–7.

68. Dinarello, C.A. Maxwell, R. and Shaldon, S. (1986) Rejection of human interleukin 1-inducing substances by polyamide ultrafilters. Abstracts, 23rd Congress EDTA-ERA, p. 119.

69. Bowman, F.W., Calhoum, M.P. and White M. (1967) Microbiological methods for quality control of membrane filters. J. Pharmaceut. Sc. 56: 222–225.

70. Howard, G. Jr. and Duberstein, R. (1980) A case of penetration of 0.2 $\mu$m rated membrane filters by bacteria. J. Parent. Drug. Ass. 34: 95–102.

71. Carazzone, M., Arello, D., Fava, M. and Sancin, P. (1985) A new type of positively charged filter: preliminary test results. J. Parent. Sc. Technol. 39: 69–74.

72. Canaud, B., Nguyen, Q.V., Stec, F. and Mion, C. (1986). In line production of substitution fluid in hemodiafiltration. Abstract Book: 4th Symposium of the International Society of Blood Purification, Osaka.

73. Favero, M.S. (1983) Distinguishing between high-level disinfection, reprocessing and sterilization. In *Reuse of Disposables. AAMI Technology Assessment Report*. Arlington, VA: Association for the Advancement of Medical Instrumentation, pp. 19–23.

74. Yodaiken, R.E. (1981) The uncertain consequences of formaldehyde toxicity. JAMA 246: 1677–1678.

75. Pizziconi, V.P. (1983) Hazards associated with chemical cleaning and disinfecting agents for reuse. In *Reuse of Disposables, AAMI Technology Assessment Report*. Arlington, VA: Association for the Advancement of Medical Instrumentation, pp. 29–34.

76. Gotch, F.A. and Keen, M.L. (1983) Formaldehyde kinetics in reused dialysers. Trans. Am. Soc. Artif. Intern. Organs 29: 396–400.

77. Hakim, R.M. Friedrich, R.A., Lowrie, E.G., with the technical assistance of Mantilla, J.M. and Lee, C. (1985) Formaldehyde kinetics and microbiology in dialysers. Kidney Int. 28: 936–943.

78. Canaud, B., Flavier, J.L. Polito, C., Nguyen, Q.V., Ramperez, P., Shaldon, S., Mion, C. (1984) Post dilutional hemofiltration: 5 years' experience at one center (Abstract) Blood Purif. 2: 201.

79. Emmerson, M.R. (1983) California proposed dialyser reused standards. In *Reuse of Disposables, AMMI Technology Assessment Report*. Arlington, VA: Association for the Advancement of Medical Instrumentation, pp. 83–86.

80. National Kidney Foundation. (1984) Revised standards for reuse of hemodialysers. Contemporary Dialysis 5(2): 29–37.
81. American National Standard for Hemodialysis Systems. (1981) 3.22: *Maximum Level of Chemical Contaminants*. Arlington. VA: Association for the Advancement of Medical Instrumentation, p. 3.
82. Kaye, M., Barber, E. and Gagnon, R. (1985) Residual formaldehyde in new and reused dialysers. Trans. Am. Soc. Artif. Intern. Organs 31: 644–646.
83. American Public Health Association. (1971) Section 408: Culture media. In *Standard Methods for the Examination of Water and Waste Water*. New York: American Public Health Association Inc., pp. 635–685.
84. Favero, M.S. and Petersen, N.G. (1977) Microbiologic guidelines for hemodialysis systems. Dial. Transpl. 6(11): 34–36.
85. Pearson, F.C., III and Weary, M. (1980) The limulus amebocyte lysate test for endotoxin. Bioscience 30: 461–464.
86. Mascoli, C.C. and Weary, M.E. (1979) Limulus amebocyte lysate (LAL) test for detecting pyrogens in parenteral injectable products and medical devices: advantages to manufacturers and regulatory officials. J. Parent. Drug. Assoc. 33: 81–95.
87. Pearson, F.C., III and Weary, M. (1980) The significance of limulus amebocyte lysate test specificity on the pyrogen evaluation of parenteral drugs. J. Parent. Drug. Assoc. 34: 103–108

# 13. Present clinical experience and future aspects of hemodiafiltration

Volker Wizemann

In the mid-seventies, when hemofiltration was introduced on a larger scale into clinical practice in Europe, it became apparent that hemofiltration and hemodialysis differ profoundly in respect to the size and molecular weight of substances to be removed from the plasma of uremic subjects. Conventional hemodialysis, performed with cuprophane membranes, had an excellent effect on removing small uremic solutes of less than 1,000 daltons by diffusive transport. However, larger substances like 'middle molecules' were extracted from the blood only in neglectable amounts.

On the other hand, convective transport of hemofiltration did not discriminate between smaller or larger substances as long as the sieving coefficient of the hemofiltration membrane was 1 for the solutes to be removed. Thus, during hemofiltration, the same clearance was measured for small substances like urea (60 daltons) and inulin (5.200 daltons). When hemofiltration with the polyacrylnitrile membrane RP 6 was used clinically, it became apparent that in the presence of an excellent middle molecule extraction the removal of small uremic solutes like urea, creatinine, and uric acid was comparatively low.

By balancing the advantages the disadvantages of hemofiltration and hemodialysis, both methods appeared unsatisfactory since the nature and molecular size of the majority of uremic toxins was unknown — and still is — and the goal of an elimination of a broad spectrum of potential toxins could not achieved by either renal replacement method. In order to combine the advantages of hemodialysis and hemofiltration, and thereby avoid the disadvantages of each single method, a combination of both renal replacement systems was introduced in 1976 by several groups [1–4].

## Definition of hemodiafiltration

Hemodialysis is defined as solute removal by diffusion. Ultrafiltration implies removal of plasma water and solutes by convection without concomitant substitution. Ultrafiltration plus simultaneous substitution is termed hemofiltration. Hemodiafiltration, which combines hemodialysis and hemofiltration

*Vincenzo Cambi (editor) Professor of Nephrology*
© *1987 Martinus Nijhoff Publishing, Boston. ISBN 0-89838-858-9. Printed in The United States.*

by the use of one device and one membrane, can be described as simultaneous hemofiltration and dialysis. From the practicable point of view, hemodiafiltration is a hemodialysis, where a permeable membrane is used and ultrafiltration rate is so high that substitution fluid has to be given. Thus, in hemodiafiltration, dialysate as well as replacement fluid is necessary used.


**Rationale for hemodiafiltration**

Hemodiafiltration is the only renal replacement method that allows a separate control of removal for small and larger toxins from uremic blood. Depending on the surface of the dialyzer/hemodiafilter and dialysate flow, the efficiency of the dialysis part can be altered as can be the hemofiltration part and thereby larger molecule removal by changing the filtration rate. The composition of the substitute and dialysate (sodium, calcium, potassium, bicarbonate concentrations) allows an additional individualization of the patients' treatment.


**Hemodiafiltration methods**

*Manual balancing of fluid*

Hemodiafiltration can be carried out with every single-pass dialysis machine, provided that a bed-scale, a hemodiafilter, an extra pump, and substitution fluid is available. As depicted in figure 13–1A, hemodiafiltration is primarily a single-pass hemodialysis where a highly permeable membrane is used. As dialysate buffer either acetate or bicarbonate can be used. When a high transmembraneous pressure is applied, ultrafiltration during the dialysis process will be as high as during a hemofiltration with the same membrane (60–120 ml/min). In the presence of such a high ultrafiltration, substitution fluid has to be replaced continuously, which can be done by an extra pump adjusted to infuse substitution fluid into the bubble catcher at nearly the same rate as ultrafiltration. A bed-scale for following the patient's weight constantly is necessary to control all fluid movements and to obtain the precalculated weight loss. As infusate we use 4.5 l plastic bags (commercially available in the (Federal Republic of Germany) containing (in mM/l): sodium 140, chloride 112, potassium 2.0, calcium 2.125, magnesium 0.75, lactate 35.75. Osmolarity is 301 mOsmol/l.

The manual balancing has the disadvantage that considerable experience is necessary to adjust the pump velocity for the substitution fluid. Frequent control of body weight and readjustment of the infusate is necessary to obtain linear volume loss. Since misbalancing cannot be totally avoided, we prefer the hemodiafiltration device with automatic fluid control as depicted in figure 13–1B.

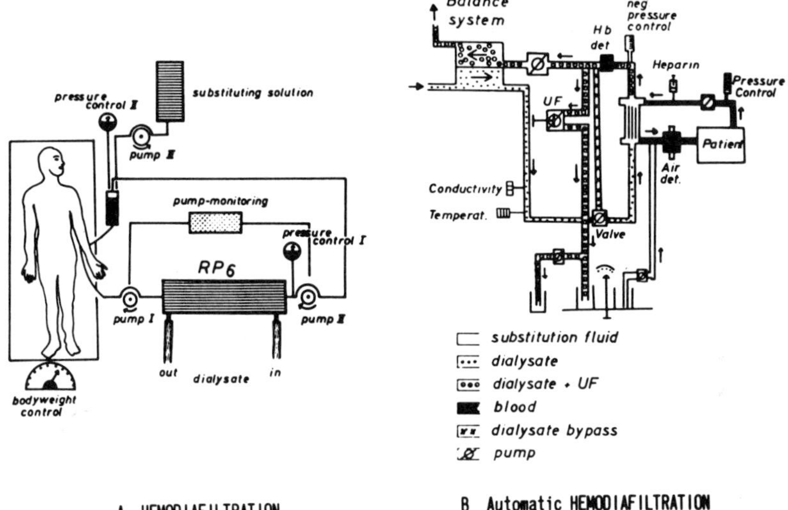


*Figure 13–1.* Hemodiafiltration devices. *A* = manual balancing of fluid (replacement solution). *B* = Automatic replacement of substitution fluid with volumetrical control of ultrafiltration and gravimetrical control of substitution fluid. This system is based on the 2008 C dialysis machine (Fresenius Co, FRG).

## Automatic balancing of fluid

For this system a specially designed hemodialysis machine is necessary (Fresenius Co, Bad Homburg, Federal Republic of Germany). In a chamber (balance system) fresh and used dialysate are balanced 1:1. Though an open circuit, this balancing system has the characteristics of a closed circuit allowing excellent volumetric control of ultrafiltration irrespective of the hydraulic permeability of the dialysis membrane. An additional gravimetrical balancing device for the substitution fluid makes hemodiafiltration possible (figure 13–1B). Since the maximal capacity of the ultrafiltration pump is limited to 4 l/h, the hemofiltration part of hemodiafiltration cannot be further increased.

## Hemodiafiltration with on-line preparation of substitution fluid from dialysate

So far, two technical devices have been described for the on-line preparation of replacement fluid from bicarbonate dialysate during hemodiafiltration. The apparatus used by Miller and coworkers [5] and the device proposed by Canaud and associates [6] are similar in the design of a balancing system for volumetric control of ultrafiltration. A matched set of cylinders or balancing chambers remove exactly the same volume from the dialyzer circuit as is freshly put into it by the dialysate proportioning system. Since there is zero net ultrafiltration, net weight loss is controllable by a separate adjustable ultrafiltration pump removing the desired fluid. The system used by Canaud [6] is based on the Fresenius 2008 C dialysis machine described in figure 13–1B. Supposing that dialysate flow is high enough and dialysate passes one or two pyrogen filters, the now sterile fluid can be divided into dialysate and replacement fluid. The device used in our center is also based on the Fresenius 2008 C dialysis machine and can be used for hemodiafiltration, hemofiltration, and peritoneal dialysis purposes. The advantage of those systems for on-line preparation of substitution fluid lies in the availability of inexpensive large amounts of replacement fluid. Furthermore, the electrolyte composition is identical in dialysate and substituate, and consequently, bicarbonate containing substitution fluid can be produced. The potential dangers of such a system consist in microbiological problems [7] and in the quality of pretreatment of tap water. The fluid, which is infused into the patients' blood, has to be sterile and free of heavy metals.

*Hypertonic hemodiafiltration*

Due to the fact that dialysate and substituate are separated, hemodiafiltration allows a unique individualization of the patients' treatment. Thus, bicarbonate and calcium can be applied separately in two different fluids; different sodium concentrations in the dialysate and the replacement fluid can be modified to achieve a better hemodynamic stability and solute removal — preferentially from the intracellular compartment — can be improved. An attempt to use the full potential of hemodiafiltration for individual therapy was made by Cambi and coworkers [8]. Hypertonic hemodiafiltration consists of a simultaneous hypertonic low volume (7.2 l of replacing solution) hemofiltration part and a hypotonic hemodialysis part, which is performed for 180 minutes [8]. In order to avoid a high serum sodium at the end of the session, the sodium concentration of the substitution fluid is reduced from 275 mM/l to 125 mM/l in the last 30 minutes of the hemodiafiltration treatment. The hypotonic dialysis solution contains a sodium concentration of 120 mM/l [8].

A future approach to use the two variable sites of fluid, electrolyte, and acid-base variation in hemodiafiltration can consist in a computer-assisted modeling of the intracellular and extracellular compartments as described for hemodialysis [9–11] and hemofiltration [12].

*Low-efficiency hemodiafiltration: biofiltration*

Based on the idea that correction of acidosis by bicarbonate infusion and the detoxification advantages of low-efficiency hemodiafiltration should be combined in a comparatively simple technical device, biofiltration was created [13–15]. By definition, biofiltration is a hemodiafiltration because infusion of a substitution fluid is necessary. In principle, a hemodialysis machine with built-in ultrafiltration control, a membrane with a relatively high hydraulic permeability, and three liters of high sodium (natrium = 145 mM/l) and high bicarbonate (100 mM/l) is used. The hourly ultrafiltration schedule is set up by adding the quantity of 1 l per hour to the desired body weight loss. Composition of the dialysate is usually identical to that used in standard dialysis and contains acetate. Dialysate flow is 500 ml/min and blood flow 300 ml/min. Prevailingly, the method was employed for short-duration purposes [13, 14].

*High-efficiency hemodiafiltration*

At present, both systems for on-line preparation of substitution fluid from the dialysate have been introduced for high-efficiency hemodiafiltration. Albertini and coworkers [16, 17] used either two dialyzers made of cellulose acetate (total surface area 3.6 m$^2$) in a serial configuration in the extracorporeal circuit [17] or a polysulphone F60 and a F40 in the same arrangement [16]. Mean blood flow was 504 + 8 ml/min and dialysate flow averaged 1,007 ml/min. Total filtrate removed per treatment averaged 13 l and a 140 mM/l sodium, and a 35 mM/l bicarbonate concentration in the dialysate was used. Mean treatment time in the 4 patients studied was 3 × 115 min/week. Measured whole blood clearances were: BUN 407 + 15; creatinine 322 + 51; and phosphate 289 + 40 ml/min [16]. The goal of the study was to more than halving standard treatment time of 3 × 4 hours/week and simultaneously to maintain the adequacy of small molecular detoxifiction, based solely on an optimal weekly urea clearance [18].

In contrast, Wizemann and coworkers [19] chose a different approach. Based on a 9-year experience with short-duration hemodiafiltration (3 × 2–3 hours/week) and on cardiac findings in dialysis patients, they avoided to shorten treatment time and designed a high-efficiency hemodiafiltration treatment with a duration of 3 × 4 hours/week. Two polysulphone F60 dialyzers in the blood line were used as hemodiafilters (total membrane surface 2.5 m$^2$), and 60 l of plasma water were ultrafiltrated per patient and per session. Consequently, 60 l of substitution fluid had to be replaced (between the first and the second dialyzer as well as after the second dialyzer = middilution and postdilution). The device used was similar to that depicted in figure 13–2. Blood flow was 300 ml/min. Measured whole blood clearances (n = 10) were: urea 275 + 8.5; creatinine 240 + 22; phosphate 225 + 22; inulin 125 + 15; $\beta_2$-microglobulin 100 + 36 ml/min.

**Comparison of hemodiafiltration efficiency to other renal replacement methods**

It can be seen from figure 13–2 that hemodiafiltration is the most effective method for removing solutes of different molecular weight. Depending on the cut-off of the membrane used, the clearance for larger substances like $\beta_2$-microglobulin (mw 11.000 daltons) or — in an extremely permeable

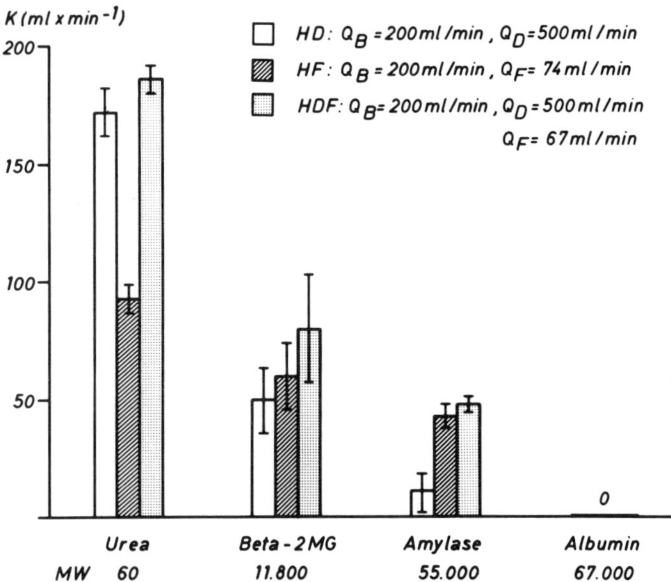


*Figure 13–2.* Comparison of clearances (K) in 10 patients during hemodialysis (HD), hemofiltration (HF), and hemodiafiltration (HDF). Blood flow was standardized (200 ml/min), and a highly permeable polysulphone membrane F60 was used during all treatments. Since net ultrafiltration in HD was zero, it cannot be excluded that the major part of $\beta_2$-microglobulin and amylase clearances in HD result from convection in the first part of the dialyzer (and back-filtration of fluid from the dialysate accounts for net zero ultrafiltration). Thus, in HD, clearances for larger solutes might be falsely too high.

membrane — alpha-amylase (mw 57.000 daltons) is higher during hemodiafiltration as compared to hemofiltration, provided that standard conditions like identical blood flows are used. When hemodiafiltration is compared to hemodialysis in the same membrane, it is evident that both methods share high transport rates for low-molecular uremic solutes (figure 13–2).

Blood flow rates of 300–600 ml/min provided, is conceivable that an identical solute removal (urea, creatinine) can be achieved by hemodiafiltration in 115–130 minutes as obtained by a standard dialysis in 240–300 minutes [16, 17, 20, 21], whereas in respect to elimination of substances with higher molecular weight, short-duration hemodiafiltration is by far superior to conventional hemodialysis. Von Albertini and associates obtained an increase in efficiency (hemodiafiltration) about 2 and one-half times over that of conventional hemodialysis by a better utilization of blood flow and the technique of simultaneous high diffusion and convection [17]. Since part of the improved efficiency derives from the development of new membranes with a high hydraulic permeability, the question arises whether those membranes should be used for hemodialysis purposes (with control of ultrafiltration), for hemofiltration, or for hemodiafiltration. Taking into account that the whole potential of such a membrane can only be utilized if diffusive and convective transport is present simultaneously (figure 13–2), use for hemodialysis purposes would imply a renunciation of an effective removal of larger substances. It is, therefore, not surprising that in a study involving 10 patients, no detectable benefit was observed when the patients were dialyzed 3 × 4 hours/week over a polysulphone F60 membrane for 4 months. Compared to a standard dialysis (3 × 4 hours/week) involving a cuprophane dialyzer with the same surface area, there was no difference in predialysis values for small uremic solutes or larger substances like alpha-amylase [22].

## Acute hemodynamic reactions during hemodiafiltration: comparison to hemodialysis and hemofiltration

Evaluation of acute hemodynamic reactions during hemodiafiltration in comparison to other renal replacement methods was performed in one invasive [23] and one noninvasive study [24] employing echocardiography. Wizemann and coworkers [23] performed five different dialysis procedures serially (hemodialysis with a bath sodium of 138 mM/l and acetate, hemodialysis with a bath sodium of 138 mM/l and bicarbonate, hemodialysis with a bath sodium of 154 mM/l and acetate, hemodiafiltration-sodium in the bath and substitute 138 mM/l, hemofiltration-sodium in the substitute 138 mM/l).

The fluid removal rate was standardized per patient and therefore was identical during all treatments. The study was performed in 5 patients with acute renal failure, who were classified as hemodynamically unstable since hypotension occurred during ultrafiltration by conventional hemodialysis. Cardiac output and total vascular peripheral resistance were measured by Fick's principle.

In healthy persons, total vascular peripheral resistance (TVPR) and cardiac output (CO) are interrelated. An increase in cardiac output usually leads to a decrease in total vascular peripheral resistance; and reversely, a decrease in cardiac output — as often observed during volume removal — is followed by a compensatory increase in total vascular peripheral resistance. Thus, blood pressure, which is the product of cardiac output times total vascular peripheral resistance, can be maintained. It can be deducted from figure 13–3 that during hemodialysis with acetate buffer and a 138 mM/l bath sodium, decrease in cardiac output is not adequately followed by a compensatory augmentation of total vascular peripheral resistance. When the same patients are treated by acetate dialysis but a higher sodium in the dialysate (154 mM/l), total vascular peripheral resistance reacts somewhat more favorable as it does during bicarbonate dialysis with 138 mM/l sodium. However, during hemofiltration, and to a slightly lesser degree during hemodiafiltration, total vascular peripheral resistance increased in the presence of a diminished cardiac output.

Schmidt and associates [24] studied 14 hemodynamically stable patients on

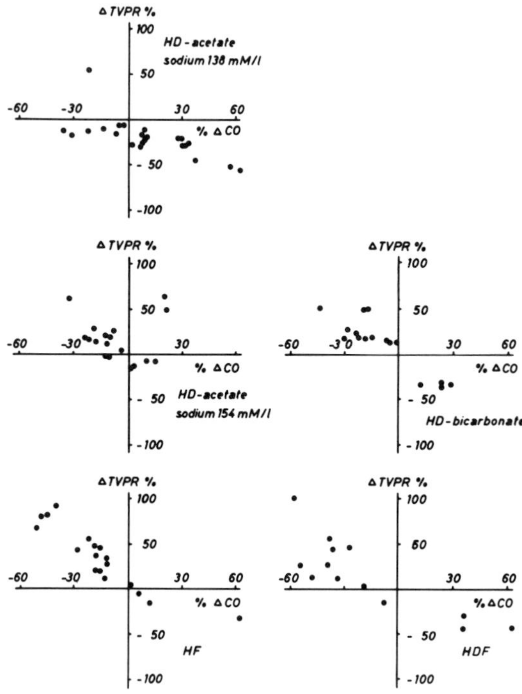

*Figure 13–3.* Hemodynamic measurements in 5 patients, who were treated by 5 different dialysis methods in sequence. For details, see text.

maintenance hemodialysis by echocardiography. Patients were treated in sequence by hemodialysis, high-flux hemodialysis, hemodiafiltration, and hemofiltration. Conditions were kept constant during all treatments: comparable weight loss, 35 mM/l acetate in the dialysate or substituate, 140 mM/l sodium in both fluids, comparable control systems for linear weight loss, and identical clearances for small solutes in all treatment regimes. Thus, nontreatment specific factors were greatly limited. There was a significant difference in posttreatment mean arterial blood pressure, which was higher after hemodiafiltration and hemofiltration as compared to hemodialysis. In respect to left ventricular and diastolic or endsystolic dimensions, fractional shortening and velocity of circumferential fiber shortening, there were no intertreatment differences.

Both studies indicate that maintenance of blood pressure during extracorporeal fluid removal might be better tolerated when performed by hemodiafiltration or hemofiltration. In hemodynamically unstable patients, this effect becomes even more apparent. Thus, it seems that hemodiafiltration might share the favorable hemodynamic effect as it was described for hemofiltration [23, 24–29].

300

## Clinical experience with hemodiafiltration

*Treatment of acute renal failure by hemodiafiltration*

Experience with hemodiafiltration in acute renal failure is limited [23] since arteriovenous (a.v.) hemofiltration and intermittent hemofiltration are usually the preferred methods. However, a considerable proportion of patients with multiorgan failure is catabolic and might be underdialysed by (a.v.) hemofiltration or intermittent hemofiltration with a daily exchange of 9–20 l of plasma water. Since hemodiafiltration by far exceeds the detoxification efficacy of both mentioned methods and hemodiafiltration — as depicted above — shares some of the favorable vascular reactions of hemofiltration, we apply daily hemofiltration to hypercatabolic patients with acute renal failure. As dialysate buffer we use bicarbonate and a biocompatible membrane like polysulphone or polyacrylnitrile for prevention of complement activation and sequent augmentation of right heart workload as observed experimentally in sheep [30].

It has been described that hemodialysis per se acts as a catabolic stimulus [31–33], which cannot solely be explained by loss of amino acids [34]. Although one study implies that hemofiltration induces catabolisms comparable to that observed in hemodialysis [35], in the last few years it has become apparent that membrane-blood interaction may play an important role in inducing catabolism [36]. So-called biocompatible membranes such as polyacrylnitrile or polysulphone release less leucocyte elastase [37] or interleukin-1 [38] than cuprophane. Since most membranes used for hemofiltration or hemodiafiltration purposes are based on biocompatible material, application of those membranes to critically ill patients might be preferable. Furthermore, besides the membrane effects on catabolism, generation of interleukin-1 and thereby activation of local prostaglandin $E_2$-release might account for hemodialysis hypotension [39].

No data exist concerning the value of hemodiafiltration as a detoxification method in exogenous poisoning. In theory [40], however, hemodiafiltration should be superior to hemodialysis in removing water soluble substances (see also figure 13–2). For the same reason, hemodiafiltration might be preferable to hemodialysis and hemofiltration in endogenous poisoning presuming that there is a place for such extracorporeal methods in the therapeutical approach.

*Treatment of chronic renal failure by short-duration hemodiafiltration*

One of the critical questions pertaining to an effective detoxification method is the dose of therapy to be applied. Having the choice between a potential qualitative improvement — provided that the duration of a hemodiafiltration session is the same as with hemodialysis — or a shortening of treatment time and maintaining the current treatment quality of hemodialysis, we [1, 20, 41] and others [8, 13, 16, 17, 42, 43] chose the latter. Before discussing the clinical experience with short-duration hemodiafiltration, the expression 'short' has to be defined.

In the 1970s dialysis duration was subsequently reduced from approximately 30 hours per week to less than the half [43]. However, in 1979 a weekly dialysis duration of 11.2 hours was termed 'ultrashort dialysis' [44] which became standard for the majority of registered dialysis patients of Europe in 1981 [45]. We, therefore, would like to consider a 4-hour dialysis, performed 3 times per week, as standard duration, and we are not willing to define such a strategy as short-duration renal replacement therapy. Three hours' duration or less, performed twice weekly, can be clearly distinguished from standard dialysis duration. In the following, we define such a strategy as short treatment.

So far, we have avoided the aspect of adequacy. Without doubt, a standard treatment of 12 hours per week or even a much longer — can be inadequate in individuals. We would, therefore, like to relate adequacy of treatment — including duration — to the preexisting status of individual patients. In the following, we will focus on two aspects: first, on detoxification parameters by short hemodiafiltration and second, on the preexisting cardiovascular state of the patients and the impact of volume removal by hemodiafiltration.

*Clinical experience with detoxification parameters under short hemodiafiltration treatment* Cioni and coworkers [46] studied 8 patients on a hemodiafiltration regime over 15 months. Treatment time was reduced to 160 minutes and afterwards to 130 minutes (3 times/week). Blood flow rate was 400 ml/min, dialysate flow 500 ml/min and 27, respectively, 18 liters of plasma water were exchanged. Urea whole blood clearance was $305 \pm 9.2$ ml/min. The follow-up of prehemodiafiltration plasma parameters showed lower values for urea, creatinine, and phosphate as compared to the preceding standard hemodialysis therapy ($3 \times 240$ min, cuprophane $1.3 \text{ m}^2$ hollow fiber dialyzer). Although the data are not present in the publication [46], the magnitude of renal replacement therapy can be estimated as the product of the dialyzer urea clearance (K, l/min) and treatment time (t, min) divided by the body urea distribution volume (V, l) as proposed by Gotch and associates [47]. Assuming a body urea distribution volume of 40 liters, $K \times t/V$ equals 0.99 for short hemodiafiltration as compared to 0.93 for standard dialysis. Thus, removal of small uremic solutes appears to be adequate in 130 min of hemodiafiltration.

Wizemann and associates [41] made an early attempt [1976] to reduce treatment time by employment of the hemodiafiltration technique. As hemodiafilter, the RP6 polyacrylnitrile membrane was used, and 9 liters of substitute were infused per session. Blood flow was 200–250 ml/min. In a comparison of intraindividual biochemical parameters from 9 patients who had been treated by hemodialysis ($1.2 \text{ m}^2$ cuprophane dialyzers, $3 \times 4$ hours/ week or longer) or hemodiafiltration ($3 \times 3$ hours/week) for 2.5 years in each period, there was no difference in pretreatment plasma values (urea, creatinine, phosphate) and hemoglobin. Velocity of motoric and sensible nerve conductivity as well as the latency-time of the H-reflex did not differ when measured at the end of the hemodialysis and hemodiafiltration period. In the light of a weekly inulin clearance of 43 liters during the hemodiafiltration period, which can be calculated from the clearance data, an increase of middle molecule clearance by at least the factor 10 during hemodiafiltration (as compared to hemodialysis) can be assumed. In accordance with the findings of most authors (for review see reference [48]), there was no apparent clinical benefit of such a high middle molecule removal, especially no effect on renal anemia or polyneuropathy. However, despite no changes in prehemodiafiltration plasma values, removal of small uremic solutes did not fulfill the present standard for adequacy ($K \times t/V = 0.81$), which may counterbalance the effects of a better middle molecule removal.

In a second study, the same group [20] shortened treatment time from $3 \times 240$ minutes of hemodialysis to $3 \times 105$ minutes of hemodiafiltration in 6 patients over a period of 6 months. A 2.1 m$^2$ polymethylmetacrylate hollow fiber or a 1.6 m$^2$ polyacrylnitrile hollow fiber hemodiafilter where applied in a device identical with that described in figure 13–1A. Blood flow was 400 ml/min, dialysate flow 500 ml/min, and 9 liters of substitution fluid were infused. Again, plasma concentrations of urea, creatinine, electrolytes, and total protein did not differ from the preceding dialysis period with the exception of plasma phosphate, which increased from $2.1 \pm 0.6$ to $2.6 \pm 1.0$ mM/l during short hemodiafiltration. Hemoglobin was unchanged. However, despite a low index for urea detoxification ($K \times t/V = 0.65$), symptoms of uremic intoxification were not observed.

Cambi and coworkers [8] performed hypertonic hemodiafiltration in 4 anuric patients over a period of 8 months ($3 \times 180$ min/week), which was compared to standard hemodialysis (1 m$^2$ hemodialyzer, blood flow 300 ml/min, dialysate flow 500 ml/min). For hemodiafiltration purposes, a 1.8 m$^2$ hemodiafilter at a blood flow of 300 ml/min, a dialysate flow of 500 ml/min was used. Ultrafiltration rate was 61 ml-min, and reinfusion rate 40 ml/min. Extraction rates for urea and middle molecules were significantly higher during hypertonic hemodiafiltration as compared to standard hemodialysis (56 versus 51%, $p < 0.05$, respectively, 52 versus 29%, $p < 0.05$). Metabolic acidosis was better controlled during hemodiafiltration, and it is of special interest that large amounts of solutes were removed during the first hours of treatment.

Zucchelli and associates [13, 14] performed short biofiltration in 5 patients. In comparison to the preceeding standard dialysis period, pretreatment plasma values (BUN, creatinine, uric acid, total protein, cholesterol) and hematocrit did not deteriorate. Metabolic acidosis was significantly better controlled during biofiltration. However, assuming a 70 kg standard weight of the patients, removal of small uremic solutes ($K \times t/V = 0.66$) did not fulfill the present standard [18].

von Albertini [17] employed the device for high-efficiency hemodiafiltration as described above and obtained solute clearances in 4 patients, which exceeded the previous by reported values. Using two polysulphone F60 dialyzers, urea clearances could even be increased to 514 ml/min at a mean blood flow of 630 ml/min [16]. Despite a high urea removal in 115 minutes of hemodiafiltration, signs of dialysis-disequilibrium syndrome were not observed (von Albertini, personal communication), which is in accordance with the findings of Wizemann and Wizemann, who did not observe changes in EEG, density of brain CT, and intraocular pressure during high urea removal rates [91]. Thus, the almost threefold gain in efficiency over standard hemodialysis allowed to shorten treatment time to $3 \times 115$ min/week without neglecting the recommendations of the National Cooperative Study [18] for small solute removal. At present, however, it is unclear if a larger group of patients has been followed up since the initial report of the study.

In conclusion, a similar or even a better quality of detoxification in chronic dialysis patients can be achieved by hemodiafiltration in a considerably shorter time than by hemodialysis, provided that extracorporeal blood flow is high enough, the diafilter surface is large, and convection is high. The main argument for short hemodiafiltration and other short renal replacement methods is the improvement of socioeconomical factors. However, we observed a considerable amount of of nurse stress when performing short hemodiafiltration [49]. It has to be kept in mind that the basis for high-efficiency treatment is a constantly high blood flow and a reliable device guaranteeing high solute removal rates. Thus, the question of controllability of those factors arises. A mistake, occurring in a highly efficient 2-hour treatment, might cause considerably higher damage as compared to a 4-hour session.

*Effect of short-duration treatment on the cardiovascular systems* Although not a short-treatment as defined above, Sprenger and associates [50] found in an ABA study in 6 patients, where 6 months of hemodiafiltration (B) was followed by 3 months of hemodialysis (A), that the occurrence of discomfort syndrome was lower in the hemodiafiltration period despite a reduction of treatment time by one-third. The observation that symptoms, which can be related to fluid removal, occur less frequently during hemodiafiltration as compared to standard dialysis [23, 46, 52–54] was confirmed.

However, despite an improved tolerance of fluid withdrawal, as observed in hemofiltration, which at present cannot be explained for both methods on a pathophysiological basis [55, 56], the cardiac status of the patients on maintenance hemodialysis has to be taken into account. It is of similar importance to ensure a safe detoxification in a short time as well as to select patients on the basis of cardiac findings in order to select those in whom a comparatively rapid fluid removal can be performed safely. There is evidence from the EDTA registry [57] that death rates are higher in dialysis patients who have been treated by short dialysis, and the statistics indicate, that — though still disputed — cardiac deaths may be more frequent in that group. Arterial hypertension is considered to be the most important factor in dialysis patients associated with the development of atherosclerosis [58]. Thus, not only the cardiac status of the patients and the duration and mode of renal replacement therapy might be of interest but there additionally is the question of how efficient a short-duration dialysis, diafiltration, or hemofiltration can be in controlling water and salt balance. It should be kept in mind that chronic dialysis patients spend only approximately 10% of their lifetime in a dialysis unit. Although the incidence of hypotension during dialysis is important, control of arterial hypertension by a dialysis method might be of even more importance in the light of the findings, that in an analysis of more than 50,000 deaths in dialysis patients, the majority can be referred to cardiovascular complications [59]. The following chapters will therefore focus on cardiovascular findings in dialysis patients and on the incidence of arterial hypotension and hypertension depending on dialysis duration.

*Cardiac findings in chronic dialysis patients — an important parameter for selecting renal replacement duration*

In an unselected population of chronic dialysis patients, the prevalence of coronary artery disease (CAD) was 26% [60]. In our center, 16 out of 43 dialysis patients (37%) had CAD assessed by angiography and 7/43 had three vessel disease. Although in 7 patients confirmed with CAD but without symptomatic dialysis hypotension, identical fluid removal in a 4-hours and 2-hour dialysis (the fluid removal rate was twice as high in 2 hours) resulted into an improvement of myocardial perfusion, left ventricular function (figure 13–4), exercise duration, and angina symptomatology [61], the pathophysiological basis of such a finding is a reduction of cardiac preload by correction of hyperhydration. However, in a regular 2-hour hemodiafiltration treatment over 6 months, we observed an increase in weight gain between hemodiafiltration sessions as compared to a standard dialysis period [20]. Since achievement of the lowest possible 'dry weight' and prevention of excessive hyperhydration in dialysis patients suffering from CAD are important therapeutical goals, we consider short hemodiafiltration or any other short-dialysis method as contraindicated in patients with CAD. A positive sodium balance can stabilize blood pressure during dialysis [62, 63] and might be one cause of the positive hemodynamic action of hemodiafiltration. On the other hand, an inadequate removal of ingested sodium by any short-dialysis therapy can induce hyperhydration and thereby might compromise CAD patients.

Cardiac arrhythmias are frequent albeit mostly not dangerous in dialysis patients [64–70]. Arrhythmias are often associated with CAD [69]. Two studies [69, 70] indicate that the incidence of ventricular ectopies is not dependent on the dialysis method, dialysate buffer, or biocompatibility of membranes, as long as dialysis hypotension can be avoided. Thus, in a normotensive dialysis patient with arrhythmias but exclusion of CAD —

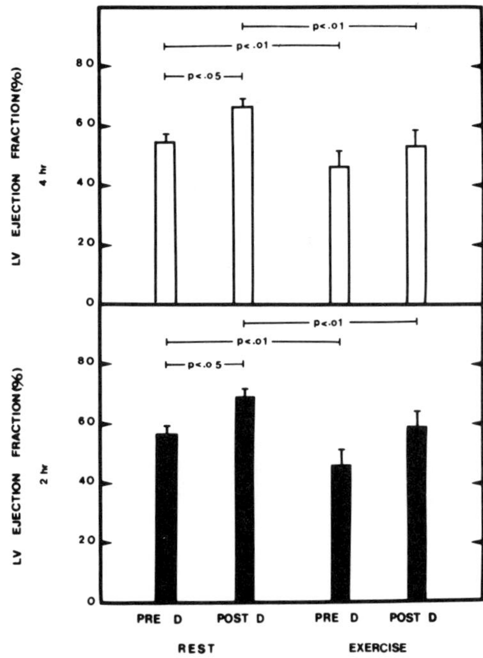


*Figure 13–4.* Left ventricular ejection fractions during rest and exercise conditions in 7 patients with confirmed coronary artery disease. All patients were treated by a 4-hour dialysis (fluid removal rate 1 kg/hour) or by a 2-hour dialysis (fluid removal rate 2 kg/hour). It can be seen that irrespective of dialysis duration, left ventricular ejection fraction was improved after dialysis, which is a consequence of a reduction in cardiac preload.

which admittedly is a rare situation — short-dialysis treatment might not be a contraindication.

Left ventricular hypertrophy, assessed by echocardiography, is a frequent finding in patients on maintenance hemodialysis [61, 71–79] with a prevalence of about 57%. Functionally, by relating left ventricular muscle mass to enddiastolic volume and referring the data to endsystolic left ventricular pressures, in approximately 30% of all dialysis patients a secondary form of hypertrophic cardiomyopathy can be diagnosed [61]. By evaluating pressure-volume relations of the left ventricle throughout 300 subsequent cardiac cycles, it can be seen from figure 13–5 that after occlusion of the arteriovenous fistula, and thereby reduction of enddiastolic volume, primarily elevated left ventricular enddiastolic pressure did not decrease. This finding indicates a disturbance of diasystolic compliance of the left ventricle, which is present in nearly all patients in whom a left ventricular hypertrophy can be diagnosed by echocardiography. Apparently, the left ventricle in dialysis patients needs an elevated diastolic pressure to fulfill its pump function.

Thus, in dialysis patients, there might be a fatal pathophysiological setting: on the one hand, compromised diastolic compliance is very sensitive to rapid

306

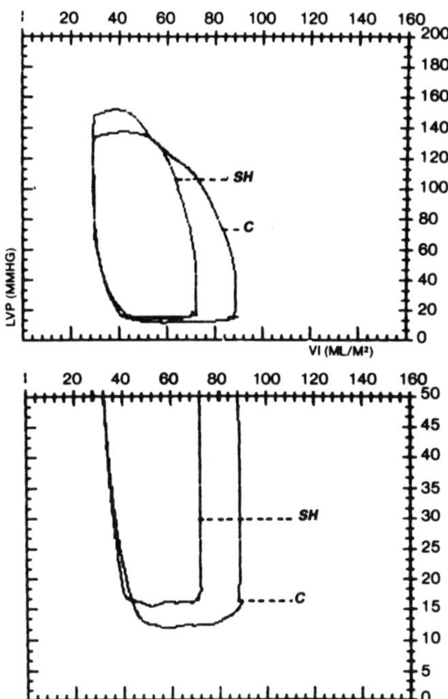


*Figure 13–5. Above*: Volume-pressure relationship in the left ventricle of chronic hemodialysis patients (control = C). The computer curve was derived from 300 subsequent cardiac circles in each of 11 patients. *Below*: Enlargement of volume-pressure relationship during the diastole. Occlusion of the a.-v. dialysis fistula (SH) results into a pronounced reduction of end diastolic volume but not in a reduction of enddiastolic pressure. This finding signifies a disturbance of diastolic compliance of left ventricles in dialysis patients.

changes in diastolic volume, which is influenced by a more or less rapid fluid removal rate. Additionally, inotropic stimulation, as induced by dialysis-dependent changes in ionized calcium [80] or simultaneous calcium/potassium changes in the plasma [81], may be hazardous in the presence of hypertrophic cardiomyopathy. On the other hand, fluid removal and augmentation of inotropism cannot be avoided in hemodialysis patients. However, the rapidity of those changes can be well controlled by the prescription of a slower and longer or a faster and shorter dialysis.

Sudden death is one of the features of hypertrophic cardiomyopathy (*Harrison's Principles of Internal Medicine*, 10th ed. pp. 1452–1453), and sudden death has been described in [non-renal patients] with hypertrophic cardiomyopathy following vasodilator therapy [82]. Changes in cardiac workload — induced by hemodialysis methods, especially by short dialysis — are much more prominent as compared to vasodilator therapy. We, therefore, consider the findings of left ventricular hypertrophy a contraindication to any kind of short blood purification method. In the light of those findings it can be speculated whether the high incidence of sudden deaths in the dialysis population [59, 83] might be due to an inadequately short dialysis.

Studying 131 patients on maintenance dialysis by echocardiography, we observed that the incidence of left ventricular hypertrophy could not be related to the degree of renal anemia, mean arterial blood pressure, and iPTH plasma concentrations. However, left ventricular hypertrophy was associated to time on dialysis. In the first year, the incidence was 26%, and after 5 years on dialysis it was 49%. It can be therefore suspected that some unique features in dialysis patients, e.g., a high arteriovenous fistula, might contribute to be development of left ventricular hypertrophy. In 11 dialysis patients, in whom CAD was excluded angiographically, we measured the effects of fistula occlusion by left heart catheterization. Fistula occlusion was followed by significant reduction in cardiac index (4.1 versus 3.0 1/min/m$^2$, p < 0.01) and left ventricular stroke work (8.2 versus 6.6 kg $\times$ min$^{-1}$/m$^2$, p < 0.05). For short-duration therapy, presence of a mature dialysis fistula is one of the prerequisites. However, designing a high fistula shunt volume for short-therapy purposes by intent would imply an uncalculable cardiac risk by increasing left ventricular workload constantly.

In conclusion, in the vast majority of chronic dialysis patients there are serious cardiac findings, which are an obstacle toward short renal replacement therapy (table 13–1). Cardiac status, therefore, has to be defined precisely before shortening treatment time. CAD, left ventricular hypertrophy, and hypertrophic cardiomyopathy cannot be diagnosed in dialysis patients by ECG and chest x-ray. CAD can be confirmed noninvasively by simultaneous isotope thallium perfusion imaging and technetium ventriculography, and left ventricular hypertrophy can be diagnosed by echocardiography. Left atrial dilatation in the presence of left ventricular hypertrophy may indicate compromised left ventricular diastolic compliance, and an excellent pump function of the left ventricle in the presence of left ventricular hypertrophy and a small cavum may arise suspicion of hypertrophic cardiomyopathy. Thus, the old rule in medicine, that diagnosis has to be made first and then followed by an adequate therapy, is also true for the description of a dialysis regime (table 13–2). Yet, the main argument against short dialysis in the presence of the described cardiac disorders is the necessity of a more rapid fluid and salt withdrawal by a shorter dialysis regime. In the following we will, therefore, discuss the impact of dialysis duration on water and salt balance.

*Table 13–1.* Contraindications for short renal replacement therapy, based on cardiac findings

| Findings | Estimated Prevalence in the Dialysis Population |
| --- | --- |
| Left ventricular hypertrophy | 50–70% |
| Left ventricular hypertrophy with left atrial dilatation | 30–50% |
| Secondary hypertrophic cardiomyopathy | 20–40% |
| Significant coronary artery disease | 25–40% |

308

*Table 13–2.* Prerequisites for short-duration renal replacement therapy

1. Extracorporeal blood flow exceeding 300 ml/min
2. Use of high-flux membranes and volumetrically controlled ultrafiltration
3. Absence of symptomatic hypotension
4. Absence of arterial hypertension
5. Absence of left ventricular hypertrophy (controlled by echocardiography)
6. No need for removing fluid exceeding 1% of dry weight per hour

*Effects of renal replacement duration on the hydration state and arterial blood pressure*

In both hemodiafiltration studies [17, 20], where patients were with treated less than 2 hours per session, a significant increase in weight gain between hemodiafiltration sessions was reported. A similar observation was made when short hemofiltration [46, 84] or short bicarbonate hemodialysis was studied [84].

Based on our cardiological findings, in the last few years we abandoned the concept of short-duration hemodiafiltration as a standard treatment for end-stage renal failure. Thus, we made the probably unique experience that a dialysis center prolonged treatment time substantially in the majority of its patients. In 1981, at the height of our short hemodiafiltration concept, mean treatment time in all our patients was 2.7 hours 3 times per week (n = 51). In 1985, mean treatment time was 4.1 hours (figure 13–6), and patients were treated prevailingly by acetate or bicarbonate hemodialysis or by long-duration hemofiltration (n = 127). Comparing the percentage of patients who had to take antihypertensive drugs or digitalis between the two dialysis strategies, there was a pronounced effect during the longer treatment time. As depicted in figure 13–6, percentage of patients taking antihypertensives dropped from 72% to 19.7%, and those taking digitalis from 35% to 5.5%.

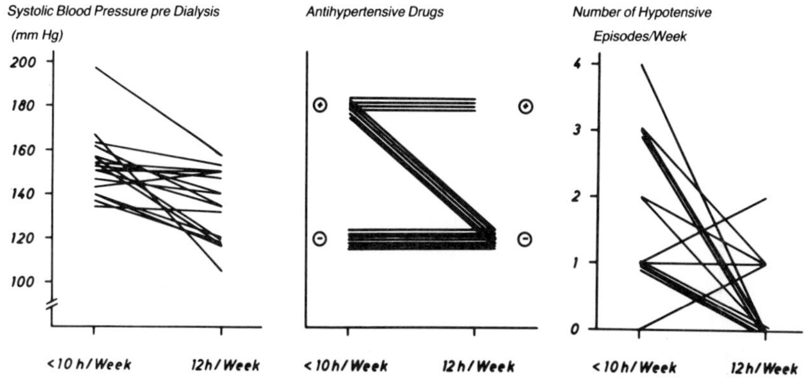


*Figure 13–6.* Consequences of a change in dialysis duration (Giessen dialysis unit).

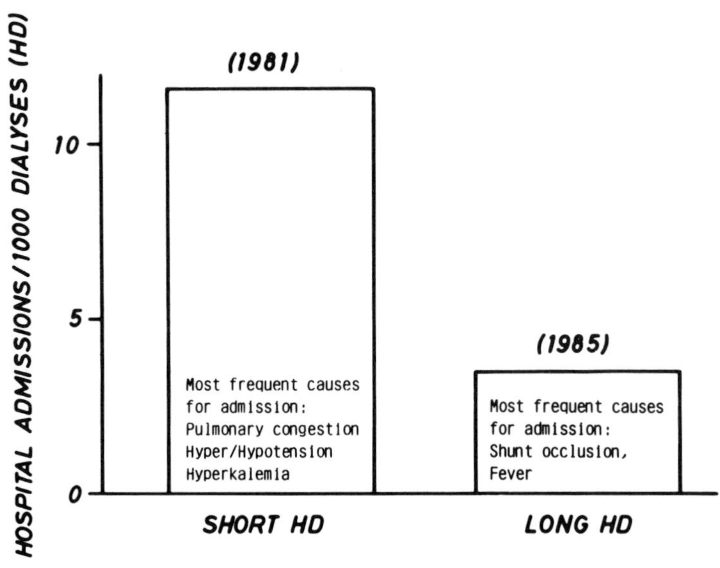


*Figure 13–7.* Rate of hospital admissions during short (mean duration 2.7 hours) and long (mean duration 4.1 hours) dialysis (Giessen dialysis unit).

In same period, there was also a pronounced fall in morbidity (figure 13–7). During the short treatment regime, 12 patients per 1.000 dialyses had to be admitted to the hospital, whereas during the longer treatment regime admission rate dropped to one-fourth. An analysis of the causes for admission might allow a discrimination of treatment-related effects. During short-duration therapy, causes for admission like pulmonary congestion, hypertension, and hypotension indicate an underlying defect in the control of hyperhydration and blood pressure control. Hyperkalemia indicates a nonsufficient potassium removal, inadequate control of metabolic acidosis, or an effect on potassium intake. In 1985, when patients were treated 52% longer as compared to 1981, causes for hospital admission were 'normal' ones like fistula occlusion or infection. Since the same physicians controlled dialysis therapy in both periods, treatment-related changes are more probable than changes in medical approach.

Seventeen patients could be studied intraindividually during both periods (figure 13–8). Predialysis systolic blood pressure was significantly lower ($p < 0.01$) when treatment time was longer. In 5 from 9 patients taking antihypertensives, this kind of drug therapy could be discontinued when treated for a longer time. Despite reduction in predialysis blood pressure observed during a longer treatment regime, there were less hypotensive episodes during longer renal replacement therapy.

In conclusion, duration of dialysis therapy might have pronounced long-term effects on water and sodium balance. Arterial hypertension and over-hydration may be direct long-term consequences of short-dialysis therapy,

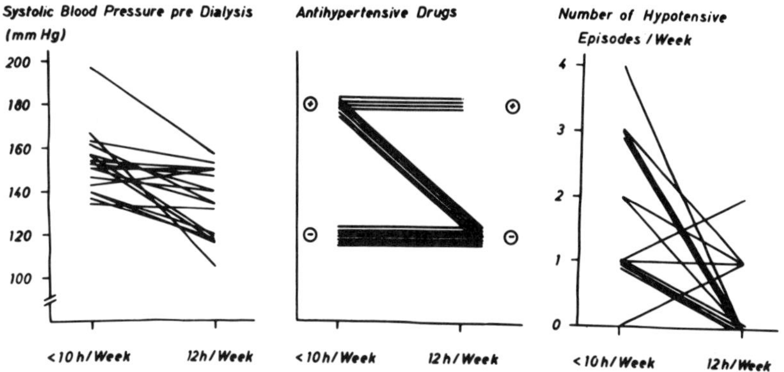


*Figure 13–8.* Intraindividual comparison of 17 patients, who were treated by short or longer dialysis therapy. Each dialysis period lasted at least 2 year.

when applied routinely. In the light of the prognostical prevalence of the risk factor hypertension, we feel that any kind of short-dialysis therapy in nonhand-picked patients can be too short and inadequate. In might be argued that the problem of overhydration and insufficient salt balance in short dialysis can be overcome by dietary control of sodium and water intake. In our experience, however, we were unsuccessful in increasing patients' compliance despite extensive dietary advice. In the future, a better modeling of fluid and sodium removal by extracorporeal blood purification methods might be helpful, but the problem of removing large amounts of water and sodium and simultaneously maintaining cardiac function blood pressure adequately still has to be demonstrated over a long period.

## Experience with high-efficiency hemodiafiltration with long duration (3 × 4 hours/week) — improvement of dialysis quality?

The availability of a new generation of membranes with a high hydraulic permeability and sievieny coefficients, which are similar to the glomerular basement membrane [85], may create a new perspective in the treatment of end-stage renal failure. So far, by standard dialysis with cuprophane membranes or even newer ones, primarily substances with a molecular weight below 5,000 daltons have been removed. Thus, not excretory renal function has been replaced, but essentially excretion of very small solutes like creatinine, urea, and electrolytes. The kidneys, however, play an important role in the excretion of peptides, peptide hormones, and low molecular weight-proteins below 50.000 daltons. For example, light chain components of gamma-globulin have a molecular weight of 22.000 daltons and are filtrated by a rate of about 8% of the GRF [86]. Glomerular clearance of $\beta_2$-microglobulin (molecular weight 11.000 daltons) is even higher. Since only a

311

very small fraction of those proteins appears in the urine, reabsorption and subsequent catabolism by the tubular cells can be suspected. Thus, the kidneys are an important catabolic site for small proteins like lysozyme, ribonuclease, $\beta_2$-microglobulin, retinol-binding protein, insulin, glucagon, parathyroid hormone, growth hormone, and Bence-Jones protein (for review see reference [86]). All those substances cannot pass the pores of cuprophane membranes, and consequently, small molecular proteins are retained in the plasma of dialysis patients. When more permeable membranes are used in dialysis, removal of those proteins is still ineffective since diffusion is dependent on the molecular radius (see also figure 13–2). Removal of larger solutes can only be performed effectively by convection in the presence of a permeable membrane. The pathophysiological significance of low-molecular protein retention in the uremic syndrome is still unclear. Yet, in 1985 it has been reported that amyloid-laden tissue obtained from dialysis patients with carpal tunnel syndrome was identical to $\beta_2$-microglobulin [87], and in uremic subjects it has been demonstrated that urinary matrix concretions are derived from $\beta_2$-microglobulin [88]. Though data are not available, removal of peptides, hormones, and small proteins has to be low in biofiltration or hemodiafiltration involving the exchange of 9 liters of plasma water. The same is true for standard hemofiltration, where only minimal effects on the plasma concentrations of small peptide hormons have been described [89].

Provided that there are high diffusive and convective transport rates over a highly permeable membrane, hemodiafiltration — if only performed long enough — can be the method of choice to test the hypothesis that a blood purification method can imitate excretory kidney function over the whole spectrum of plasma substances filtrated by the glomeruli. We, therefore, have used high-efficiency hemodiafiltration, as described above, in 3 × 4 hour/week sessions. From figure 13–9 it can be seen that in 10 patients treated for 1 week by standard hemodialysis and a second week by high-efficient hemodiafiltration, plasma concentrations of $\beta_2$-microglobulin and amylase can only be influenced by the latter method. The same is true for myoglobin and iPTH fragments (figure 13–10).

In July 1985, we have started an ABA study in 7 patients involving (1) a standard dialysis period (3 × 4 hours/week) and (2) a high-efficiency hemodiafiltration period (3 × 4 hours/week). In contrast to the standard dialysis period, after 6 months of hemodiafiltration $\beta_2$-microglobulin plasma concentrations were decreased (figure 13–11, $p < 0.01$), and albumin was increased ($p < 0.01$), whereas urea, creatinine) and phosphate concentrations did not change. There was also no effect of high-efficiency hemodiafiltration on the degree of renal anemia (Hbg 10.1 during HD versus 10.3 after 6 months HDF, $p < 0.05$), but polyneuropathy was positively influenced clinically as was velocity of nerve conduction (figure 13–12), as observed by Civati and associates [90] in high-efficient hemofiltration.

312

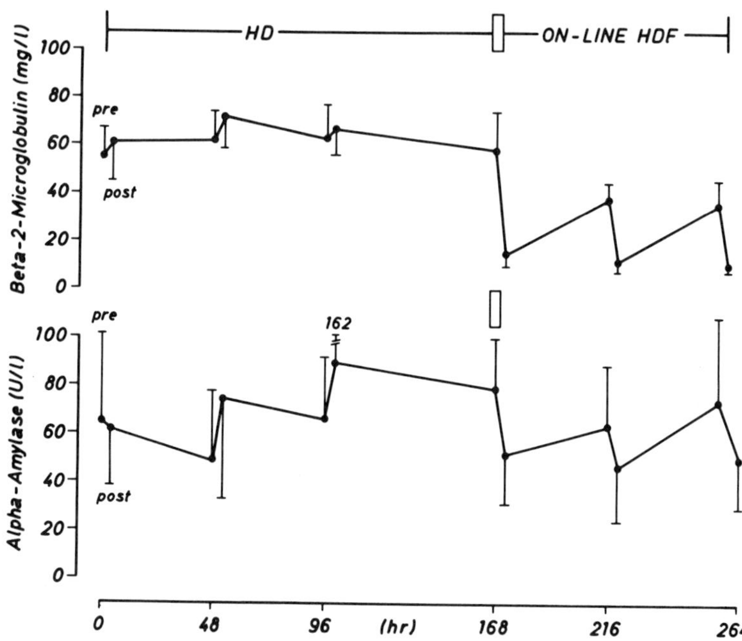



*Figure 13–9.* Plasma biochemistry in 10 patients, who were treated for 1 week by standard dialysis (HD) and the following week by high-efficiency hemodiafiltration (on-line HDF). For details, see text.

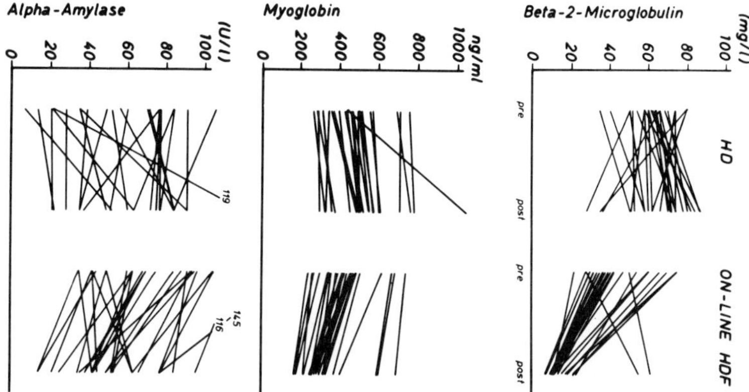



*Figure 13–10.* Plasma concentration of $\beta_2$-microglobulin (mw 11.000 daltons), myoglobin (mw 17.000 daltons) and alpha-amylase (mw 55.000 daltons) in individuals, following standard hemodialysis (HD) or high-efficiency hemodiafiltration (on-line HDF).

313

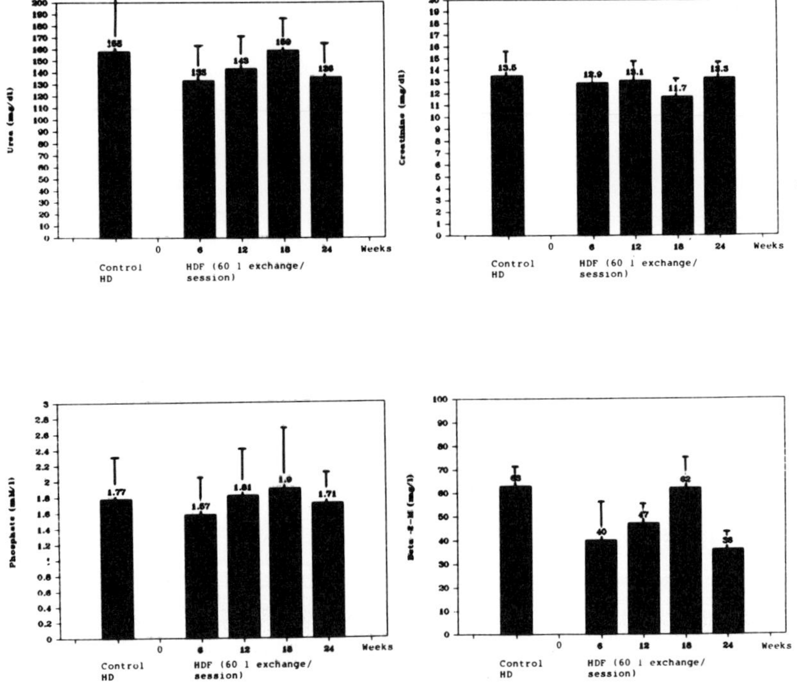

*Figure 13-11.* Plasma biochemistry in 7 patients, who were treated by high-efficiency hemodiafiltration (HDF) in comparison to the preceding standard dialysis period (HD). Following HDF treatment, there was a significant (p 0.01) reduction in pretreatment $\beta_2$-microglobulin values.

## Indications for hemodiafiltration and future aspects

It has not yet been decided by a positive definition, what adequacy of renal replacement therapy would include. In theory, hemodiafiltration is the most effective blood purification method available, but as long as the nature and molecular size of uremic toxins are not precisely defined, the clinical benefit of such an approach remains largely hypothetical. Hemodynamic tolerance of fluid removal and dialysis-related discomfort syndrome are improved in hemodiafiltration, comparable to hemofiltration. Therefore, hemodiafiltration can be used in hemodynamically unstable patients, provided that treatment time is not reduced. However, it is still unclear as to which amount of convection is necessary to achieve those effects and how sodium balances will be influenced. In our hands, hemodiafiltration employed as a short-duration method has proven to be a failure since long-term side effects related to sodium and water balance resulted in overhydration and arterial hypertension. Since patient-related cardiac findings, as described in detail, represent severe contraindications to any short-dialysis schedule, we do not

314

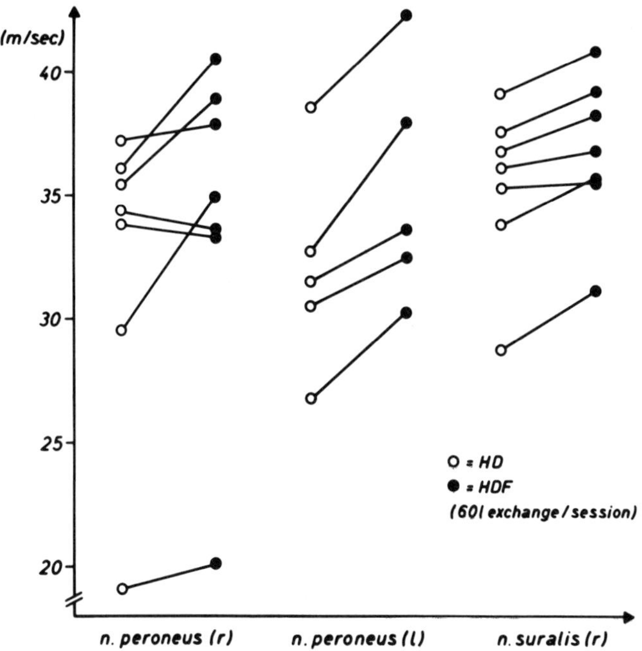


*Figure 13–12.* Velocity of nerve conduction in seven patients during standard hemodialysis (HD) and following a 6-month period of hemodiafiltration (HDF).

believe that differences related to kidney replacement methods can counter-balance the deficiencies in the patients' status (table 13–3).

At present, hemodiafiltration is indicated in the elderly, who are hemodynamically unstable and who — due to a poor fistula — cannot be treated adequately by hemodialysis or hemofiltration. In case dialysis membranes with a high hydraulic permeability are used for hemodialysis purposes, backfiltration of dialysis fluid within the dialyzer [48] can be safely prevented by hemodiafiltration. In centers where hemofiltration cannot be performed, hemodiafiltration is the second best method for preventing dialysis hypotension.

As for future aspects, development of safe devices for on-line preparation of sterile dialysate and substitution fluid could give hemodiafiltration a new dimension in terms of efficiency, which may help to prevent renal anemia, polyneuropathy, carpal-tunnel syndrome, and osteodystrophy. Furthermore, with a better control of sodium and water fluxes during hemodiafiltration, hypotension during water removal might be prevented without risking overhydration or sodium overloading. Thus, hemodiafiltration appears to have a bright future, since it will always be the most efficient blood purification method which provides unique sites for intervention (dialysate, substituate) to design an individual kidney replacement.

315

*Table 13–3.* Indications for hemodiafiltration (HDF)

| HDF Method | Indications | Potential Method-Related Risks |
| --- | --- | --- |
| Biofiltration | Prevention of back-filtration Metabolic acidosis, hypotension in case, other HDF methods are not available | Underdialysis, when used as short treatment Positive sodium balance — hypertension, hyperhydration |
| Hypertonic HDF | Dialysis hypotension<br><br>Short-HDF in stable patients | Positive sodium balance — hypertension, hyperhydration Underdialysis |
| HDF with 9 l exchange | Dialysis hypotension In elderly, when low blood flow does not allow hemofiltration | Underdialysis, when used as short treatment Positive sodium balance-hypertension, hyperhydration |
| High efficiency short HDF | Reduction of treatment time | So far, unknown long-term effects Positive sodium balance — hypertension, hyperhydration Sudden death in patients with hypertrophic cardiomyopathy Myocardial infarction in patients with coronary artery disease Bacterial or pyrogen contamination by self-prepared substitution fluid |
| High efficiency long HDF | Polyneuropathy Metabolic acidosis Symptoms potentially related to small protein retention in the plasma | So far, unknown long-term effects Bacterial or pyrogen contamination (or by unknown water-products) by self-prepared substitution fluid |

# References


1. Leber, W.W, Wizemann, V., Goubeaud, G., Rawer, P. and Schütterle, G. (1978) Simultaneous hemofiltration/hemodialysis: An effective alternative to hemofiltration and conventional hemodialysis in the treatment of uremic patients. Clin. Nephrology 9: 115.
2. Kunitomo, T., Lowrie, E.G., Kumazwa, S., O'Brian, M., Lazarus, J.M., Gottlieb, M.N. and Merrill, J.P. (1977) Controlled ultrafiltration (UF) with hemodialysis (HD): analysis of coupling between convective and diffuse mass transfer in a new HD-UF system. Trans. Am. Soc. Artif. Intern. Organs 23: 234.
3. Dieter, K., Franz, H.E., Breitig, D., Meyer, C. and Schmidt-Wiederkehr, P. (1977) Blutdetoxifikation durch simultane dialyse und diafiltration. Biochem. Techn. 22: 277.
4. Ota, K., Suzuki, T., Ozkau, Y., Era, K., Agishi, T., Sugino, N., Haraguchi, M., Mitani, N. and Kumazawa, S. (1978) Clinical evaluation of a pre-set ultrafiltration rate controller available for single pass and hemodiafiltration systems.
5. Miller, J.H., von Albertini, B., Gardner, P.W. and Shinaberger, J.H. (1984) Technical aspects of high-flux hemodiafiltration for adequate short (under 2 hours) treatment. Trans. Am. Soc. Artif. Intern. Organs XXX: 377.
6. Canaud, B., N'Guyen, O., Lagarde, C., Stec, F., Polaschegg, H. and Mion, C. (1985) Clinical evaluation of a multipurpose dialysis system adequate for hemodialysis or for

postdilution hemofiltration/hemodiafiltration with on-line preparation of substitution fluid from dialysate. Contr. Nephrol. 46: 184.

7. Mayr, H.U., Stec, F., Canaud, B., Mion, C. and Shaldon, S. (1984) Microbiological aspects of the batch preparation of replacement fluid for hemofiltration. Blood Purification 2: 158.

8. Cambi, V., Buzio, G., Arisi, L., Calderini, C., David, S., Manari, A., Bono, E. and Zanelli, P. (1981) Vascular stability and middle molecule removal in hypertonic haemodiafiltration. Proc. Europ. Dial. Transpl. Ass. 18: 681.

9. Petitclerc, T. Man, N.K., Castillon, J., Rocard, P., Boisvieux, J.F. (1982) Simplified modelling of sodium transfer during hemodialysis. Proc. Int. Symp. Kinetic Mod. Artificial Organs. Rostock-Warnemünde.

10. Raja, R., Kramer, M., Barber, K. and Chen, S. (1983) Sequential changes in dialysate sodium during hemodialysis. Trans. Am. Soc. Artif. Intern. Organs XXIX: 649.

11. Kimura, G., van Stone, J.C., Bauer, J. (1983) Prediction of postdialysis serum sodium concentration and transcellular fluid shifts without measuring body fluid volumes. Artificial Organs 7: 410.

12. Kimura, G., Satani, M., Schunich, K., Kuroda, K., Itoh, K., Ikeda, M. (1982) A computerized model to analyze transcellular fluid shifts during hemofiltration. Artificial Organs 6: 31.

13. Zucchelli, P., Santoro, A., Ragiotto, G., Degli, Esposti, E., Sturani, A. and Capecchi, V. (1984) Biofiltration in uremia: preliminary observations. Blood Purification 2: 187.

14. Zucchelli, P., Santoro, A., Fusarolil, M., Borghi, M., Sasdelli, M., Montanari, A., Pecchini, F. (1985) Biofiltration versus hemodialysis in uremia: biochemical and cardiovascular evaluations. Abstract. Contemporary management of renal failure. Marrakech, Nov. 10–15, p. 41.

15. Mioli, V., Ragaiolo, M., Buonchirstiani, U., Taccone, G., Tarchini, R. et al. (1985) Polycentric study of 384 months of biofiltration with PAN. Abstract. Contemporary management of renal failure. Marrakech, Nov. 10–15, p. 42.

16. von Albertini, B., Miller, H.J., Gardner, P.W. and Shinaberger, J.H. (1985) Performance characteristics of the hemoflow F60 in high-flux hemodiafiltration. Contr. Nephrol. 46: 169.

17. von Albertini, B. Miller, J.H., Gardner, P.W. and Shinaberger, J.H. (1984) High-flux hemodiafiltration: under six hours/week treatment. Trans. Am. Soc. Artif. Intern. Organs XXX: 227.

18. Cooperative Dialysis Study. (1983) E.G. Lowrie (guest ed.) and N.M. Laird. Kidney Int. 23: Suppl. 13.

19. Wizemann, V., Techert, F., Schütterle, G. (1985) High-efficiency on-line hemofiltration or hemodiafiltration performed with a dialysis machine. International workshop on hemofiltration. New York, October 9–10.

20. Wizemann, V., Kramer, W., Knopp, G., Rawer, P., Mueller, K. and Schütterle, G. (1983) Ultrashort hemodiafiltration: Efficiency and hemodynamic tolerance. Clinc. Nephrology 19: 24.

21. Wizemann, V. and Kramer, W. (in press) Short-term dialysis — long term complications. Nine years experience with short-duration renal replacement therapy.

22. Wizemann, V., Velcovsky, H.G., Bleyl, H. and Brünning, S. (1985) Removal of hormones by hemofiltration and hemodialysis with a highly permeable polysulphone membrane. Contr. Nephrol. 46: 61.

23. Wizemann, V., Sychla, M., Leber, H.W. and Schütterle, G. (1982) Hemodynamics during five different techniques in the treatment of acute renal failure. In *Acute Renal Failure*, H.E. Eliahaou (ed.) London: John Libbey and Co, p. 176.

24. Schmidt, M., Schoeppe, W. and Baldamus, C.A. (1985) Hemodynamics during hemodialysis with dialysers of high hydraulic permeability. Contr. Nephrol. 46: 1227.

25. Baldamus, C.A., Ernst, W., Frei, K. and Koch, K.M. (1982) Sympathetic and hemodynamic response to volume removal during different forms of renal replacement therapy. Nephron 31: 324.

26. Quellhorst, E., Schuenemann, B. and Hildebrand, U. (1985) Hemofiltration — an improved

method of treatment for chronic renal failure. Contr. Nephrol. 44: 194.

27. Bergström, J., Asaba, H., Fürst, P. and Oules, R. (1976) Dialysis, ultrafiltration, and blood pressure. Proc. Eur. Dial. Transplant. Ass. 13: 293.

28. Shaldon, S., Bean, M., Claret, G., Deschodt, G., Oules, R., Ramperez, P., Mion, H. and Mion, C. (1978) Haemofiltration with sorbent regeneration of ultrafiltrate. First clinical experience in end-stage renal disease. Proc. Eur. Dial. Transplant. Ass. 15: 120.

29. Quellhorst, E., Schuemann, B. and Hildebrand, U. (1981) How to prevent vascular instability. Proc. Eur. Dial. Transplant. Ass. 18: 243.

30. Walker, J.F. Lindsay, R.M., Peters, S.D., Sibbald, W.J. and Linton, A.L. (1983) A sheep model to examine the cardiopulmonary manifestations of blood-dialyser interactions. ASAIO-Journal 6: 123.

31. Borah, M.F., Schoenfeld, P.Y., Gotch, F.A., Sargent, J.A., Wolfson, M. and Hymphreys, M.H. (1978) Nitrogen balance during intermittent dialysis therapy of uremia. Kidney Int. 14: 491.

32. Ward, R.A., Shirlow, M.J., Hayes, J.M., Chapman, G.V., Farrell, P.C. (1979) Protein catabolism during hemodialysis. Am. J. Clin. Nutr. 32: 2443.

33. Farrell, P.C. and Hone, P.W. (1980) Dialysis induced catabolism. Am. J. Clin. Nutr. 33: 1417.

34. Ono, K., Sasaki, T. and Waki, Y. (1984) Glucose in the dialysate does not reduce the free amino acid loss during routine hemodialysis of non-fasting patients. Clin. Nephrol. 21: 106.

35. Canaud, B., Mayr, H., Araujo, A., Garred, L., Farrell, P., Minon, C. (1983) Catabolic changes induced by postdilution hemofiltration (abstract). Blood Purification 1: 42.

36. Bergström, J. (1985) Protein catabolic factors in patients on renal replacement therapy. Blood Purification 3: 215.

37. Schaefer, R.M., Heidland, A. and Hörl WH. (1985) Release of leucocyte elastase during hemodialysis. Effect of different membranes. Contr. Nephrol. 46: 109.

38. Shaldon, S. (1986) Guest lecture at the Symposium of Urology, April 17–18, Moscow.

39. Henderson, L., Koch, K., Dinarello, C. and Shaldon, S. (1983) Hemodialysis hypotension: the interleukin hypothesis. Blood Purification 1: 3.

40. Sprenger, K., Stephan, A., Kratz, W., Huber, K. and Franz, H. (1985) Optimizing of hemodiafiltration with modern membranes? Contr. Nephrol. 46: 43.

41. Wizemann, V., Rawer, P., Schmidt, H., Techert, F. and Schütterle, G. (1982) Efficiency of hemodialysis, hemofiltration, hemodiafiltration. In *Hemodiafiltration*, G. Schütterle; V. Wizemann and G. Seyffart (eds.) Oberursel/Ts., FRG: Verlag Hygieneplan, p. 25.

42. Cambi, V., Arisi L., David, S., Bono, F. and Gardini, G. (1985) 2-h dialysis: A realistic goal? Contr. Nephrol. 44: 40.

43. Cambi, V., Garini, G., Savazzi, G., Arisi, L., David, S., Zanelli, P., Bono, F. and Gardini, F. (1983) Short dialysis. Proc. Europ. Dial. Transpl. Ass. 20: 111.

44. Trafford, S., Sharpstone, P., Evans, R., Ireland, R. (1979) Evaluation of ultra-short dialysis. Br. Med. J. 1: 518.

45. Kramer, P., Broyer, M., Brunner, F.P., Brynger, H., Donckerwolcke, R.A., Jacobs, C., Selwood, N.H., Wing, A.J. (1982) Combined report on regular dialysis and transplantation in Europe, XII, 1981. Proc. Europ. Dial. Transpl. Ass. 19: 4.

46. Cioni, L., Palmarini, D., Pilone, N., Rindi, P. (1984) Hemodiafiltration: better efficiency with respect to hemodialysis and hemofiltration. Blood Purification 2: 30.

47. Gotch, F. and Gee, C. (1984) Urea kinetic modelling: a noncomputerized quantitative guide to individualize the dialysis prescription. Council on renal nutrition. National Kidney Foundation, December 8, Washington D.C.

48. Stiller, S., Mann, H. and Brunner, H. (1985) Rückfiltration von Dialyseflüssigkeit bei der Dialyse und hochpermeablen Membranen (Back filtration of dialysis fluid in the dialysis with high permeable membranes, in German). Nieren- und Hochdruckkrankheiten 14: 41.

49. Techert, F. and Wizemann, V. (1986) Ten years experience with short dialysis — a decade of staff stress (Abstract). 25th Congress of the EDTA-ERA-EDTNA, Budapest.

50. Sprenger, K.B.G., Bundschu, D., Figuerora, P. and Franz, H.E. (1981) Vergleich von

Hämodiafiltration gegenüber Hämodialysis mit kontrollierter Ultrafiltration in einer ABA Langzeitstudie. Nieren- und Hochdruckkrankheiten 10: 226.

51. Leber, H.W., Wizemann, V. and Rawer, P. (1981) Kurzzeitbehandlung dialysepflichtiger urämischer Patienten mittels simultaner Hämofiltration/Hämodialyse (in German). Verlag Carl Bindernagel, p. 13.

52. Vanholder, R., Verbanck, J., Schelstraete, J., de Smet, R. and Ringoir, S. (1982) Unipuncture simultaneous hemofiltration and dialysis. In *Hemodiafiltration*, G. Schütterle, V. Wizemann and G. Seyffart (eds.) Oberursel/Ts., FRG: Verlag Hygieneplan, p. 89.

53. Leber, H.W., Wizemann, V. and Techert, F. (1980) Simultaneous hemofiltration/hemodialysis: short-and-long term tolerance. Introduction of a system for automatic fluid replacement. Artif. Organs 4: 108.

54. Mazzitello, G., Candito, C., Grandinetti, F., Pugliesi, G. and Rondanini, V. (1984), Intolerance to hemodialysis and hemodiafiltration (Abstract). Blood Purification 2: 56.

55. Shaldon, S., Baldmus, C.A. and Koch, K.M. (1983) Of sodium, symptomatology and syllogism. Blood Purification 1: 16.

56. Henderson, L. (1980) Symptomatic hypotension during hemodialysis. Kidney Int. 17: 571.

57. Kramer, P., Boyer, M., Brunner, F.P., Brynger, H., Donckerwolcke, R.A., Jacobs, C., Selwood, N.H., Wing, A.J. (1982) Combined report on regular dialysis and transplantation in Europe, XII, 1981. Proc. Europ. Dial. Trans. Ass. 19: 4.

58. Rostand, S.J. Gretes, J.C., Kirk, K.A., Rutsky, E.A. and Andreoli, T.E. (1979) Ischemic heart disease in patients with uremic undergoing maintenance hemodialysis. Kidney Int. 16: 600.

59. Wing, A.J., Brunner, F.P., Brynger, H., Jacobs, C., Kramer, P., Selwood, N.H. and Gretz, N. (1984) Cardiovascular-related causes of death and the fate of patients with renovascular disease. Contr. Nephrol. 41: 306.

60. Rostand, S.G., Kirk, K.A., Rutsky, E.A. (1984) Dialysis-associated ischemic heart disease: insides from coronary angiography. Kidney Int. 25: 653.

61. Kramer, W., Wizemann, V., Kindler, M. and Thormann, J. (1985) Urämische Herzkrankheit. Inzidenz und klinische Wertigkeit nicht invasiver kardialer Befunde bei dialysepflichtiger Niereninsuffizienz (I). Med. Welt 36: 1228.

62. Gotch, F.A. and Sargent, J.A. (1983) Hemofiltration: an unnecessarily complex method to achieve hypotonic sodium removal and controlled ultrafiltration. Blood Purification 1: 16.

63. Basile, C., di Maggio, A., Longo, S. and Scatizzi, A. (1984) Sodium balance in hypertonic hemodiafiltration. Blood Purification 2: 70.

64. de Mello, V.R., Malone, D., Thanavaro S., Kleiger, R.E., Kessler, G. and Oliver, G.C. (1981) Cardiac arrhythmias in end-stage renal disease. Southern Medical J. 74: 178.

65. Blumberg, A., Häusermann, M., Strub, B. and Jenzer, H.R. (1983) Cardiac arrhythmias in patients on maintainance hemodialysis. Nephron 33: 91.

66. Avram, M.M., Edson, J., Gan, A. and Edson, J.N. (1978) Continuous monitoring of cardiac rhythm in hemodialysis patients. Dialysis and Transplantation 7: 516.

67. Morrison, G., Michelson, E.L., Brown, S. and Morganroth, J. (1980) Mechanism and prevention of cardiac arrhythmias in chronic hemodialysis patients. Kidney Int. 17: 811.

68. Macdonald, I.L., Uldall, R. and Buda, A.J. (1981) The effect of hemodialysis on cardiac rhythm and performance. Clinical Nephrology 15: 321.

69. Wizemann, V., Kramer, W., Funke, T. and Schütterle, G. (1985) Dialysis-induced cardiac arrhythmias: fact or fiction? Importance of pre-existing cardiac disease in the induction of arrhythmias during renal replacement therapy. Nephron 39: 356.

70. Quellhorst, E. (1984) Herzrhythmusstörungen während und nach Hämodialyse, Hämofiltration und Hämodiafiltration bei Patienten mit chronischer Niereninsuffizienz — vergleichende Langzeig-EKG-Untersuchungen. Aus: Die Behandlung von Herzrhythmusstörungen bei Nierenkranken (in German). Basel: Karger, p. 23.

71. Stegaru-Hellring, B., Buss, J. and Strauch, M. (1984) Urämische Kardiomyopathie — echokardiographische Untersuchungen der linksventrikulären Dynamik (in German) Nieren- und Hochdruckkrankheiten 13: 396.

72. Madsen, B.R., Alpert, M.A., Whiting, R.B., van Stone, J., Ahmad, M. and Kelly, D.L. (1984) Effect of hemodialysis on left ventricular performance. Am. J. Nephrol. 4: 86.

73. Renger, A., Müller, M., Jutzler, G.A. and Bette, L. (1984) Echocardiographic evaluation of left ventricular dimensions and function in chronic hemodialysis with cardiomegaly. Clinical Nephrology 21: 164.

74. Klein, J., McLeish, K., Hodsen, J. and Lordon, R. (1983) Hypertrophic cardiomyopathy: an acquired disorder of endstage renal disease. Trans. Am. Soc. Artif. Intern Organs 24: 120.

75. Mc Gonigle, R.J.S., Fowler, M.R., Timmis, A.B., Weston, M.J. and Parsons, V. (1984) Uremic cardiomyopathy: potential role of vitamin D and parathyroid hormone. Nephron 36: 94.

76. Ireland, M.A., Mehta, B.R. and Shiu, M.F. (1981) Acute effects of haemodialysis on left heart dimensions and left ventricular function: an echocardiographic study. Nephron 29: 73.

77. Bernadi, D., Bernini, L., Cini, G., Ghione, S., Bonechi, I. (1985) Asymmetric septal hypertrophy and sympathetic overactivity in normotensive hemodialyzed patients. American Heart J. 109: 539.

78. Bullock, R.E., Amer, H.A., Simpson, I., Ward, M.K. and Hall, R. (1985) Cardiac abnormalities and exercise tolerance in patients receiving renal replacement therapy. Brit. Med. J. 289: 1479.

79. Großmann, R. and Albert, F.W. (1984) Echokardiographische Befunde bei terminal niereninsuffizienten Patienten unter chron. intermittierender Dialysebehandlung (in German). Nieren- und Hochdruckkrankheiten 13: 401.

80. Henrich, W.L., Hunt, J.M., Nixon, J.V. (1984) Increased ionized calcium and left ventricular contractility during hemodialysis. N. Engl. J. Med. 310: 19.

81. Kramer, W., Wizemann, V., Thormann, J., Bechthold, A., Schütterle, G. and Lasch, H.G. (1985) Mechanism of altered myocardial contractility during hemodialysis: Importance of changes in the ionized calcium to plasma potassium ratio. Klin. Wochenschr. 63: 272.

82. Topol, E.C. Traill, T.A., and Fortain, N.C. (1985) Hypertensive hypertrophic cardiomyopathy in the elderly. New Engl. J. Med. 312: 277.

83. Brunner, F.P., Brynger, H., Chandler, C. Donckerwolcke, R.A. Hethway, R.A. Jacobs, C., Selwood, N.H. and Wing, A.J. (1979) Combined report on regular dialysis and transplantation in Europe. Proc. Eur. Dial. Transplant. Ass. 16: 4.

84. Keshaviah, P., Berkseth, R., Ilstrup, K., McMichael, C. and Collins, A. (1985) Reduced treatment time: hemodialysis versus hemofiltration. Symposium of the American Society of Artificial Organs, May 1–4, Atlanta, U.S.A.

85. Schneider, H., Liomin, E. and Streicher, E. (1985) Hemodynamic study of diffusive and convective procedures using a polysulphone membrane. Contr. Nephrol. 46: 151.

86. Klahr, S. (1983) Renal metabolism of plasma proteins and peptide hormones. In *The Kidney and Body Fluids in Health and Disease*, S. Klahr (ed.). New York: Plenum Publishing Corp.

87. Gejyo, F., Yamada, T., Odani, S. et al. (1985) A new form of amyloid protein associated with chronic hemodialysis was identified as $\beta_2$-microglobulin. Biochem. Biophys. Research Communications 129: 701.

88. Bommer, J., Waldherr, R., Ritz, E. (1985) Kidney lesions in uraemic patients and $\beta_2$-microglobulin derived amyloid. Lancet: December, p. 1438.

89. Matthaei, D., Ludwig-Köhn, H., Kramer, P., Holzmann, H., Morsches, E., Benes, P., von Henning, V., Klug, P. and Scheler, F. (1983) Changes of plasma hormon levels in hemofiltration. Artificial Organs 6: 21.

90. Civati, G., Guastoni, C., Perego, A., Teatini, U., Zoppi, F. and Minetti, L. (1983) Long-term clinical results with high-efficiency hemofiltration. Blood Purification 1: 184.

91. Wizemann, V. and Wizemann, A. (1984) Letter to the editor. Am. J. Nephrol. 4: 134.

# 14. Cardiovascular stability in hemodialysis and hemofiltration

C.A. Baldamus, S. Shaldon, and K. M. Koch

Hemodynamic disturbances during end-stage renal disease (ESRD) treatment manifest objectively as changes in blood pressure, predominantly hypotension. The incidence of symptomatic hypotension during hemodialysis has increased over the recent years in spite of the fact that dialysis regimes changed to 3 times weekly. The French dialysis registry reports a rise from 15% in 1973 to 25% in 1979 [1, 2, 3]. This increased risk of hypotension is associated with various factors. Rapid fluid withdrawal during shortened treatment time seems to be the most important cause, but increasing age and nonrenal diseases of the dialysis population also contribute. In fact from 1973 to 1980 patients' mean age increased from 41 to 48 years, and mean treatment time decreased from 19 to 12 hours weekly [4, 5].

In the mid-seventies when other treatment modalities with improved vascular stability like hemofiltration became available, scientific interest started to focus on hemodynamics in hemodialysis, and alternative regimes. However, before analyzing these different treatment modalities and discussing the various proposed mechanisms, the physiology of blood pressure maintenance has to be reviewed. Following Ohm's law, blood pressure is the resultant product of total peripheral vascular resistance and cardiac output which is determined by stroke volume and heart rate. Stroke volume is dependent on myocardial contractility and vascular volume.

Maintenance of blood pressure is such a crucial vital function that it is maintained even at the expense of organ perfusion which is sacrificed in an inverse rank order of vital importance.

The circulatory control to maintain blood pressure is regulated by about 400 basic physiologic phenomena, and their interdependence was identified by Guyton and associates [6] in a classic report on circulatory control. Several mechanisms, largely neural and humoral, have the capacity to modulate vascular resistance independent of local control and to influence the mechanisms by which it is adjusted to meet peripheral metabolic demands. Cardiac output itself is strongly determined by peripheral vascular resistance. Cardiac output will increase and remain elevated if total peripheral resistance (TPR) decreases as occurs, for instance, with creation of an arteriovenous fistula for dialysis vascular access. The second determinant of cardiac output

*Vincenzo Cambi (editor) Professor of Nephrology*
© *1987 Martinus Nijhoff Publishing, Boston. ISBN 0-89838-858-9. Printed in The United States.*

is venous return. This relates to blood volume and to the capacitance of the systemic venous system. Cardiac output then may drop due either to a decrease of total blood volume or to reduction of venous tone, thereby increasing the capacitance of the systemic venous bed.

The time course of blood pressure regulation is staggered from seconds to days (figure 14–1). Of these regulatory systems shown, the neural and humoral mechanisms respond within seconds and minutes [7]. Only aldosterone secretion occurs late and can be left out of consideration when discussing blood pressure regulation during intermittent dialysis and hemofiltration.


## Literature review

A literature review of blood pressure regulation during hemodialysis and related therapies is complicated by the fact that operating conditions of the various renal replacement therapies are difficult to keep comparable. But even when investigating in a single form of treatment the change of one outcome measure in response to one test parameter, additional variables have seldom been maintained constant. There are a great number of publications

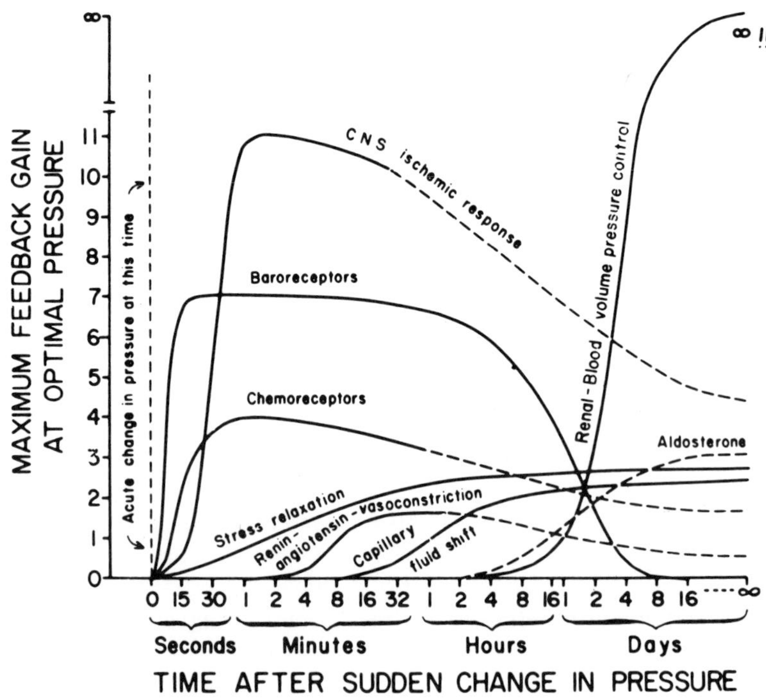


*Figure 14–1.* Degree of activation, expressed in terms of feedback gain, of different pressure control mechanisms following a sudden change in arterial pressure [7]. Note the rapid activation of nervous mechanisms followed within minutes by hormonal reactions.

322

reporting only on the incidence of drop in blood pressure during treatment. These reports are incomplete if one is describing hemodynamic regulation of blood pressure during treatment. To obtain a deeper insight it is necessary to measure blood pressure, cardiac output, and heart rate. These measurements permit a calculation of the total peripheral vascular resistance. There are only a few publications available in which, along with hemodynamic parameters, hormonal or other outcome measures are reported.

The observation that ultrafiltration causes only rarely symptomatic hypotension was first reported by Kobayashi and coworkers [8] in 1972 and was later confirmed by Ing and colleagues [9] in 1975. It was Bergström in 1976 [10] who compared ultrafiltration with hemodialysis; he found that ultrafiltration alone was hemodynamically well tolerated but not when combined with diffusive solute transport. As a dialysate buffer he used acetate. At the same meeting Quellhorst and associates [11] reported their first clinical experience with postdilution hemofiltration using lactate as buffer substance. Beside other benefits they found an excellent tolerance to fluid removal of up to 5 kg/4 hours without hypotension or muscle cramps. This improved tolerance to fluid withdrawal during hemofiltration, when compared to hemodialysis, was confirmed by several investigators [12, 13, 14, 15, 16, 17].

In 1977 Graefe and coworkers [18] observed a reduced intratreatment morbidity when replacing the acetate dialysate buffer by bicarbonate. In a systematic study this group then substantiated their initial observation and showed that in a given time more fluid can be withdrawn without symptoma- tology during bicarbonate than during acetate hemodialysis [19]. In view of Bergström's data [10] they discussed acetate as a major contributing factor for vascular instability, whereas Bergström [20] denied this point and related it more to changes in serum osmolality. Shaldon and associates [17] in 1979 were the first who investigated the hemodynamic changes during hemofiltration and hemodialysis under comparable conditions. At a maximal drop in mean arterial blood pressure of 5 mmHg in contrast to 32 mmHg in hemodialysis, they found a significant increase in total peripheral vascular resistance during hemofiltration but not during hemodialysis. They showed also that the change in serum osmolality was not the causative factor for the differences found [2]. Baldamus and coworkers [12] in 1980 reported on hemodynamics in a study comparing ultrafiltration, acetate hemodialysis, bicarbonate hemodialysis, and acetate hemofiltration. They measured also intratreatment changes of catecholamines. Other operating conditions like weight loss, treatment time, small solute removal rates, and constitution of dialysate and hemofiltration, replacement fluid remained constant in order to achieve comparable experimental conditions. Blood pressure (figure 14–2) remained stable during ultrafiltration and hemofiltration, whereas it fell significantly during acetate dialysis and also during bicarbonate hemodialysis but here to a lesser degree. Heart rate (figure 14–2) increased in acetate hemodialysis and bicarbonate hemodialysis but not during in ultrafiltration

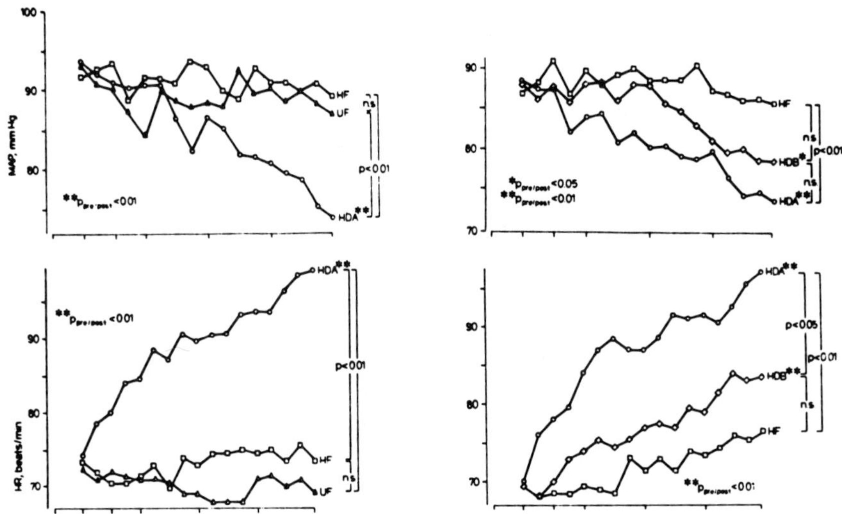

*Figure 14–2.* Mean arterial blood pressure (MAP) and heart rate (HR) during ultrafiltration (UF), hemofiltration (HF), acetate hemodialysis (HDA), and bicarbonate hemodialysis (HDB). Redrawn from 22.

and hemofiltration. Cardiac index (figure 14–3) fell during ultrafiltration and hemofiltration, and less during bicarbonate hemodialysis. The drop during acetate hemodialysis was not significantly different from all other three treatments. Total peripheral vascular resistance (figure 14–3) increased during ultrafiltration and hemofiltration, but not during acetate hemodialysis and bicarbonate dialysis. Plasma noradrenaline levels (figure 14–3) increased during ultrafiltration and hemofiltration, but not during acetate hemodialysis and bicarbonate hemodialysis.

Table 14–1 gives a brief review on hemodynamic data, reported in the literature, which in their vast majority support the described pattern shown in figures 14–2 and 14–3.

Ultrafiltration and hemofiltration are not the only treatment modalities with reported vascular stability. Improved hemodynamic stability is also reported for hemodiafiltration [47, 48] and more recently for hemodialysis using dialysis membranes with high hydraulic permeability [45, 49].

*In conclusion*

As shown in table 14–1, the majority of reports clearly show that the ESRD patient on renal replacement treatment is able to react to volume removal isolated ultrafiltration in a physiological manner, at least quantitatively, to volume removal. During hemofiltration this physiological response is maintained. In contrast, during hemodialysis the same patient fails to react adequately to fluid withdrawal with an increased vascular resistance. There

324

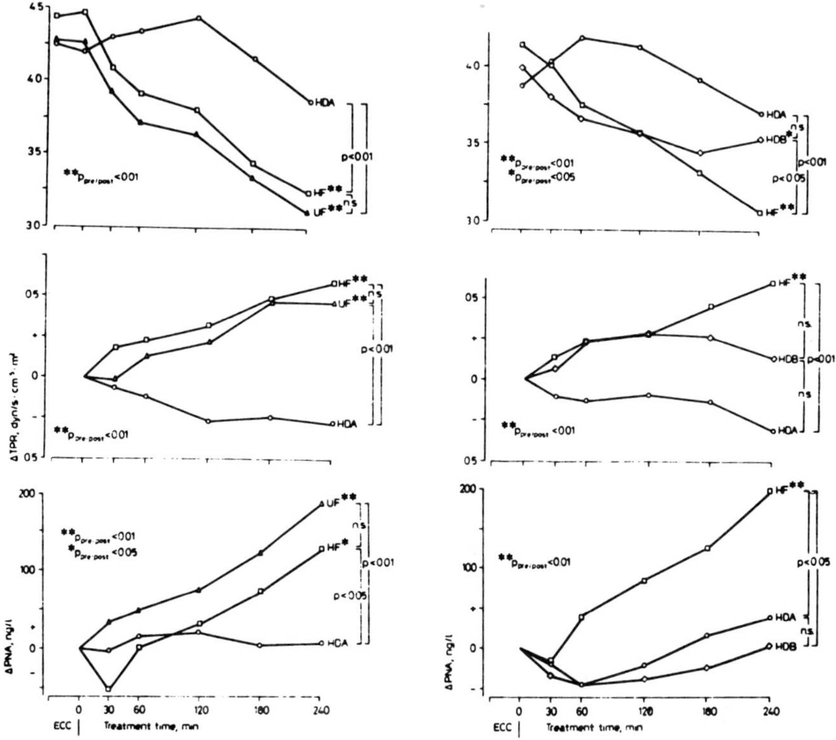

*Figure 14–3.* Cardiac output (CO), change ov total peripheral vascular resistance ($\triangle$TPR) and of plasma noradrenaline concentrations (PNA) during ultrafiltration (UF), hemofiltration (HF), acetate hemodialysis (HDA), and bicarbonate hemodialysis (HDB). Redrawn from 22.

exists some evidence that this coincides with a blunted increase of sympathetic tone. The actual cause of the different hemodynamic response, however, remains uncertain. The possible etiological factors (table 14–2 will now be discussed in detail.


## Mechanisms involved

According to Kjellstrand [50], dialysis-induced hypotension is a multifactorial event. To understand the genesis of dialysis hypotension the possible factors have been grouped into pathogenetic, mediating pathophysiologic, and underlying pathological factors. Pathogenetic factors are directly related to the treatment itself. Mediators are initiated by pathogenic factors. Both pathogeneic mechanisms and/or mediators act on pathophysiological pathways which might be altered by underlying pathological factors. In an attempt to explain the different hemodynamics in hemofiltration and hemodialysis, these different factors are listed in table 14–2 as completely as possible.

325

*Table 14–1.* Hemodynamic changes during different extracorporeal treatment for uremia

| First Author | Reference | Year | Treatment | Pre — Post Treatment Change | | | | |
|---|---|---|---|---|---|---|---|---|
| | | | | BP | HR | CO | TPR | PNA |
| Bergström | 10 | 1976 | HD·A | − | + | | | |
| | | | UF | c | c | | | |
| Brecht | 23 | 1976 | HD·A | | | | | c |
| Graefe | 18 | 1977 | UF | c | | | | |
| | | | HD·A, Na 133 | − − | | | | |
| | | | HD·B, Na 133 | − | | | | |
| Bergström | 20 | 1978 | UF/HD·A | c/− | | −/+ | +/− | |
| | 24 | | HD·A/UF | −/c | | +/− | −/+ | |
| Pogglitsch | 25 | 1978 | UF/HD·A | −/− | | c/+ | +/− | |
| | | | HD·A | − | c | − | | |
| Zucchelli | 26, 27 | 1978 | HD·A | | | | c | |
| Canella | 28 | 1978 | UF | c | | | | + |
| | | | HD·A | − | | | | c |
| Baldamus | 14 | 1978 | HD·A | − | + | | | |
| | | | HF·A | c | (+) | | | |
| Shaldon | 17 | 1979 | HD·A | − | + | + | c | |
| | | | HF·A | c | c | − | + | |
| Quellhorst | 29 | 1979 | HD·A | − | | | | |
| | 30 | | HF·A | c | | | | |
| Hampl | 31 | 1979 | HD·A | − | + | (−) | c | |
| | 32 | 1980 | UF/HD·A | c/− | c/+ | −/c | +/c | |
| | | | HF·L | c | c | − | + | |
| Baldamus | 12 | 1980 | HF·A | c | (+) | − | + | + |
| | 22 | 1982 | UF | c | (+) | − | + | + |
| | | | HD·A | − | + | + | − | c |
| | | | HD·B | − | (+) | + | c | c |
| Quellhorst | 13 | 1980 | HD·L | − | + | + | c | c |
| | | | HF·L | c | + | − | + | + |
| Shaldon | 33 | 1980 | HD·A | − − | + | | − | |
| | | | HD·B | − | + | | c | |
| | | | HF·A | c | (+) | | + | |
| | | | HF·B | c | c | | + | |
| Keshaviah | 34 | 1980 | HD·A | − | + | − | c | |
| | | | UF/HD·A | c/− | +/c | −/c | +/− | |
| Henrich | 35 | 1980 | HD·A | − | + | | | c |
| | | | UF | c | − | | | + |
| | | | HD+Man | c | c | | | c |
| Wehle | 36 | 1981 | HD·A, Na140+U | − | | + | − | |
| | 37 | | HD·B, Na140+U | − | | + | − | |
| | | | HD·B, Na133+U | − − | | c | − | |
| Aljama | 15 | 1982 | HD·A | − | | c | − | |
| | | | HD·B | c | | − | c | |
| | | | HF·A | c | | − | + | |
| | | | HF·A | c | | − | + | |
| | | | UF | c | | − | + | |
| Cini | 38 | 1982 | UF/HD·A | c/c | c/+ | −/+ | +/− | |
| | | | HD·A/UF | c/c | +/c | +/− | c/+ | |
| Hampl | 39 | 1982 | HD·A | − | + | c | c | |
| | | | HD·B | c | c | − | + | |

326

*Table 14–1. (Continued)*

| First Author | Reference | Year | Treatment | Pre — Post Treatment Change | | | | |
|---|---|---|---|---|---|---|---|---|
| | | | | BP | HR | CO | TPR | PNA |
| Kishimoto | 40 | 1982 | HD·A | − | | c | − | |
| | | | UF | c | | − | + | |
| Vincent | 41 | 1982 | HD·A | − | + | − | c | |
| | | | HD·B | c | c | − | (+) | |
| Schick | 42 | 1983 | HD·A | − | + | c | − | c |
| | | | HD·B | c | + | c | c | c |
| Frewin | 43 | 1984 | HD·A | − | | | | − |
| Leenen | 44 | 1984 | HD·A | − | ++ | + | − | |
| | | | HD·B | c | c | c | c | |
| Schneider | 45 | 1984 | HFD·A | − | + | − | c | + |
| | | | HFD·B | c | + | + | c | (−) |
| | | | HDF·A | c | + | − | + | + |
| | | | HDF·B | c | + | + | − | − |
| | | | HF·A | c | + | − | + | + |
| | | | HF·B | c | (+) | + | − | c |
| Freyschuss | 46 | 1984 | UF | c | c | − | + | |
| | | | HD·A | c | ++ | (+) | − | |
| Zucchelli | 16 | 1984 | HD·A | − | + | | c | c |
| | | | HF·A | c | c | | + | + |

Treatments:
| | | |
|---|---|---|
| UF | = | ultrafiltration |
| HF | = | hemofiltration |
| HD | = | hemodialysis |
| UF/HD<br>HD/UF | = | sequential therapy, UF followed by HD or vice versa |
| HDF | = | hemodiafiltration |
| HFD | = | high flux hemodialysis |
| ·A | = | acetate dialysate/replacement fluid |
| ·B | = | bicarbonate dialysate/replacement fluid |
| ·L | = | lactate dialysate/replacement fluid |
| Na 133 | = | sodium cocnentration in dialysate |
| +U | = | urea containing dialysate |
| +Man | = | mannitol containing dialysate |

Hemodynamic changes:
| | | |
|---|---|---|
| BP | = | blood pressure |
| HR | = | heart rate |
| CO | = | cardiac output |
| TPR | = | total peripheral vascular resistance |
| PNA | = | plasma noradrenaline concentration |
| c | = | pretreatment and posttreatment are comparable |
| − | = | decrease, (−) weak, −− strong |
| + | = | increase, (+) weak, ++ strong |

*Table 14–2.* Mechanisms possibly interfering with blood pressure regulation during hemofiltration and hemodialysis

| Pathogenic Factors | Mediators | Pathophysiological Factors | Underlying Pathology |
| --- | --- | --- | --- |
| Ultrafiltration | Hypovolemia | Myocardial contractility | Heart disease |
| Solute removal | Electrolyte imbalance | Heart rate | Vascular disease |
| Solute uptake | Acid base change | Vascular volume | Autonomic neuropathy |
| Membrane/blood interaction | Prostaglandines | Total peripheral resistance | Medication |
| | Complement activation | | |
| | White blood cell products | | |
| | Platelet products | | |
| | A D H | | |
| | Atrial natriuretic factor | | |
| | Interleukin-1 | | |
| | Catecholamines | | |

**Hypovolemia**

Hypotension during dialysis is primarily attributed to intravascular hypovolemia caused by ultrafiltration. Ultrafiltration leads to an increase to plasma protein concentration and of colloid osmotic pressure, which increases the volume of fluid shifted from the interstitial into the intravascular space. Hypotension occurs only if the ultrafiltration rate exceeds the vascular refilling rate,while at the same time vascular resistance or heart rate do not increase. Vascular refilling in dialysis patients exceeds that of normal patients after hemorrhage [51] and was found to be in the order of 300 ml/hr [52, 53]. According to a study of Kim and colleagues [52], the critical time when systemic hypotension occurs is at a plasma volume of or below 50 ml/kg body weight (bw). Hemodynamic consequences of hypovolemia do not depend only on the absolute blood volume reduction but also on the mobility of blood from the venous capacitance vessels mainly in the lung [54]. Chaigon and coworkers [53] concluded from their measurements of blood volume distribution and cardiac output in hemodialysis that the postdialysis reduction of cardiac output might be related more to the relocation of blood volume than to the absolute degree of blood volume contraction. Compliance of these venous capacitance vessels very much depends on sympathetic venous tone, and this might be impaired by autonomic neuropathy. Nothing is known in uremic patients about sympathetic regulation of the intrathoracic blood volume in response to ultrafiltration. Hypovolemia may result in shock with all its deleterious consequences [7] when the circulation fails to meet the needs of vital organ perfusion. However, this is not entirely a function of circulatory volume alone but also of cardiac function and of total peripheral vascular resistance.

*In conclusion*

Intravascular hypovolemia occurs if ultrafiltration, an inevitable event of intermittent dialysis treatment, exceeds vascular refilling. It leads to intra-treatment hypotension and shock if compensatory mechanisms like mobilization of blood from venous capacitance vessels, increase in total peripheral resistance, heart rate, and myocardial contractility are overstressed.

**Osmotic changes**

Hypotension has frequently been associated with a drop in serum osmolality [10, 18, 55, 35, 56] and has been linked to the dysequilibrium syndrome [35, 36]. The connection between changes in osmolality and symptoms of hypotension was further substantiated in 1976 by Bergström [10]. He observed that in the same patients fluid removal by ultrafiltration with no change in serum osmolality was well tolerated, but that the identical weight loss during conventional dialysis (acetate buffer) led to hypotension. Shaldon [58] then drew attention to the potential benefit of separating ultrafiltration from solute exchange by sequencing both treatment steps. Subsequently the improved tolerance to ultrafiltration, which was initially observed by Kobayashi and associates in 1972 [8], was confirmed by several investigators (table 14–1). Bergström and his group indicated in their initial report [10] that the change in serum osmolality might be a causative factor. They then conducted an experiment where they omitted or mitigated the drop in osmolality by increasing the sodium concentration of the dialysate [36, 37]. They found as others [18, 55] had, an improved vascular stability with increasing dialysate sodium concentration, and attributed this to better or no change in serum osmolality. In contrast to this interpretation, Shaldon [21] compared hemodynamic stability in the same patient population at low and high efficiency treatment in a crossover study. Patients had reached a metabolic steady state with increased serum urea concentrations during the low efficiency treatment phase. Due to identical intratreatment removal of waste products, mainly urea, low and high efficiency treatments resulted in identical changes of serum osmolality but symptomatology varied: hypotension occurred much more frequently during high than during low efficiency hemodialysis. Therefore Shaldon and coworkers concluded that the absolute change in osmolality can not be the major contributing factor to hypotension during hemodialysis. Berström's observation, therefore, has to be reinterpreted. The difference between both studies is that the fall in serum osmolality is omitted in Bergström's acute experiment by sodium. In contrast in Shaldon's steady state study, the change in serum osmolality was comparable since he used identical dialysate sodium concentrations. Changes of body urea and sodium content, however, affect body compartments differently and, because of this, lead to different hemodynamic consequences. This view is supported by studies by Wehle and associates [36, 59] who prevented a change in osmolality by adding urea to the dialysate, or alternatively by increasing dialysate sodium concentration. Only with high sodium dialysate were they able to prevent hypotensive reactions. Hemodynamic stability can also be achieved if osmolality is maintained by solutes, like mannitol, with which the distribution volume is restricted to intravascular and/or interstitial space [35].

Urea disequilibrium does not occur during routine hemodialysis or hemofiltration as urea equilibrates in total body water instantaneously. This is due to urea's high transcellular mass transfer coefficient [60, 61, 62, 63] so that it does not build up an intra- to extracellular concentration gradient. In contrast, sodium is mainly distributed in the extracellular volume. Sodium diffusing into the cell is actively transported outward into the extracellular compartment in exchange with potassium. This 'restriction' to the interstitial space makes sodium an osmotically active substance causing clinically relevant volume shifts across the cellular membrane. An increase of extracellular sodium concentration as in hemodialysis with dialysate of high

330

sodium concentrate (>142 meq/l) causes an extracellular volume shift. At low dialysate sodium (<138 meq/l) concentration an opposite fluid transport occurs from the extracellular to the intracellular compartment. The latter condition aggravates the interstitial and intravascular hypovolemia caused by ultrafiltration (figure 14–4). The dialysate sodium concentration at zero net diffusive sodium flux ($D_{Na} = 0$) is dependent on the Donnan effect ($a$) which was found to be: $a = 1\text{-}0{,}0073 \times C_{TPP}$ for the operating conditions of hemodialysis [64]. It is further dependent on serum sodium concentration ($C_{Na}$)

$$D_{Na=0} = \frac{C_{Na=0}\,(1 - 0{,}0073 \times C_{Tpp})}{1 - 0{,}01 \times C_{TPP}}$$

$C_{TPP}$ represents plasma total protein concentration in $g/dl$.

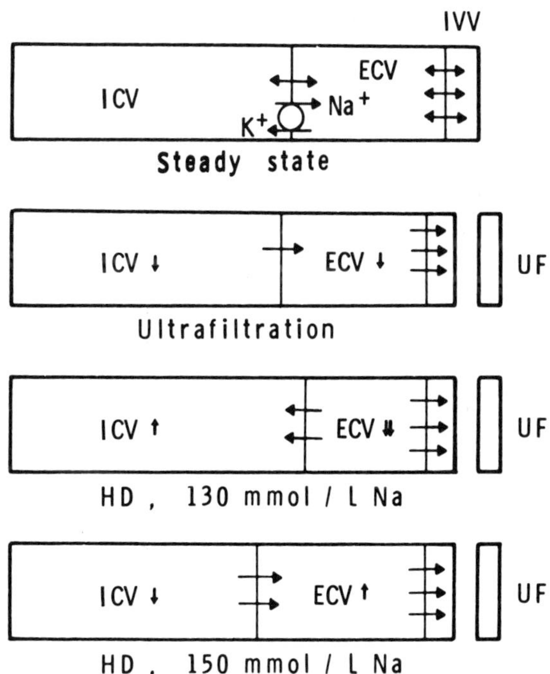


*Figure 14–4.* Volume shifts during hemodialysis. In steady state body compartments are constant. Intravascular volume (IVV) is maintained mainly by the colloid oncotic pressure of proteins. Equilibrium of intracellular (ICV) and extracellular volume (ECV) is regulated mainly by the sodium-potassium pump, and by the passive permeability of the cell membrane. Ultrafiltration (UF) leads to a redistribution: ICV, ECV, and IVV decrease. During hemodialysis with low sodium concentration in dialysate the interstitial sodium concentration decreases. This leads to a volume flux from the ECV to the ICV and aggravates intravascular hypovolemia caused by UF. In contrast during high sodium dialysis interstitial sodium concentration rises. This then causes a volume flux from ICV to ECV and improves intravascular hypovolemia.

For clinical conditions this dialysate sodium concentration $(D_{Na=0})$ is approximately 3 meq/l higher than serum sodium concentration.

In view of these data the hemodynamic differences described in Wehle's [36, 37] and Shaldon's [21] experiments are easily understood. In Shaldon's study, ultrafiltration was not partially compensated for by an intracellular to extracellular volume shift as was the case in Wehle's study, where the intratreatment osmotic change was prevented by increasing dialysate sodium concentration. The magnitude of the intracellular fluid shift induced by a sodium dialysate of 135 meg/l was found to be 1–1,51 [55, 65]. Keshaviah and associates [66] in dog experiments found a reduction of 800 ml in extracellular volume in excess to 800 ml ultrafiltrate which was lost from intravascular and extracellular colume. Van Stone and associates [67] studied the effect of dialysate sodium concentration on body fluid compartments in patients and came to similar results as Keshaviah [66] had in dogs. At a total weight loss of 0 and of 2.0 kg they varied dialysate sodium concentration to 7% above and below pretreatment serum sodium concentration. Serum osmolality decreased in all groups, and a significant inverse correlation between changes in intracellular volume and total serum osmolality existed. This correlation (figure 14–5) appeared to be due entirely to changes in serum sodium concentration as there was no significant correlation between changes in intracellular volume and changes in serum urea concentration, the other major determinant of serum osmolality.

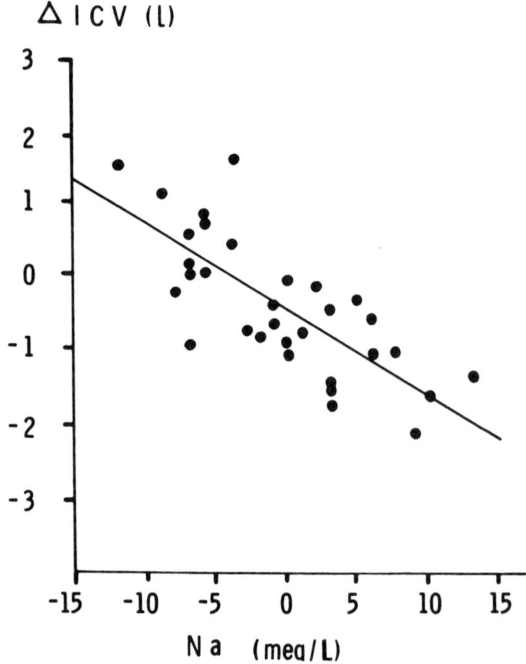


*Figure 14–5.* Correlation between change of plasma sodium concentration and change of intracellular volume (ΔICV). This figure derives from references number [68].

The discussion as to whether the hemodynamic benefits of hemofiltration were simply sodium related was initated by Gotch and coworkers [64, 69, 79, 71] who, based on theoretical calculations, postulated that during hemofiltration, protein concentration within the hemofilter increased due to ultrafiltration along the device and that therefore the Donnan factor would also increase. As a consequence the sodium concentration of the ultrafiltrate would decrease with the increasing plasma filtration fraction. This is in contrast to several reports demonstrating that filtrate sodium concentration is independent of plasma protein concentration [72, 73, 74]. Additional data [75, 76] at single values of protein concentration have been presented showing no net sodium holdback, i.e., filtrate and retentate sodium concentration are approximately equal. In an in vivo study Lysaght and associate [77] were able to demonstrate that the ratio of sodium concentration in the filtrate to that in the plasma (βm) increases. These results were confirmed in a careful in vitro model study by the same investigators [75]. In an albumin sodium chloride

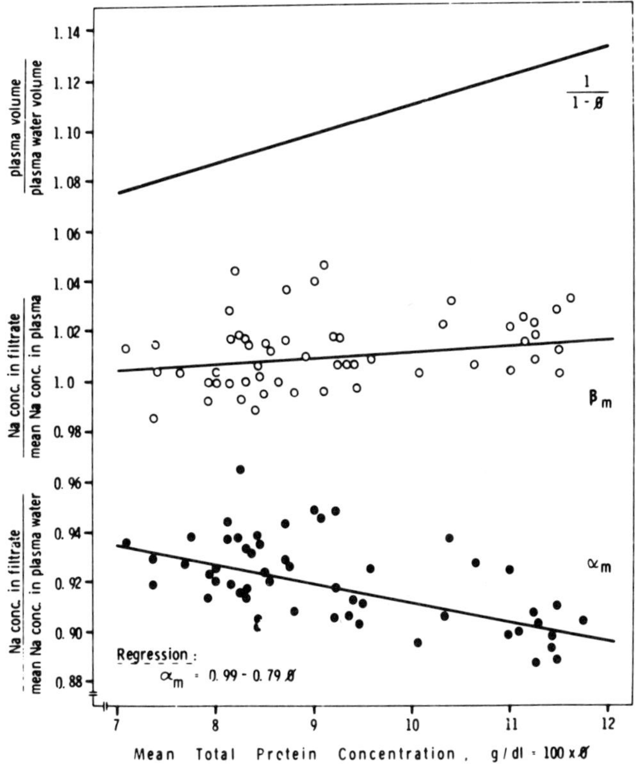



*Figure 14-6.* In vivo sodium sieving coefficient, measured during hemofiltration [77]. Plasma volume relative to plasma water $\left(\dfrac{1}{1-\varnothing}\right)$ volume increases with increasing plasma protein concentration. The ratio of sodium concentration in filtrate to mean sodium concentration in plasma water ($\alpha_m$) decreases with increasing protein concentration. As a result of these the ratio of sodium concentration in filtrate to mean sodium concentration in plasma ($\beta_m$) is practically not influenced by mean total protein concentration.

333

solution sodium plasma water sieving coefficient decreased with increasing protein concentration by only 1% (figure 14–6). This effect was counterbalanced by an increase in sodium plasma water concentration. The relative magnitude of these two oppositely directed effects differed from that of blood, so that the overall sieving coefficient changed slightly with plasma albumin level. Nevertheless the same basic phenomenon was clearly operating in vitro as in vivo

To further clarify this controversial issue, sodium balance was compared during hemodialysis and hemofiltration under defined and comparable experimental conditions [78]. Sodium balance was measured in hemofiltration but could only be calculated following the Gotch model in hemodialysis [64]. The results showed essentially no difference in sodium flux between hemodialysis and hemofiltration using an identical sodium concentration of 140 meq/l in dialysate as well as hemofiltration replacement fluid. The hemodynamic benefit of hemofiltration remain valid also for these experiments.

In order to compare the hemodynamic consequences of a changing sodium balance in hemodialysis and hemofiltration, Baldamus and his group [79, 80] measured the individual sodium loss (meq/kg weight loss) and correlated it to the individual change in blood pressure and total peripheral vascular resistance (figure 14–7), under controlled conditions. Blood pressure remained stable in hemofiltration throughout, while it decreased during hemodialysis with increasing sodium loss. The corresponding total peripheral resistance rose with increasing sodium loss only during hemofiltration but decreased in hemodialysis with increasing sodium loss. The latter observation is possibly explained by the stimulation of prostaglandinE production as shown by Schultze and his group in hemodialysis with low dialysate sodium concentration [81]. Decreased ADH secretion might be another explanation.

The difficulty in measuring an exact sodium balance during hemodialysis results from multiplication of two high numbers (volume × sodium concentraction) and from the imprecision of sodium determination ($\pm 2$–3 meq/l). Therefore it is difficult to prove or disprove Gotch's hypothesis. The strongest argument against the hypothesis is the experimental observations by Henderson and colleagues [82]. They were able to show in a predilution hemofiltration experiment that hemodynamic stability was still greater than in a comparable hemodialysis. During predilution hemofiltration, according to Gotch [64], blood plasma protein concentration decreases and therefore the sodium sieving coefficient should increase, resulting in the more negative balance than in hemodialysis.


*In conclusion*

As long as changes in serum osmolality during hemodialysis and hemofiltration are due to removal of solutes which equilibrate in total body water and have a high transcellular mass transfer coefficient (urea), these changes do

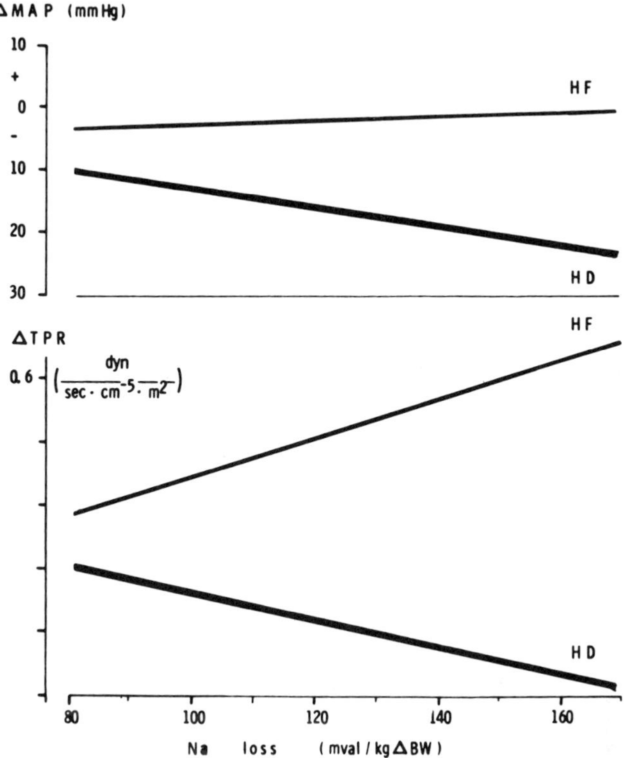


*Figure 14–7.* Correlation of change in mean arterial blood pressure (△MAP) and total peripheral vascular resistance (△TPR) with individual sodium loss, given as mval/kg weight loss (80) per treatment (Na loss). The same patients underwent hemodialysis (HD) and hemofiltration (HF) at standardized working conditions: 3 kg linear weight loss, identical small solute clearances and treatment time. Even at high sodium loss, i.e., a decrease in interstitial sodium concentration, blood pressure is maintained in HF by an increased TPR. In contrast TPR even decreases with increasing sodium loss and, as a result of this, blood pressure falls.

not affect blood pressure. However, if solutes are removed selectively from, or substituted to, the intravascular or interstitial space, this causes a fluid shift from the extracellular to the intracellular compartment or vice versa. This fluid shift then compensates or aggravates the hypovolemia caused by the unavoidable ultrafiltration. These fluid shifts are hemodynamically more effective during hemodialysis because the physiologic regulation of total peripheral vascular resistance is impaired. In contrast, during hemofiltration the physiological response is not impaired.

## Electrolyte changes

Intermittent end-stage renal disease treatment inevitably results in fast electrolyte changes. In addition, treatment-related acid base changes cause an electrolyte shift at the cellular level.

335

*Potassium*

Extracellular potassium is rapidly removed during treatment by the dialysis procedure and by an intracellular shift parallel with normalization of uremic metabolic acidosis. These fast potassium concentration changes have been discussed as one causative factor for the increased incidence of cardiac arrhythmia during treatment. Quellhorst and associates [83] studied the effect of potassium on intratreatment and posttreatment cardiac arrhythmia. They investigated the same patients during hemodialysis, hemofiltration, and hemodiafiltration. They reported a higher incidence of arrhythmias Lown class IV and V in all treatment regimes when patients were exposed to low potassium bath concentration. This was independent of the buffer source (acetate or bicarbonate). The incidence was low in hemofiltration, increased in hemodiafiltration, and became frequent in hemodialysis. In addition, hypotension appeared to be a predisposing factor. Morrison and associates [84] observed an increase in ventricular arrhythmia at low dialysate potassium concentration. Intratreatment arrhythmia occurred more frequently in patients with ventricular hypertrophy and in those on digitalis medication.

Potassium itself is a vasoactive substance [85, 86]. A decrease in extracellular potassium concentration causes vasoconstriction [87]. This vasoactivity appears to result from actions on the sarcolemmal NA-K-ATPase.

*Sodium*

According to loss, net sodium balance during the dialytic procedure is negative. Depending on the sodium concentration in the dialysate or in the hemofiltration replacement fluid, extracellular sodium concentration increases or decreases. Sodium, beyond being a potent osmotic agent and causing intracellular or extracellular fluid shifts is known to induce vascular smooth muscle contraction [88, 89].

An increase of extracellular sodium increases passive intracellular sodium flux and hence reduces membrane potential. This sodium influx, however, depends upon intracellular ionic calcium. Whether the small changes of extracellular sodium concentration during hemodialysis or hemofiltration have an effect on total peripheral vascular resistance is still controversial.

Interstitial sodium concentration influences vascular resistance indirectly by its influence on vasopressin secretion. Vasopressin secretion is enhanced at increased sodium concentration as well as by a decreased extracellular volume [90]. Measurements of changes in plasma vasopressin concentration during end-stage renal disease treatment are still lacking.

Sodium influences total peripheral vascular resistance also indirectly by its effect on the renin/angiotension system. Lowering serum sodium con-

336

centration in an isovolemic dialysis increases the renin release and leads to an increase in blood pressure [91].

*Calcium*

One object of intermittent dialysis treatment is a positive calcium balance. A rise of ionized calcium increases peripheral vascular resistance [92, 93] and improves cardiac contractility [94, 95]. Acidosis blunts this response [96]. So far the effect of calcium on total peripheral resistance during end-stage renal disease treatment has not been studied. It has recently been suggested that calcium improves left ventricular contractivility. In isovolemic hemodialysis left ventricular contractility increased if plasma ionized calcium concentration was raised by 0,25 mmol/l [97, 98].

The mechanism might involve parathyroid hormone [99]. Calcium balance during different ESRD treatments are difficult to monitor [100]. Here again hemofiltration is superior to hemodialysis because of the simplicity to measure input and output. Comparative hemodynamic studies comparing hemodialysis and hemofiltration under controlled conditions of intratreatment calcium balance are missing.

*Magnesium*

Magnesium overload is a consequence of chronic renal failure. It is removed by renal replacement therapy. Decreasing plasma magnesium concentration increases vascular reactivity and concomitantly vascular resistance [101], but vascular response differs from organ to organ and is tightly linked to other ions, calcium in particular. Competition between magnesium and calcium is reported for the vascular smooth muscle cells [101] as well as for the heart [102, 103]. Studies of the effect of magnesium on cardiocirculatory parameters during dialysis are missing.

*In conclusion*

Electrolyte changes influence hemodynamics in many ways. They cause fluid shifts between intracellular and extracellular compartments, and consequently they change blood volume (sodium). They act directly on the peripheral vasculature and change total peripheral vascular resistance (sodium, potassium, etc.). In addition, they modulate cardiac performance (calcium).

**Buffer-related changes**

One essential requirement of end-stage renal disease treatment is the removal of hydrogen ions which cause the metababolic hypochloremic acidosis of chronic renal failure. These hydrogen ions are mainly generated from protein metabolism. At a standard daily protein intake of 1 g/kg bw 60 meq hydrogen ions are formed per day [104, 105]. During each renal replacement therapy these hydrogen ions have to be removed or neutralized.

*Acetate/bicarbonate*

Up to 1964 acid base balance during hemodialysis was achieved with bicarbonate as dialysate buffer. It was Mion and his group (106) who replaced bicarbonate in dialysate by acetate to calculate proportioning of dialysis fluid with only one concentrate, as bicarbonate necessitates separation of calcium from bicarbonate in concentrated form. Acetate has been used with great success and without major complications as dialysate buffer. Graefe and associates in 1976 [19, 108] drew attention to the fact that acetate may play a role in the etiology of dialysis-induced hypotension and intradialytic symptomatology. Since then a great number of investigations have focused on the metabolism of acetate and its cardiovascular effects.

Already in 1928 Bauer and Richards [109] were able to demonstrate that acetate is a potent vasodilator. This effect was subsequently confirmed by others [110, 111, 112]. While the vascular effect of acetate, decreasing peripheral vascular resistance, is unopposed, there exists controversy on the effect of acetate on myocardial contractility. Kirkendol and associates [113] found in anesthetized dogs a dose-dependent decrease in myocardial contractility and a fall in mean arterial pressure following a bolus injection of acetate. They postulated that acetate was a myocardial depressant. This view was supported by data of Aizawa and colleagus [114, 115] showing that the ratio of the pre-ejection period to left ventricular ejection time (PEP/LVET) calculated from electrocardiogram increased during acetate infusion as well as during dialysis, indicating myocardial depression. Criticism of these data derived from the methodology. Based on echocardiography, Chen [116] was able to demonstrate during dialysis that PEP/LVET ratio is an unreliable parameter for myocardial function. Their data showed a reduction of preload as well as afterload at an increased heart rate. They interpreted this as a sign for improved myocardial contractility. This was also found in a study by Liang and Löwenstein [117] who infused acetate in an increasing dosage into anesthetized dogs. As a consequence of this acetate application, cardiac output increased due to increase in heart rate as well as in stroke volume. Total peripheral vascular resistance decreased. This positive inotropic effect of acetate was confirmed in a later investigation by Kirkendol and associates [118] when they infused acetate instead of giving it as a bolus. Only at a high dosage of 1 mmol/min/kg bw they registered in dogs a fall in blood pressure.

Similar results were obtained by Keshaviah [119]. In anesthetized dogs acetate infusion was immediately followed by a rise in cardiac output and a fall in total peripheral resistance (figure 14–8). Mean arterial pressure fell and pulmonary artery pressure rose.

From the effects of acetate, namely an increase of cardiac output and a

338

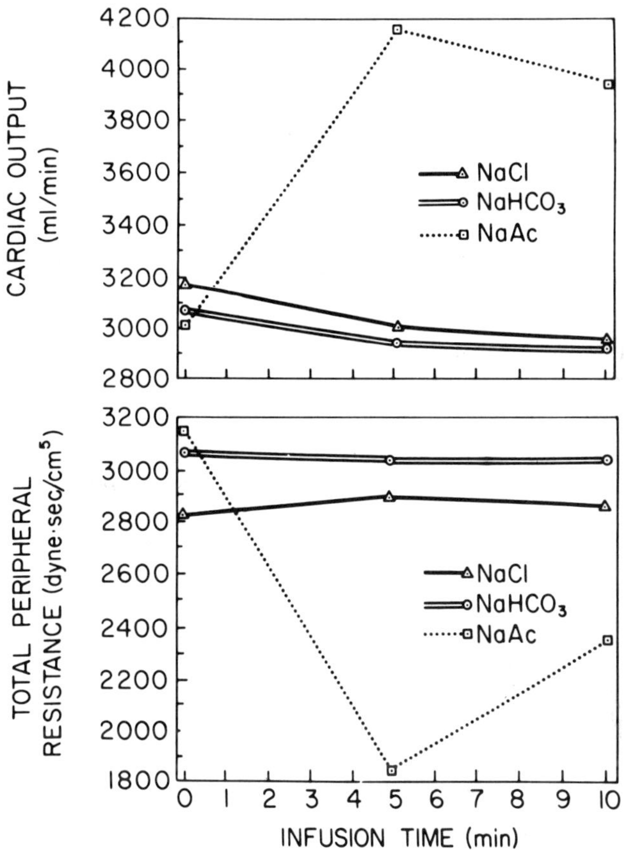


*Figure 14–8.* Changes in cardiac output and in total peripheral vascular resistance during infusion of sodium acetate, sodium chloride or sodium bicarbonate (2, 4 mmol/min) in anesthetized dogs [119].

decrease of total peripheral resistance, it is easy to explain the great variance of reported data on hemodynamics during hemodialysis [12, 5, 18, 22, 33, 36, 37, 39, 42, 44, 45]. In regular uncomplicated patients no hemodynamic complications can be observed. Increase of cardiac output compensates for the fall in total vascular resistance. However, patients with impaired cardiac function are unable to further increase cardiac output, and hypotension is the result of peripheral vasodilatation.

Cardiac performance can also be negatively influenced by high acetate load during dialysis when plasma acetate concentration increases to toxic levels. It is therefore important to discuss acetate metabolism briefly.

Acetate plasma concentration depends on acetate load and on acetate metabolic rate. Acetate load during standard hemodialysis amounts to 1,100–1,200 meq per treatment leading to an increased mean plasma acetate concentration of 5 meq/l ranging from 2,5–12 meq/l. As plasma acetate concentration rises, acetate metabolism reaches a maximum. The kinetics fit best the Michaelis Menton model from which a maximal metabolic rate can be calculated (V max. 8,1 meq/min) as well as the plasma concentration at which metabolic rate is half maximal (Km = 8,6 meq/l) [105]. These are only mean figures with a great interindividual variance from acetate-intolerant patients with V max. of only 5,6 meq/min and a Km of 2,3 meq/l to patients with high metabolic rates (V max = 50 meq/min; Km = 24 meq/l). From this great variability it can be concluded that there exists a substantial number of patients who only have a limited capacity to metabolize acetate and who may suffer from the resultant but unwanted alteration of acid base homeostasis and who also may experience hemodynamic complications due to the direct acetate effects.

In view of acetate kinetic data [120, 121, 122] it is hard to accept that at identical small solute removal rates the acetate load would be higher in hemodialysis than in hemofiltration. Shaldon and associates [17] were the only investigators who measured plasma acetate concentrations during acetate hemodialysis and acetate hemofiltration under matched operating conditions. They could not observe a difference in plasma acetate concentrations. At a dialysance of more than 2 ml/min/kg bw bicarbonate loss (about equal to acetate gain) exceeds metabolic production of bicarbonate. This is an important point since modern dialysis equipment allows high acetate dialysance of far beyond this critical figure [123]. Here acetate as dialysis buffer must be replaced by bicarbonate.

There exists some experimental evidence that acetate metabolism differs between hemodialysis and hemofiltration. Kishimoto and associates [191] were able to show an improved acetate metabolism in hemofiltration. They attribute this improvement to the better liver organ blood flow in hemofiltration when compared to hemodialysis [124, 219].

Besides, the fact that acetate is a potent vasodilator, it is important to note that acetate might induce hypotension by a further mechanism. At blood acetate concentration of 10 meq/l and more [104] during hemodialysis, acetate stimulates interleukin-I production from monocytes [125]. The role of interleukin-I in the pathogenesis of hemodialysis will be discussed in a later section.

Several investigators have studied the incidence of hypotension and other intratreatment symptomatology during acetate hemodialysis and compared it to bicarbonate dialysis. Graefe was the first who saw fewer hypotensive episodes during bicarbonate dialysis than during acetate dialysis [108, 19]. These findings were supported by a number of authors [22, 42, 44, 126]. Others found no differences [68, 127], and Aizawa even noticed a significant decrease in blood pressure during bicarbonate but not during acetate dialysis [115]. In few publications differences were only detectable in specific situations and in particular patients [39]. A detailed analysis might help to understand the underlying mechanisms. Wehle [59] reported no differences at dialysate sodium concentration of 140 meq/l. At 133 meq/l, however, hypotension occurred more frequently during acetate than during bicarbonate dialysis. In an additional series of experiments [68] they performed isovolemic dialysis at different dialysate sodium concentration, and with acetate and bicarbonate as the buffer source. They counterbalanced the change in osmolality by urea. Total peripheral vascular resistance decreased significantly in acetate dialysis and to a minor degree in bicarbonate dialysis. Neither urea nor sodium had an effect on total peripheral vascular resistance. But sodium still had an effect on blood pressure, most likely by its effect on the extracellular volume shift. Similar data were reported by Raya and associates [128]. These reports indicate that acetate decreases vascular resistance which then is counterbalanced by an increased cardiac output. Only if critical volume loss, caused either by ultrafiltration or by an intracellular volume shift (low sodium dialysate), stresses the compensatory mechanisms to a maximum, clinical differences between acetate and bicarbonate dialysis become detectable. Comparing the hemodynamic data of acetate and bicarbonate hemodialysis with those of hemofiltration, the majority of authors report a decrease in vascular resistance during acetate dialysis but a missing increase during bicarbonate dialysis [12, 13, 22, 33, 29, 44]. In contrast, during hemofiltration total peripheral resistance increases in a physiological way [12, 13, 33]. Only one report shows an increase in vascular resistance in acetate hemodialysis and hemofiltration, but an unchanged or even decreased vascular resistance in bicarbonate dialysis [45].

*Hypoxemia/hypocapnia*

Acetate might have an additional indirect effect on hemodynamics via hypoxemia. Hypoxemia occurs immediately after start of hemodialysis and, using acetate dialysate, it persists throughout. According to a literature review [129, 130], $pO_2$ drops for a mean of 14,5 mmHg. Several mechanisms have been discussed:

1. Increased oxygen consumption due to either acetate metabolism [131] or to the stress situation of a treatment with increased caloric turnover [132].

2. Decreased oxygen delivery due to the Bohr effect, the acid base dependent change of oxygen affinity of the hemoglobin molecules [133]. The other possibility is related to membrane bioincompatibility (see below) of cellulosic membranes with complement activation and leucocytic sequestration in pulmonary capillaries [134, 135].

3. Depressed ventilatory drive due to the $CO_2$ loss across the dialyzer [136, 137] or as a direct consequence of acetate metabolism [130, 135, 137, 138, 139].

Acetate, besides its effect on hypoxemia, might negatively influence cardiac performance in an additional way. Hampl and associates [39] have demonstrated clinical evidence in patients prone to hypotension that the low $pCO_2$ (30,4 mmHg) during acetate dialysis, when compared in the same patients to bicarbonate dialysis (pCO2 38,2 mmHg), was associated with significant EEG changes and with an increased incidence of hypotension. The EEG disturbance are thought to be a result of decreased cerebral bloodflow which is partially regulated by pCO2 [140, 141]. Hypocapnia leads to a decrease, of cerebral bloodflow, whereas hypercapnia results in an increase.

Differences in pCO2 were reported for acetate hemodialysis and hemofiltration [142]. A low pCO2 could be explained by generation of CO2 within the dialyzer [143, 144], which, however, is not fully accepted [145]. A reduced pCO2 decreases cerebral bloodflow which leads to reduction of sympathetic activity [28, 146, 147, 148] with the consequence of an impaired increase in peripheral vascular resistance during acetate hemodialysis. But it does not explain why during bicarbonate dialysis the peripheral resistance and plasma noradrenaline concentrations do not increase. Keshaviah [119] speculated, based on a report by Lian and Löwenstein [117] that byproducts of acetate metabolism like adenine nucleotides of adenosine were inadequately removed during acetate hemodialysis and that this may play a role in etiology of dialysis-induced hypotension. Here again the missing increase of total peripheral vascular resistance during bicarbonate hemodialysis remains unexplained.

*In conclusion*

The use of acetate as dialysate buffer source is associated with vasodilatation, with increased cardiac output, with hypoxemia, and with hypocapnia. Negative introposm may occur if a very high acetate load is given [123] and its maximal metabolic rate is exceeded. This situation can occur today with hyperefficient modern dialysis treatment. In regular stable hemodialysis patients, the vasodilating action of acetate is compensated for by an increase in cardiac output. Only in patients with impaired cardiac and circulatory function can acetate lead to hemodynamic instability. Studies of acetate metabolism and its effect on the cardiovacular system explain why total peripheral vascular resistance decreases during acetate hemodialysis. However, it remains unclear why resistance increases during hemofiltration in spite of the fact that acetate load is comparable. Furthermore, it is still unexplained why during bicarbonate hemodialysis total peripheral vascular resistance does not increase.


**Hormonal changes**

Differences in removal of vasoactive substances have been discussed to explain the hemodynamic differences observed between hemodialysis and hemofiltration [22, 28]. Generation of one or more substances interfering with sympathetic activity during dialysis treatment, but being removed during hemofiltration and not during hemodialysis, or being formed only during hemodialysis but not hemofiltration, would explain all established findings, i.e., increase of sympathetic activity and total peripheral resistance during ultrafiltration and hemofiltration but no response during hemodialysis.

*Catecholamines*

Catecholamines are the most discussed vasoactive substances. The failure of noradrenaline concentration to increase [23, 26] during hemodialysis has been explained by its removal during dialysis. In hemofiltration the increase [13, 27] was explained by a higher removal rate during hemodialysis. This argument was invalidated when catecholamine dialysance was measured during hemodialysis and hemofiltration [22]. The ratio of noradrenaline to urea clearance was found to be 0.6 in hemodialysis versus 0.9 in hemofiltration (figure 14–9). Therefore, at matched small solute removal rates the observed increase in plasma noradrenaline during hemofiltration but not during hemodialysis cannot be explained by an increased removal in hemodialysis [22]. The increase in sympathetic tone during hemofiltration and ultrafiltration and not during hemodialysis remains as yet unexplained.

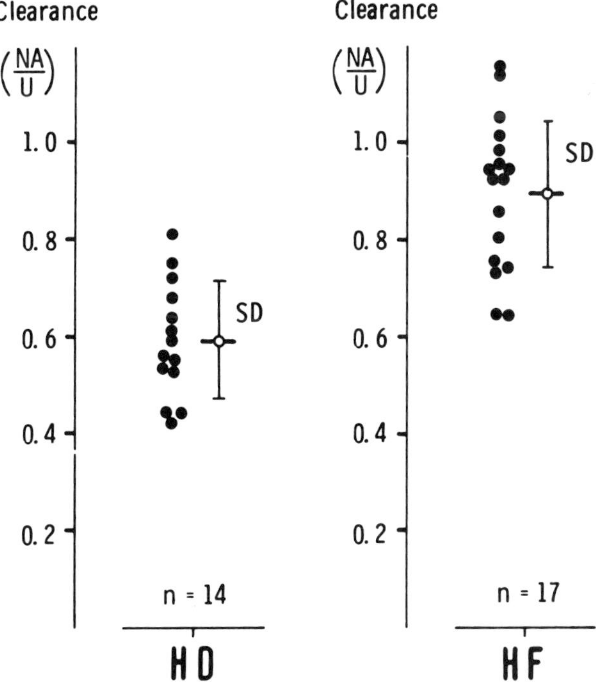


*Figure 14–9.* Transmembraneous noradrenaline (NA) transport relative to that of urea (U), expressed as fractional clearance during hemodialysis (HD), and hemofiltration (HF). Mean values of HD and HF are significantly different.

*Vasopressin*

Vasopressin was discussed by Gotch and Sargent [64] as a contributing factor to vascular stability since it is a strong vasoconstrictor. Secretion is stimulated by even small changes in osmolality, sensed in the hypothalamus (osmoreceptors). When plasma osmolality is increased by urea, a solute rapidly equilibrating between intracellular and extracellular fluid, ADH release is not enhanced. If, however, sodium or mannitol, solutes which remain in the extracellular space, are infused, ADH is released (figure 14–10) [149]. Therefore, ADH secretion has to be discussed in connection with intracellular extracellular volume shifts (see earlier discussion). In view of the observed hemodynamic changes during different therapeutic modalities, ADH secretion might help to explain why during hemodialysis at high sodium loss, i.e., decrease of interstitial sodium concentration, total peripheral resistance decreases (figure 14–7). This question, however, remains still to be answered: Why at identical high sodium loss are the same patients able to increase vascular resistance during hemofiltration but not during hemodialysis?

Comparative studies on ADH secretion during hemodialysis and hemofiltration are lacking.

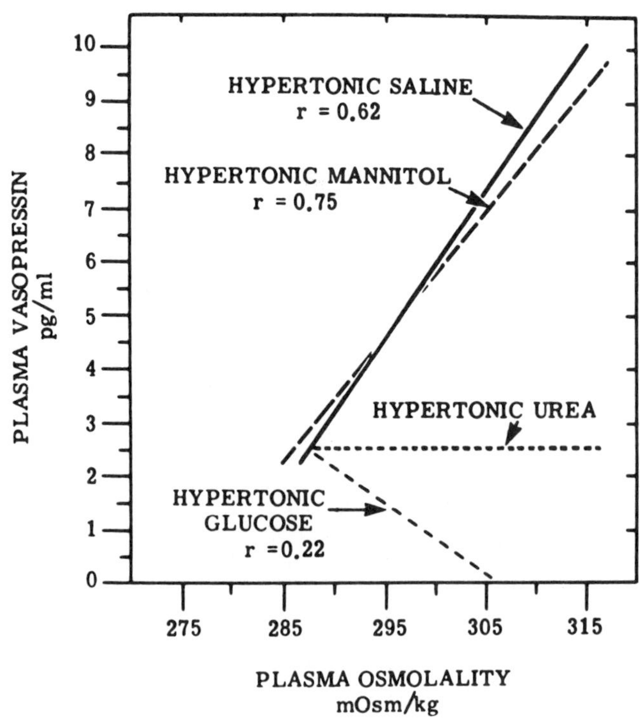


*Figure 14–10.* Relationship of plasma vasopression to osmolality [49] in healthy adults infused intravenously with hypertonic solutions of saline, mannitol, glucose, and urea.

344

*Atrial natriuretic factor*

Atrial natriuretic factor is a potent vasodilating hormone, which is secreted following artrial dilatation [150] stimulated by volume loading [151]. As a polypeptide containing 28 amino acids, its molecular size was calculated to be of about 3.000 daltons [152]. This size range of molecule is removed effectively only during hemofiltration but not during hemodialysis. It is reasonable to assume increased secretion during the interdialytic period as a result of intertreatment fluid intake. During hemofiltration this vasodilator substance is removed but not during hemodialysis. Thus in long-term hemodialysis therapy it will maintain a high plasma concentration if the endogeneous half-life of this polypeptide is sufficiently long or prolonged in uremia. Increased susceptibility to hypotension in patients with cardiac impairment would also fit this hypothesis.

No studies on atrial natriuretic factor exist so far in uremic patients.

*Prostaglandins*

Prostaglandins have to be separated into those with vasodilating and those with vasoconstricting potency. In addition, they may act differently on the peripheral systemic and pulmonary vasculature. To date there exist only few references that relate to hemodialysis, none so far focusing on hemofiltration. Preliminary data suggest an increase in plasma prostaglandine (PGE 2) levels when using cellulosic membranes for hemodialysis. This is not observed with polyacrylonitrile membranes [153]. This increase correlated with complement activation by cellulosic material and the consequent forming of leucocytic lung aggregates. Borges and associates [154] speculated about a connection between increased incidence of intratreatment symptomatology and with increased PGE 2 production. The only direct evidence that plasma PGE 2 rises during hemodialysis derives from data by Schultze and associates [81]. They were able to demonstrate an increase only if dialysis was performed at dialysate sodium concentrations of 125 meq/l. Together with the rise of PGE 2 plasma renin activity (PRA) increased, too. An interaction of PGE 2 synthesis and renin secretion is also known from other disease states [155, 156, 157]. A ratio of PGE/PRA correlated well with a decrease in systemic blood pressure. A principal argument against the direct influence of PGE 2 on peripheral vascular tone, which the authors discussed, is the high pulmonary clearance rate for PGE 2. Pulmonary clearance, however, might severely be altered as a result of sequestration of leucocytes, although this would be an early event and hypotension usually occurs late during dialysis.

Prostacyclin, a second prostanoid vasodilator, is released during hemodialysis [158]. Using a cellulosic membrane, an early rise is seen which coincides with the peak of hypoxemia.

Thromboxane, a potent vasoconstrictor, also increases during the early phase of dialysis [159, 218, 219]. This can be shown in sheep to be induced by complement activation and pulmonary leucostasis [160].

So far these data do not contribute to the explanation of the different hemodynamics during hemodialysis and hemofiltration. Local secretion of prostaglandins may, however, play a role in the context of the interleukin-I hypothesis [16] (see section on blood device interaction).

*In conclusion*

ProstaglandinE 2, a potent vasodilator, is secreted early during hemodialysis with cellulosic membranes as a direct and/or indirect result of complement activation and pulmonary leucostasis. Prostacyclin and thromboxane are also stimulated. This does not occur if dialysis is performed with synthetic, 'biocompatible' membranes. If the interleukin-I hypothesis proves to be true, late and local prostaglandinE 2 stimulation might help to explain dialysis hypotension.

**Extracorporeal temperature**

Maggiore and associates [162] found that hemodynamic stability seen during ultrafiltration was abolished when returning extracorporeal blood was rewarmed to body core temperature. On the other hand, they were able to improve vascular stability during hemodialysis by decreasing temperature of returning extracorporeal blood. They suggested that intratreatment vascular stability was at least partly a temperature-related phenomen. Their finding could be confirmed by several authors [163, 167]. In an extended study Maggiore investigated hemodialysis and hemofiltration, and found that hemodynamic differences between cold hemodialysis and cold hemofiltration became partly abolished [168, 169, 170]. However, the maximal drop of blood pressure in warm hemofiltration was less than in warm hemodialysis. Schäfer and colleagues [171, 172] in similar experiments compared two situations in hemofiltration with either 35°C or 40°C replacement fluid and found no significant difference in hemodynamic stability. It appears that hemodialysis is more sensitive to temperature changes than hemofiltration. This might be related to temperature-dependent reactions within the dialyzer, the point of greatest heat exchange [173]. Membrane-related complement activation is prevented by decreasing dialysate temperature [174]. The fact that hemo-dynamics during hemodialysis are especially temperature-dependent in con-trast to hemofiltration would fit the interleukin-I hypothesis (see upcoming section on interleukin-I): complement activation as well as macrophage IL-I production are temperature sensitive [175]

*In conclusion*

Hemodynamic stability during dialysis and hemofiltration can be diminished by increasing core body temperature. This lowers total peripheral vascular resistance. Temperature sensitivity seems to be higher during hemodialysis than during hemofiltration. This is in agreement with the interleukin-I hypothesis since complement activation and macrophage interleukin-I production are both temperature sensitive.


**Blood device interaction**

In every extracorporeal treatment, blood comes in contact with the foreign material of dialyzer or filter, of blood lines, of connections, etc. In addition, sterilants and plasticizers may be leached out by blood with its lipophilic properties as these substances cannot be rinsed out with saline.

*Complement activation*

One of the best investigated phenomena of blood/device interaction is the complement activation of cellulosic membranes which occurs immediately after blood membrane contact [176, 134]. The sequence of events is a membrane-initiated complement activation, via the alternate pathway, with generation of complement products, one of which is C 5a [177]. As a result of complement activation, the peripheral leucocyte count drops; pulmonary leucostasis occurs with its impairment of circulation and function [178]. Leucostasis, with increased formation of platelet aggregates, initates prostaglandin release [176]. The entire sequence of events following complement activation by cellulosic membrane is reviewed in detail elsewhere [179]. It should be mentioned that complement activation in hemodialysis [174] seems to be temperature sensitive (see earlier section). In relation to dialysis: associated hypotension it is important to note that complement is activated immediately following the first blood membrane contact. In contrast, however, hypotension occurs late during treatment

*Interleukin-I*

Henderson and associates [161] offered a very stimulating hypothesis. Based on several clinical observations in chronic dialysis patients, like temperature increment during treatment, low plasma zink levels [180], increased plasma levels of acute phase response proteins, etc., they postulated that interleukin-I is activated during dialysis. One pathway by which it can be activated is by complement factor C 5a. This complement component binds to macrophages and induces interleukin-I production [181, 182]. Once monocytes become activated they release interleukin-I after 3–4 hours [183], a time lag that coincides with the peak incidence of hypotensive episodes during hemodialysis. A second way of interleukin-I activation can derive from dialysate containing endotoxin [188]. These exogenous pyrogens, which are extensively absorbed to dialysis membranes, either penetrate the membrane and gain access to the bloodstream or they remain bound to the membrane but stimulate adherent monocytes to produce interleukin-I.

Interleukin-I, besides having other effects (figure 14–11), induces prostaglandin E 2 release, which then leads to hypotension by its vasodilating potency. Another vasodilating effect is to be expected from interleukin-I-induced prostacyclin release [184].

Meanwhile, first experimental data seem to support the interleukin-I hypothesis [125]: hemodialysis generates C 5a [186, 187] at correct concentrations for IL-I induction in vivo [179]. The temperature dependency of complement activation [174] and the improved vascular stability for cold hemodialysis [162, 168, 209, 213, 215, 216] may be interpreted as indirect support of the interleukin-I hypothesis.

In an ex vivo extracorporeal hemodialysis circuit, Lonnemann and associates [125] were able to demonstrate monocytic IL-I production if the dialysate was contaminated with endotoxin. Hemodialysis raises circulating IL-I plasma levels in end-stage renal disease patients postdialysis [183]. Muscle protein catabolism occurs during sham hemodialysis and peaks at 3 hours after start of dialysis. It is blocked by the prostaglandin inhibitor indomethacin [186]. Acetate in concentrations routinely used in hemodialysis induce monocytes in vitro to produce IL-I [125].

Induction of interleukin-I production is speculated to be less during

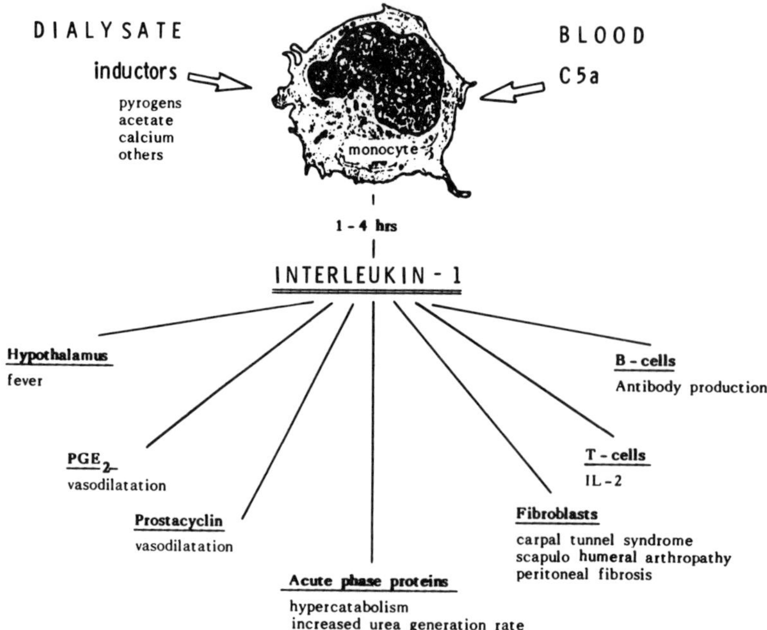



*Figure 14–11.* Possible consequences of dialysis associated interleukin-I production from activated monocytes.

hemofiltration because of the following reasons. In hemofiltration, noncellulosic synthetic membranes are used. They do not activate the complement system. Second, replacement fluid is pyrogen-free in contrast to dialysate which regularly contains major contamination with exogenous pyrogen. Third, monocytes adherent to the membrane are not exposed to high concentrations of IL-I inductors as is the case in hemodialysis. Indirect experimental support in vivo derives from a study by Minetti and associates [189] who found hemofiltration (HF) less catabolic than comparable hemodialysis (HD).

*In conclusion*

Direct experimental evidence that blood/device interaction interferes with the physiologic response to volume removal is still limited. The interleukin I hypothesis, however, offers a stimulating explanation for a great number of adverse dialysis-related phenomena, one of which is intratreatment hypotension. Several factors which might initiate interleukin-I production in HD are not apparent during HF. Time will show whether the interleukin-I hypothesis proves to be correct.

## Underlying pathology

*Autonomic neuropathy*

Hypohidrosis, impotence, reduction in heart rate, beat-to-beat variation, and severe hypotension during HD treatment indicate an impaired autonomic system [190–194] in many dialysis patients. In regard to hypotension during HD, the baroreflex with its baroreceptors, the afferent limb, the central intersection, the vagal and sympathetic efferent limb, and the end organ response are the critical determinants of acute blood pressure regulation. Lilley and associates [193] investigated a group of HD patients with frequent hypotensive episodes and compared it to a group without hypotensive complications

They studied the entire baroreflex by analyzing the baroreflex sensitivity from beat-to-beat changes of pulse interval and of arterial pressure following an amylnitrite inhalation. Plasma dopamine-β-hydroxylase activity and cold pressure test served as indicators for the efferent sympathetic nervous system. Their results suggested that hypotension may result from a lesion in the baroreceptors, cardiopulmonary receptors, or the visceral afferent nerves. Nies and associates [195] as well as others [191, 196–198] confirmed the lesions of the baroreflex to be located at the baroreceptor site or in the afferent limb. They found this autonomic nervous lesion to highly correlate with incidence of intratreatment hypotension. The blunted response of heart rate to a hypotensive stimulus and, more specifically, the pathologic diving

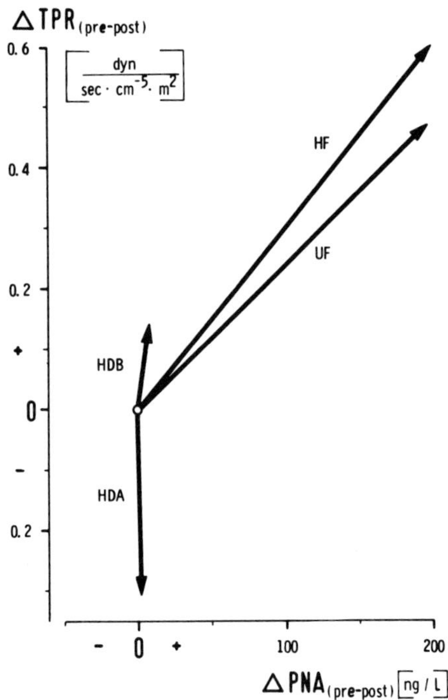



*Figure 14–12.* Relation between intratreatment change in total peripheral vascular resistance (△TPR) and change in plasma noradrenaline concentration (△PNA) during ultrafiltration (UF), hemofiltration (HF), acetate (HDA), and bicarbonate hemodialyse (HDB). Pretreatment to posttreatment changes are drawn as vectors [78].

test [27] were interpreted as indicators for an efferent vagal lesion. Uremic disturbance of end organ responsiveness are controversial. Kersh and co-workers [197] and Nies and coworkers [195] noted an adequate increase in blood pressure following a noradrenalin infusion, whereas Romoff and colleagues [199] interpreted the normal increase of plasma noradrenaline concentration after orthostasis in combination with an inadequate rise of blood pressure as an indicator for diminished end organ responsiveness. This view is supported by Rascher and his researchers [198] who in uremic rats demonstrated a diminished increase of hind leg total peripheral resistance following peripheral noradreanline application (table 14–2).

In addition to an impaired baroreflex, uremia-related abnormalities in catecholamine metabolism like altered biosynthesis [200], reuptake [201], and density of sympathetic innervation [202] have been described, and could explain the increased basal plasma noradrenaline levels in uremic patients [27, 199, 203–205].

Although autonomic neuropathy is a common finding in uremia and although severe lesions seem to provoke hypotension during treatment, the hemodynamic difference between hemodialysis and hemofiltration, as des-

350

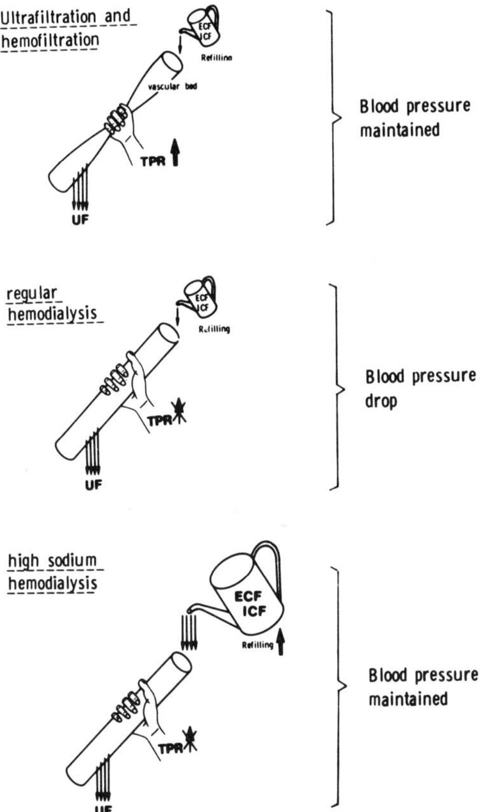


*Figure 14–13.* Hemodynamic response to weight removal [78]. In ultrafiltration and hemofiltration blood pressure is maintained by an increase in total peripheral vascular resistance (TPR). If weight removal rate (UF) exceeds vascular refilling from extracellular (ECF) and intracellular (ICF) compartments, blood pressure drops during hemodialysis because here the same patient is unable to increase TPR. Only if vascular refilling rate increases, as in high sodium dialysis, and counterbalances ultrafiltration can blood pressure remain stable.

cribed above, cannot be explained by alterations of the autonomic nervous system. In controlled studies the same patients behaved hemodynamically different during hemodialysis and hemofiltration [12, 13, 15, 16, 17, 22, 40]. Only an acute impairment of the baroreflex during hemodialysis can explain the lost ability to increase vascular resistance which remains intact, at least qualitativly, during ultrafiltration and hemofiltration (table 14–3). Early studies of baroreflex sensitivity by Pickering [192] and more recent studies of the different segments of the baroreflex arc performed by Baldamus and associates [206] during hemodialysis and hemofiltration were unable to identify any acute changes during hemodialysis and hemofiltration. Baroreflex sensitivity was the only parameter that improved during hemofiltration. These data are supported by Zucchelli and colleagues [16]. They in addition

351

found an increase in Valsalv ratio during hemodialysis and hemofiltration, but significantly more pronounced in hemofiltration. So far end organ responsiveness has not been tested comparatively during hemodialysis and hemofiltration. Even if end organ responsiveness were to deteriorate during hemodialysis, this would enhance sympathetic tone resulting in high plasma noradrenaline levels, whereas the opposite has been found in hemodialysis [13, 22].

*In conclusion*

Autonomic neuropathy frequently exists in uremic patients [190–194, 207, 208] and predisposes to intratreatment hypotension [191, 193, 195–197] Hemodynamic differences between hemodialysis and hemofiltration cannot be explained by autonomic insufficiency because the same patient reacts differently during hemodialysis and hemofiltration. Acute treatment-induced impairment of baroreflex, however, cannot be demonstrated [206]. Differences in end organ responsiveness, not tested so far, seem unlikely to explain the hemodynamic differences.

*Cardiovascular disorders*

In end-stage renal disease patients, maintained on hemodialysis, the heart is usually damaged, and the term uremic cardiomyopathy [209, 215] reflects myocardial dysfunction which becomes evident during the course of the renal failure. The etiology is multifactorial. Among the etiologic factors hypertension, atherosclerosis, anemia, and hypovolemia are the most important ones. Abnormal acid base status and electrolyte metabolism as well as hyperparathyroidism, diabetes mellitus, and nutritional deficiency contribute also. Uremic toxins usually are listed but not specifically identified. Regardless of the etiology patients suffering clinically from cardiomyopathy run a high risk of intra-treatment-related hypotension. This can easily be explained by their very limited capacity to compensate an acute additional workload.

In this critical situation the treatment modality with the least adverse effect should be applied. Hampl [32] and others [12] clearly showed that these patients benefit from hemofiltration. Comparative hemodynamic studies in these patients might help to amplify the effect of variants, which in uncomplicated patients are completely compensated.

According to Hung and associates [209] patients with impaired cardiac function benefit from hemodialysis by lowering preload as well as afterload. This effect is not restricted to volume overload but was validated also for patients with impaired left ventricular function. Patient with normal cardiac function did not increase ejection fraction. Nixon and associates [216] tried to separate the effect of volume removal from that of removal of uremic toxins. Ultrafiltration produced a pure Frank Starling effect. In contrast, hemodialysis with and without volume loss produced a shift in the ventricular function curve to the left, which indicates an increase in left ventricular contractility. In a subsequent study the same group [97] was able to demonstrate that the increase of left ventricular contractile state was due to an increase of ionized calcium. Comparable detailed investigations of the cardiac state during hemofiltration are not available.

Differences in patients' cardiac status might explain the different hemodynamic results reported by different authors [32, 12, 22] and beyond that it clearly shows that studies comparing two treatment regimes should always be performed in the same patients.

*In conclusion*

Patients with 'uremic cardiomyopathy' or any other form of cardiac impairment are especially sensitive to volume removal. Intratreatment hypotension then is the most frequent result. These are especially the patients who benefit from hemofiltration. Because of their high sensitivity, future studies in these patients might help to clarify specific pathogenic aspects of hemodialysis-associated hypotension.

*Medication*

Patients on regular renal replacement therapy very often receive drugs effecting the cardio circulatory system such as antihypertensives, glycosides, antiarrhythmics, and bronchodilators. In addition, analgesics, narcotics, and psychotherapeutics may interfere with hemodynamic compensatory mechanisms. Very little is known so far about pharmacokinetics and pharmacodynamics during hemofiltration. Differences are expected for drugs which are water soluble and of a size too big for efficient elimination during hemodialysis (>1 KD) but still small enough to be filtered effectively during hemofiltration (<15 KD).

## References


1. Degoulet, P., Reach, I., Rozenbaum, W., Aime, F., Devries, C., Berger, C., Rojas, P., Jacobs, C. and Legrain, M. (1979) Programme Dialyse-informatique. VI. — Survie et facteurs de risque. J. Urol. Nephrol. 85: 909–962.
2. Degoulet, P., Proulx, J., Aime, F., Berger, C., Bloch, P., Goupy, F. and Legrain, M. (1976) Programme Dialyse — Informatique. III. — Donnees epidemiologiques. Stragegies de dialyse et resultats biologiques. J. Urol. Nephrol. 82:1001.
3. Degoulet, P., Réach, I., Di Giulio, S., Devriés, C., Rouby, J.J., Aimé, F. and Vonlanthen, M. (1981) Epidemiology of dialysis induced hypotension. Proc. EDTA 18: 133.
4. Brynger, H, Brunner, F.P., Chantler, C., Donckerwolcke, R.A., Jacobs, C., Kramer, P., Selwood, N.H. and Wing, A.J. (1979) Combined report on regular dialysis and transplantation in Europe 17: 4.
5. Brunner, F.P., Giesecke, B., Gurland, H.J., Jacobs, C., Parsons, F.M., Schärer, K., Seyffart, G., Spies, G. and Wing, A.J. (1974) Combined report on regular dialysis and

transplantation in Europe. Proc. Europ. Dial. Transpl. Ass. 12: 3.

6. Guyton, A.C., Coleman, T.G. and Granger, H.J. (1972) Circulation: overall regulation. Ann. Rev. Physiol. 34: 13.

7. Guyton, A.C. (1980) In *Circulatory Physiology III: Arterial Pressure and Hypertension.* Saunders Company. Philadelphia, London, Toronto: W.B.

8. Kobayashi, K., Shibata, M., Kato, K. et al. (1972) Studies on the development of a new method of controlling the amount and contents of body fluids (extracorporeal ultrafiltration method ECUM and the application of this method for patients receiving long term hemodialysis. Jap. J. Nephrol. 14:1

9. Ing, T., Ashbach, D.L., Kanter, A. et al. (1975) Fluid removal and negative-pressure hydrostaticultrafiltration using a partial vacuum. Nephron 14: 451.

10. Bergström, J., Asaba, H., Fürst, P. and Oulés, R. (1976) Dialysis, ultrafiltration and blood pressure. Proc. EDTA 13: 293.

11. Quellhost, E., Rieger, J., Doht, B., Beckmann, H., Jacob, I., Kraft, B., Mietzsch, G. and Scheler, F. (1976) Treatment of chronic uramia by an ultrafiltration kidney — first clinical experience. Proc. EDTA 13: 314.

12. Baldamus, C.A., Ernst, W., Fassbinder, W. and Koch, K.M. (1980) Differing haemo-dynamic stability due to differing sympathetic response: comparison of ultrafiltration, haemodialysis and haemofiltration. Proc. EDTA 17: 205.

13. Quellhorst, E., Schuenemann, B., Hildebrand, U. and Falda, Z. (1980) Response of the vascular system to different modifications of haemofiltration and haemodialysis. Proc. EDTA 17: 197.

14. Baldamus, C.A., Schoeppe, W., Koch, K.M. (1978) Comparison of haemodialysis and post dilution haemofiltration on an unselected dialysis population. Proc. Europ. Dial. Transpl. Ass. 15: 228.

15. Aljama, P., Martin-Malo, A., Sanz, R., Pasalodos, J., Sancho, M., Moreno, E., Gómez, J., Pérez, R., Burdiel, L.G. and Andrés E. (1982) Left ventricular function during haemofiltration and haemodialysis: a comparative study. Proc. EDTA 19: 281.

16. Zucchelli, P., Santoro, A., Sturani, A., Degli Esposti, E., Chiarini, C. and Zuccalà, A. (1984) Effects of hemodialysis and hemofiltration on the autonomic control of circulation. Trans. Am. Soc. Artif. Intern. Organs 30: 163.

17. Shaldon, S., Deschodt, G., Beau, M.C., Claret, G., Mion, H. and Mion, C. (1979) Vascular stability during high flux haemofiltration. Proc. Eur. Dial. Transplant. Ass. 16:695.

18. Graefe, U., Milutinovich, J., Follette, W.C., Babb, A.L. and Scribner, B.H. (1977) Improved tolerance to rapid ultrafiltration with the use of bicarbonate in dialysate. Proc. EDTA 14: 153.

19. Graefe, U., Milutinovich, J., Follette, W.C., Vizzo, J.E., Babb, A.L. and Scribner, B.H. (1978) Less dialysis-induced morbidity and vascular instability with biacrbonate in dialysate. Ann. Intern. Med. 88: 332.

20. Bergström, J. (1978) Ultrafiltration without simultaneous dialysis for removal of excess fluid. Proc. EDTA 15: 260.

21. Shaldon, S., Deschodt, G., Beau, M.C., Remperez, P. and Mion, C. (1978) The importance of serum osmotic changes in symptomatic hypotension during short hemo-dialysis. Proc. Dial. Transpl. Forum 8: 184.

22. Baldamus, C.A., Ernst, W., Frei, U. and Koch, K.M. (1982) Sympathetic and hemodynamic response to volume removal during different forms of renal replacment therapy. Nephron 31:324.

23. Brecht, H.M., Schoeppe, W., Scheuermann, E., Nassauer, A, Baldamus, C. and Koch, K.M. (1978) Factors involved in hemodialysis hypotension (Abstract). 7th Congr. Int. Soc. Nephrol., Montreal.

24. Wehle, B., Asaba, H., Castenfors, J., Fürst, P., Gunnarsson, B., Shaldon, S. and Bergström, J. (1979) Hemodynamic changes during sequential ultrafiltration and dialysis. Kidney Int. 15: 411.

354

25. Pogglitsch, H., Holzer, H., Waller, J., Pristautz, H., Leopold, H. and Katschnigg, H. (1978) The cause of inadequate haemodynamic reactions during ultradiffussion. Proc. EDTA 15: 245.

26. Zucchelli, P., Catizone, L., Esposti, E.D., Fusaroli, M., Ligabue, A. and Zuccala, A. (1978) Influence of ultrafiltration on plasma renin activity and adrenergic system. Nephron 21: 317.

27. Zuccala, A., Degli Esposti, E., Sturani, A., Chiarini, C., Santoro, A., Catizone, L. and Zucchelli, P. (1978) Autonomic function in hemodialyzed patients. Int. J. Artif. Organs. 1: 76.

28. Cannella, G., Picotti, G.B., Mioni, G., Cristinelli, L. and Maiorca, R. (1978) Blood pressure behaviours during dialysis and ultrafiltration. A pathogenic hypothesis on hemodialysis-induced hypotension. Int. J. Artif. Organs 1: 69.

29. Quellhorst, E. (1979) Hämofiltration — Differentialindikation zur Hämodialyse unter Berücksichtigung hämodynamischer und metabolischer Aspekte. Klin Wochenschr 57: 1061.

30. Quellhorst, E. and Schuenemann, B. (1979) Postdilution hemofiltration is rational and preferable. Proc. Dial. Transpl. Forum 9: 54.

31. Hampl, H., Paeprer, H., Unger, V. and Kessel, M.W. (1979) Hemodynamics during hemodialysis, sequential ultrafiltration and hemofiltration. J. Dialysis 3: 51.

32. Hampl, H., Paeprer, H., Unger, V., Fischer, C., Resa, I. and Kessel, M. (1980) Hemodynamic changes during hemodialysis, sequential ultrafiltration, and hemofiltration. Kidney Int. 18: S-83.

33. Shaldon, S., Beau, M.C., Deschodt, G., Ramperez, P. and Mion, C. (1980) Vascular stability during hemofiltration. Trans. Am. Soc. Artif. Intern. Organs 26: 391.

34. Keshaviah, P., Illstrup, K., Constantini, E., Berkseth, R. and Shapiro, F. (1980) The influence of ultrafiltration and diffusion on cardiovascular parameters. Trans. Am. Soc. Artif. Intern. Organs 26: 328.

35. Henrich, W.L., Woodard, T.D., Blachley, J.D., Gomez-Sanchez, C., Pettinger, W. and Cronin, R.E. (1980) Role of osmolality in blood pressure stability after dialysis and ultrafiltration. Kidney Int. 18: 480.

36. Wehle, B., Asaba, H., Castenfors, J., Gunnarsson, B. and Bergström, J. (1981) Influence of dialysate composition on cardiovascular function in isovolaemic haemodialysis. Proc. Eur. Dial. Transpl. Ass. 18: 153.

37. Wehle, B., Asaba, H., Castenfors, J., Fürst, P., Gunnarsson, B. and Bergström, J. (1979) Hämodynamische Veränderungen während Ultrafiltration und Hämodialyse bei Urämikern. Z Urol. u Nephrol. 72: 3.

38. Cini, G., Camici, M., Pentimone, F. and Palla, R. (1982) Echocardiographic hemodynamic study during ultrafiltration sequential dialysis. Nephron 30: 124.

39. Hampl, H., Klopp, II., Wolfgruber, M., Pustelnik, A., Schiller, R., Hanefeld, F. and Kessel, M. (1982) Advantages of bicarbonate hemodialysis. Artif. Organs 6: 410.

40. Kishimoto, T. Sugimura, K., Nakatani, T., Yamagami, S., Ezaki, K., Okazaki, S. and Maekawa, M. (1982) The effects of diffusion and ultrafiltration on cardiac output and organ blood flows. Proc. Europ. Dial. Transpl. Ass. 19: 275.

41. Vincet, J.L., Vanherweghem, J.L., Degaute, J.P., Berré, J., Dufaye, P. and Kahn, R.J. (1982) Acetate-induced myocardial depression during hemodialysis for acute renal failure. Kidney Int. 22: 653.

42. Schick, E.C., Jr., Idelson, B.A., Liang, C., Redline, R.C. and Bernard, D.B. (1983) Comparison of the hemodynamic response to hemodialysis with acetate or bicarbonate. Trans. Am. Soc. Artif. Intern. Organs 29: 25.

43. Frewin, D.B., Bartholomeusz, F.D.L., Cummings, M.F., Clarkson, A.R., Barry, L.A., Furber, B., De Lorenzo, C., Jonsson, J.R. and Taylor, W.B. (1984) Changes in plasma catecholamine levels during hemodialysis. Australian N.Z. J. Med. 14: 31.

44. Leenen, F.H.H., Buda, A.J., Smith, D.L., Farrel, S., Levine, D.Z. and Uldall, P.R. (1984) Hemodynamic changes during acetate and bicarbonate hemodialysis. Artif. Organs

8: 411.

45. Schneider, H., Liomin, E. and Streicher, E. (1985) Hemodynamic studies of diffusive and convective procedures using a polysulfone membrane. Contr. Nephrol. 46: 134.

46. Freyschuss, U., Asaba, H., Danielsson, A., Bergström, J. (1984) Cardiovascular adaptation to dialysis in healthy man. Contr. Nephrol: 41: 376–379.

47. Wizemann, V., Sychla, M. and Leber, H.W. (1980) Simultaneous hemofiltration/hemodialysis versus hemofiltration and hemodialysis: Hemodynamic parameters: Proc. ESAO 7: 143.

48. Wizemann, V., Kramer, W., Knopp, G., Sychla, M., Schmidt, H., Rawer, P. and Schütterle, G. (1982). In *Hemodiafiltration*, G. Schütterle, V. Wizemann and G. Seyffart (eds.). Oberursel: Verlag Hygieneplan, p. 89.

49. Schmidt, M., Schoeppe, W. and Baldamus, C.A. (1985) Hemodynamics during hemodialysis with dialyzers of high hydraulic permeability. Contr. Nephrol. 46: 127.

50. Kjellstrand, C.M. (1980) Can hypotension during dialysis be avoided? In *Controversies in Nephrology*, G.E. Schreiner, Washington, D.C.: (ed.) Georgetown University, p. 12.

51. Skillmann, J.J., Awwad, H.K. and Moore, F.D. (1967) Plasma protein kinetics of the early transcapillary refill after hemorrhage in man. Surg. Gyn. Obst. 125: 983.

52. Kim, K.E., Neff, M., Cohen, B. et al (1970) Blood volume changes and hypotension during hemodialysis. Trans. Amer. Soc. Artif. Int. Organs 16: 508.

53. Chainon, M., Chen, W.T., Tarazi, R.C., Bravo, E.L. and Nakamoto, S. (1981) Effect of hemodialysis on blood volume distribution and cardiac output. Hypertension 3: 327.

54. Ashkar, E. and Hamilton, W.F. (1963) Cardiovascular response to graded exercise in the sympathectomized-vagotomized dog. Am. J. Physiol. 204: 291.

55. Falls, W.F., Jr., Stacy, W.K., Bear, E.S. et al. (1972) Dialysis-induced change of extracellular fluid volume in man. Proc. Dial. & Transpl. Forum 2: 155.

56. Rodrigo, R., Shideman, J., McHigh, R., Buselmeier, T. and Kjellstrand, C. (1977) Osmolality changes during hemodialysis, Ann. Intern. Med. 86: 554.

57. Port, F.K., Johnson, W.J. and Klass, D.W. (1973) Prevention of dialysis disequilibrium syndrome by use of high sodium concentration in the dialysate. Kidney Int. 3: 327.

58. Shaldon, S. (1976) Sequential ultrafiltration and dialysis. Proc. Eur. Dial. Transpl. Assoc. 13: 300.

59. Wehle, B., Asaba, H., Castenfors, J. et al. (1978) The influence of dialysis fluid composition on the blood pressure response during dialysis. Clin. Nephrol. 10:62.

60. Bell, R.L., Curtis, F.K., and Babb, A.L. (1965) Analog simulation of the patient-artificial kidney system. Trans. Am. Soc. Artif. Intern. Organs 11: 183.

61. Rastogi, R.P., Frost, T., Anderson, J., Schroft, R. and Kerr, D.N.S. (1968) The significance of disequilibrium between body compartiments in the treatment of chronic renal failure by hemodialysis. Proc. Eur. Dial. Transpl. Assoc. 5: 102.

62. Frost, T.H. and Kerr, D.N.S. (1977) Kinetics of hemodialysis: A theroretical study of the removal of solutes in chronic renalfailure compared to normal health. Kidney Int. 12: 41.

63. Borah, M.F., Schoenfeld, P.Y., Gotch, F.A., Sargent, J.A., Wolfson, M. and Humphreys, M.H. (1978) Nitrogen balance during intermittent dialysis therapy of uremia. Kidney Int. 14: 491.

64. Gotch, F.A., Sargent, J.A. (1983) Hemofiltration: an unnecessarily complex method to achieve hypotonic sodium removal and controlled ultrafiltration. Blood Purfication 1: 9.

65. Oh, M.S., Levison, S.P. and Carroll, H.J. (1975) Content and distribution of water and electrolytes in maintenance hemodialysis. Nephron 14: 421.

66. Keshaviah, P., Berkseth, R.O., Shapiro, F.L. et al. (1978) Mechanisms and control of fluid removal by ultrafiltration. Proceedings of the 11th Annual Contractor's Conference (Artificial Kidney Program, National Institutes of Arthritis, Metabolism and Digestive Disease.

67. Van Stone, J.C., Bauer, J. and Carey, J. (1980) The effect of dialysate sodium concentration on body fluid distribution during hemodialysis. Trans. Amer. Soc. Artif. Intern. Organs 26: 383.

68. Van Stone; J.C. and Cook, J. (1978) The effect of replacing acetate with bicarbonate in the dialysate of stable chronic hemodialysis patients. Proc. Clin. Dial. Transplant. Forum 9: 103.

69. Gotch, F.A., Lam, M.A., Prowitt, M. and Keen, M. (1980) Preliminary clinical results with sodium-volume modeling of hemodialysis therapy. Proc. Dial. Transpl. Forum 10: 12.

70. Gotch, F.A. (1981) Net sodium flux in post dilution hemofiltration. Kidney Int. 19: A 146.

71. Gotch, F.A. and Sargent, J.A. (1982) Hemofiltration: an unnecessarily complex method to achieve hypotonic sodium removal and controlled ultrafiltration. Contr. Nephrol. 4: 279.

72. Shaldon, S., Baldamus, C.A., Koch, K.M., Mion, C.A. and Lysaght, M.J. (1982) Is better sodium balance responsible for maintenance of blood pressure with hemofiltration? or the logical fallacy of the undistributed middle. Controversies in Nephrology 4: 267.

73. Ramenofsky, J.A., Prestidge, H., Ford, C., Sanfelippo, M.L. and Henderson, L.W. (1982) Novel applications for hemofiltration membranes. Trans. Am. Soc. Artif. Internal Organs 27: 613.

74. Bosch, J.P., Lauer, A.P., Belledone, M., Constantiner, A. and Glabman, S. (1982) Effect of protein concentration on the ultrafiltrate (Qf) electrolyte composition (Abstract). Am. Soc. Artif. Internal Organs 11: 42.

75. Lysaght, M.J. (1983) An experimental model for the ultrafiltration of sodium ion from blood or plasma. Blood Purification 1: 25.

76. Shaldon, S., Baldamus, C.A., Beau, M.C., Koch, M.K., Mion, C.M. and Lysaght, M.J. (1983) Acute and chronic studies of the relationship between sodium flux in hemodialysis and hemofiltration. Trans. Am. Soc. Artif. Internal Organs 29: 641.

77. Lysaght, M.J., Baldamus, C.A., Koch, K.M., Mion, C.A., Pusch, W. and Shaldon, S. (1982) Relevance of sodium flux to vascular stability in post dilution hemofiltration. Kidney Int. 21: A172.

78. Shaldon, S., Baldamus, C.A., Koch, K.M. and Lysaght, M.J. (1983) Of sodium, symptomatology and syllogism. Blood Purification I: 16.

79. Baldamus, C.A., Ernst, W., Lysaght, M.J., Shaldon, S. and Koch, K.M. (1983) Hemodynamics in hemofiltration. Int. J. Artif. Organs 6: 27.

80. Baldamus, C.A. (1983) Hemofiltration. In *Nephrology '83*, G. D'Amico and G. Colasanti (eds). Milano: Wichtig Editore, p. 163.

81. Schultze, G., Maiga, M., Neumayer, H–H, Wagner, K., Keller, F., Molzahn, M. and Nigam, S. (1984) Prostaglandin $E_2$ promotes hypotension on low-sodium hemodialysis. Nephron 37: 250.

82. Henderson, L.W., Sanfelippo, M.L. and Stone, R.A. (1979) Comparison of hemodialysis and hemofiltration. Proc. XII. Ann. Contractor's Conf. Artificial Kidney-Chronic Uremia Program, NIAMDO (National Institutes of Health) Bethesda.

83. Quellhorst, E. (1984) Herzrhythmusstörungen während und nach Hämodialyse, Hämofiltration und Hämodiafiltration bei Patienten mit chronischer Niereninsuffizienz — vergleichende Langzeit-EKG-Untersuchungen. In *Die Behandlung von Herzrhythmus-störungen bei Nierenkranken*. J. Braun (ed.) Basel: Karger-Verlag, p. 23.

84. Morrison, G., Michelson, E.L., Brown, S. and Morganroth, J. (1980) Mechanism and prevention of cardiac arrhythmias in chronic hemodialysis patients. Kidney Int. 17: 811.

85. Haddy, F.J. (1983) The role of potassium ions in regulating vascular resistance. In *Advances in Microcirculation*, Vol. II, B.M. Altura (ed). Basel: S. Karger, p. 43.

86. Fukuchi, S., Hanata, M., Takahashi, H., Demura, H., and Goto, K. (1965) The relationship between vascular reactivity and extracellular potassium. Tohoku J. Exp. Med. 85: 181.

87. Haddy, F.J., Scott, J.B., Emerson, T.E., Jr., Overbeck, H.W. and Daugherty, R.M. (1969) Effects of generalized changes in plasma electrolyte concentration and osmolarity on blood pressure in the anesthetized dog. Circulation Res. 24 (Suppl. 1): 59.

88. Friedman, S.M. (1983) Sodium ions and regulation of vascular tone. In *Advances in Microcirculation*, Vol. II, B.M. Altura (ed.). Basel: S. Karger, p. 20.

89. Lang, S. and Blaustein, M.P. (1980) The role of the sodium pump in the control of vascular tone in the rat. Circulation Res. 46: 463.

90. Dunn, F.L., Brennan, T.J., Neson, A.E. and Robertson, G.L. (1973) The role of blood osmolality and volume in regulating vasopressin secretion in the rat. J Clin. Invest. 52: 3212.

91. Brecht, H.M. (19  ) Wirkung der Hyponatriämie und der Hypovolämie auf die Sympathikus- und Reninaktivität bei der terminalen Niereninsuffizienz.

92. Altura, B.T. (1983) Influence of calcium ions on microvascular permeability, contractility and reactivity. In *Advances in Microcirculation*, Vol. II, B.M. Altura (ed.). Basel: S. Karger, p. 62.

93. Overbeck, H.W., Molnar, J.I. and Haddy, F.J. (1961) Resistance to blood flow through the vascular bed of the dog forelimb. Local effects of sodium, potassium, calcium, magnesium, acetate, hypertonicity and hypotonicity. Am. J. Cardiol. 8: 533.

94. Bristow, M.R., Schwartz, H.D., Binetti, G., Harrison, D.C. and Daniels, J.R. (1977) Ionized calcium and the heart: elucidation of in vivo concentration-response relationships in the open-chest dog. Circulation Res. 41: 565.

95. Connor, T.B., Rosen, B.L., Blaustein, M.P., Applefeld, M.M. and Doyle, L.A. (19  ) Hypocalcemia precipitatin congestive heart failure. N. Engl. J. Med. 307: 869.

96. Wei, E.P., Thames, M.D., Kontos, H.A. and Patterson, J.L., Jr. (1974) Inhibition of the vasodilator effect of hypercapnic acidosis by hypercalcemia in dogs and rats. Circulation Res. 35: 890.

97. Henrich, W.I., Hund, J.M. and Nixon, J.V. (1984) Increased ionized calcium and left ventricular contractility during hemodialysis. N. Engl. J. Med. 310: 19.

98. Chaignon, M., Chen, W.T., Tarazi, R.C., Nakamoto, S. and Salcedo, E. (1982) Acute effects of hemodialysis on echographic-determined cardiac performance: improved contractility resulting from serum increased calcium with reduced potassium despite hypovolemic-reduced cardiac output. Am. Heart J. 103: 374.

99. Drüecke, T., Fauchet, M. Fleury, J. et al (1980) Effect of parathyroidectomy on left-ventricular function in haemodialysis patients. Lancet I: 112.

100. Schneider, H. (1982) Die Kinetic des Kalziumtransports bei Dialyse und Filtration. In *Die adäquate Dialyse*, E. Streicher and W. Schoeppe (eds.) Berlin and Heidelberg, New York: Springer-Verlag, pp. 119–132.

101. Altura, B.M. (1983) Magnesium and regulation of contractility of vascular smooth muscle. In *Advances in Microcirculation*, Vol. II. Basel: S. Karger, p. 77.

102. Langer, G.A., Serena, S.D. and Nudd, L.M. (1974) Cation exchange in heart cell culture: correlation with effects on contractile force. J. Mol. Cell. Cardiol. 6: 149.

103. Shine, I.I. (1979) Myocardial effects of magnesium. Am. J. Physiol. 237: H413.

104. Weiner, M.W. (1982) Acetate metabolism during hemodialysis. Artif. Organs 6: 370.

105. Vreman, H.J., Assomull, V.M., Kaiser, B.A., Blaschke, T.F. and Weiner, M.W. (1980) Acetate metabolism and acid-base homeostasis during hemodialysis: influence of dialyzer efficiency and metabolic capacity for acetate metabolism. Kidney Int. 18 (Suppl 10): S62.

106. Mion, C.R., Hegstrom, R.M., Boen, S.T. and Scribner, B.H. (1964) Substitution of sodium acetate for sodium bicarbonate in the bath fluid for hemodialysis. Trans. Am. Soc. Artif. Intern. Organs 10: 110.

107. Kaiser, B.A., Assomull, V.M., Vreman, H.J., Weiner, M.W. (1979) Dialysance of acetate and bicarbonate: effect of ultrafiltration. Proc. Clin. Dial. Transplant. Forum 9: 104.

108. Graefe, U., Follette, W.C., Vizzo, J.E., Gutisman, L.D. and Scribner, B.H. (1976) Reduction in dialysis-induced morbidity and vascular instability with the use of bicarbonate in dialysate. Proc. Clin. Dial. Transpl. Forum 6: 203–206.

109. Bauer, W. and Richards, J.W. (1928) A vasodilator action of acetate. J. Phyiol. (London) 66: 371.

110. Olinger, G.N., Werner, P.H., Bonchek, L.I. and Boerboom, L.E. (1979) Vasodilator effects of the sodium acetate in pooled protein fraction. Ann. Surg. 190: 305.

111. Frohlich, E.D. (1965) Vascular effects of the Kreds intermediate metabolites. Am. J. Physiol. 208: 149.

112. Molnar, J.I., Scott, J.B., Frohlich, E.D. and Haddy, F.J. (1962) Local effects of various anious and $H^+$ on dog limb and coronary vascular resistances. Am. J. Physiol 203: 125.

113. Kirkendol, P.L., Devia, C.J., Bower, J.D. and Holbert, R.D. (1977) A comparison of the cardiovascular effects of sodium acetate, sodium bicarbonate and other potential sources of fixed base inhemodialysate solution. Trans. Am. Soc. Artif. Intern. Organs 23: 399–405.

114. Aizawa, Y. and Shibata, A. (1978) Hemodynamic effects of acetate in man. J. Dial. 2: 235.

115. Aizawa, Y., Ohmori, T., Imai, K., Nara, Y., Matsuoka, M. and Hirakawa, Y. (1977) Depressant action of acetate upon the human cardiovascular system. Clin. Nephrol. 8: 477.

116. Chen, T.S., Friedman, H.S., Del Monte, M. and Smith, A.J. (1979) Hemodynamic changes during dialysis. Proc. Clin. Dial. Transplant. Forum 9: 66.

117. Lian, C.S. and Lowenstein, J.M. (1978) Metabolic control of the circulation: effects of acetate and pyruvate. J. Clin. Invest. 62: 1029.

118. Kirkendol, P.L., Robie, N.W., Gonzalez, F.M. and Devia, C.J. (1978) Cardiac and vascular effects of infused sodium acetate in dogs. Trans. Am. Soc. Artif. Intern. Organs 24: 714.

119. Keshaviah, P.R. (1982) The role of acetate in the etiology of symptomatic hypotension. Artif. Organs 6: 378.

120. Sargent, J.A. and Gotch, F.A. (1978) Principles and biophysics of dialysis. In *Replacement of Renal Function by Dialysis*, Drukker, Parsons and Maker (eds.) The Hague-Boston: Nijhoff, pp. 38–68.

121. Gotch, F.A., Sargent, J.A., Keen, M.L., Lam, M. and Provitt, M.H. (1978) Solute kinetics of intermittent dialysis therapy. Annual progress report. Artificial Kidney — Chronic Uremia Program NIAMDD (National Institute of Health, Bethesda).

122. Gotch, F.A., Sargent, J.A. and Keen, M.L. (1982) Hydrogen ion balance in dialysis therapy Artif. Organs 6: 388.

123. Von, Albertini, B. Miller, J.H., Gardner, P.W., and Shinaberger, J.H. (1984) Performance characteristics of high flux haemodiafiltration. Proc. EDTA-ERA 21: 447.

124. Kishimoto, T., Yamamoto, K., Yamamoto, T., Mizutani, Y., Horiuchi, N., Hirata, S., Yamagami, S., Yamakawa, M. and Maekawa, M. (1983) Acetate intolerance in hemodialysis. Trans. Am. Soc. Artif. Internal Organs 29: 402.

125. Shaldon, S., Deschodt, G., Branger, B., Oulés R., Granolleras, C., Baldamus, C.A., Koch, K.M., Lysaght, M.J. and Dinarello, C.A. (1985) Haemodialysis hypotension: the interleukin hypothesis restated. Proc. EDTA 22: in press.

126. Iseki, K., Onoyama, K., Maeda, T., Shimamatsu, K., Harada, A., Fijimi, F. and Omae, T. (1980) Comparison of hemodynamics induced by conventional acetate hemodialysis, bicarbonate hemodialysis and ultrafiltration. Clin. Nephrol. 14: 294.

127. Weitzman, R.E., Gorbaty, I. and Davidson, W.D. (1978) The effect of bath composition on blood pressure and vasoactive hormone levels during hemodialysis. Am. Soc. Nephrol. (Abst.), p. 56A.

128. Raja, R. and Kramer, M. and Rosenbaum, J.L. (1980) Prevention of hypotension during iso-osmolar hemodialysis with bicarbonate dialysate. Trans. Amer. Soc. Artif. Intern. Organs 26: 375.

129. Nissenson, A.R., Kraut, J.A., and Shinaberger, J.H. (1984) Dialysis-associated hypoxemia: pathogenesis and prevention. Asaio. Journal 7: 1.

130. Davidson, W.D., Dolan, M.J., Whipp, B.J., Weitzman, R.E. and Wasserman, K. (1982) Pathogenesis of dialysis-induced hypoxemia. Artif. Organs 6: 406.

131. Ward, R.A. and Wathen, R.L. (1982) Utilization of bicarbonate for base repletion in hemodialysis. Artificial Organs 6: 396.

132. Wathen, R.L., Ward, R.A., Harding, G.B. and Myer, L.C. (1982) Acid-base and metabolic responses to anion infusion in the anesthetized dog. Kidney Int. 21: 592.

133. Wathen, R.L. (1977) The impact of acetate and bicarbonate containing dialysate on hydrogen ion balance. Proc. Renal Physicians Assoc. 1: 19.

134. Craddock, P.R., Fehr, J., Brigham, K.L., Kronenberg, R.S. and Jacob, H.S. (1977) Complement and leukocyte-mediated pulmonary dysfunction in hemodialysis. N. Engl. J. Med. 296: 769.

135. Bischel, M.D., Scoles, B.G. and Mohler, T.G. (1975) Evidence for pulmonary micro-

embolization during hemodialysis. Chest 67: 335.

136. Sherlock, J., Ledwith, J. and Letteri, J. (1977) Hypoventilation and hypoxemia during hemodialysis: reflex response to removal of $CO_2$ across dialyzer. Trans. Amer. Soc. Artif. Intern. Organs 23: 406.

137. Aurigemma, N.M., Feldman, N.T., Gottlieb, M. et al. (1977) Arterial oxygenation during hemodialysis. N. Engl. J. Med. 297: 871.

138. Oh, M.S., Uribarri, J.V., Del Monte, M.L. et al. (1979) Consumption of $CO_2$ in metabolism of acetate as an explanation for hypoventilation and hypoxemia during hemodialysis. Proc. Clin. Dial. Transpl. Forum 9: 226.

139. Romaldini, H., Rodriguez-Roisin, R., Lopez, F.A., Ziegler, T.W., Bencowitz, H.Z. and Wagner, P.D. (1984) The mechanisms of arterial hypoxemia during hemodialysis. Am. Rev. Respir. Dis. 129: 780.

140. Wasserman, A.J. and Patterson, J.L. (1961) The cerebral vascular response to reduction in arterial carbon dioxide tension. J. Clin. Invest. 40: 1297.

141. Finnerty, F.A., Jr., Witkin, L. and Fazekas, J.F. (1954) Cerebral hemodynamics during cerebral ischemia induced by acute hypotension. J. Clin. Invest. 33: 1227.

142. Hampl, H., Fischer, C.H., Resa, I., Paeprer, H. and Kessel, M. (1979) Recirculation dialysis (RD) (20 to 40 liters of dialysate) with venous bicarbonate buffering — an alternative procedure to hemofiltration (HF). Int. J. Artif. Organs 2: 235.

143. Bosch, J.P., Glabman, S., Moutoussis, G., Belledonne, M., von Albertini, B. and Kahn, t. (1984) Carbon dioxide removal in acetate hemodialysis: effects on acid base balance. Kidney Int. 25: 830.

144. Bosch, J., Constantiner, A., Belledonne, M., MacMoune, F., Glabman, s., von Albertini, B. (1981) Bicarbonate generation and red blood cell hypocapnia during acetate hemodialysis. Trans. Am. Soc. Artif. Intern. Organs 27: 172.

145. Bosch, J.P., Gotch, F.A., Kjellstrand, C.M. and Scribner, B.H. (1981) Acetate versus bicarbonate in dialysis. Trans. Am. Soc. Artif. Intern. Organs 27: 655.

146. Gregory, G.A., Egerll, E.I., Smith, N.T. and Cullen, B.F. (1974) The cardiovascular effects of carbon dioxide in man awake and during diethyl ether anesthesia. Anestesiology 40: 301.

147. Burnum, J.F., Hickam, J.B. and McIntosh, H.D. (1954) The effect of hypocapnia on arterial blood pressure. Circulation 9: 89.

148. Suutarinen, T. (1966) Cardiovascular response to changes in arterial carbon dioxide tension. Acta Physiol. Scand. 67 (Suppl. 266): 1.

149. Robertson, G.L., Athar, S. and Shelton, R.L. (1977) Disturbances in body fluid osmolality. Am. Physiol. Soc.: 133.

150. Maack, T., Marion, D.N., Camargo, M.J.F., Kleinert, H.D., Laragh, J.H., Vaughan, E.D., Jr. and Atlas, S.A. (1984) Effects of auriculin (atrial natriuretic factor) on blood pressure, renal function, and the renin-aldosterone system in dogs. Am. J. Med. 77: 1069.

151. Lang, R.E., Thoelken, H., Ganten, D., Luft, F.C., Ruskoaho, H. and Unger, T. (1985) Atrial natriuretic factor is a circulating hormone stimulated by volume loading. Nature: — in press.

152. Kangawa, J. and Matsuo, H. (1984) Purification and complete amino acid sequence of alpha-human atrial natriuretic polypeptide (alpha-hANP). Biochem. Biophys. Res. Comm. 118: 131.

153. Schmitt, G., Tobin, M., Metheson, J. and Flamenbaum, W. (1981) Prostaglandin E(PGE) blood levels during hemodialysis comparison of cellulosic and polycralonitrile membranes. Kidney Int. 19: A158.

154. Borges, H., Shideman, J. and Kjellstrand, C.M. (1981) Hypotension during chronic hemodialysis: on the effects of prostaglandin inhibition. Proc. 8th Int. Congr. Nephrol. Athens, 1981, p. 433.

155. Friedrich, T., Lichey, J., Nigam, S., Heidrich, E., Doye, K., Schultze, G., Wegscheider, K. and Priesnitz, M. (1982) Levels of prostaglandins and complement activity in plasma of patients with acute myocardial infarction. Proc. Vth Int. Conf. on Prostaglandins, Florence.

360

156. Lichey, J., Nigam, S., Friedrich, T., Maiga, M., Schultze, G., Heidrich, E., Doye, K., Wegscheider, K. and Priesnitz, M. (1982) Elevated levels of prostaglandins in arterial and venous blood of patients with pulmonary embolism. Proc. Vth Int. Conf. on Prostaglandins, Florence.

157. Dzau, V.J., Packer, M., Lilly, L.S., Swartz, S.L., Hollenberg, N.K. and Williams, G.H. (1984) Prostaglandins in severe congestive heart failure. Relation to activation of the renin-angiotensin system and hyponatremia. N. Engl. J. Med. 310: 347.

158. Leithner, C., Sinzinger, H., Silberbauer, K. and Stummvoll, H.K. (1981) Platelet microaggregates and release of endogenous prostacyclin during the initial phase of haemodialysis. Proc. Europ. Dial. Transpl. Ass. 18: 122.

159. Branger, B., Oulés R., Bonardet, A., Deschodt, G., Rey, R., Treissede, D., Granolleras, C., Balducchi, J.P., Shaldon, S., Mion, H. and Fourcade, J. (1984) Hemodynamic and prostaglandin level changes during acetate hemodialysis versus bicarbonate hemodialysis. Contr. Nephrol. 41: 388.

160. McDonald, J.W., Ali, M., Morgan, E., Townsend, E.R. and Cooper, J.D. (1983) Thromboxane synthesis by sources other than platelets in association with complement induced pulmonary leukostasis and pulmonary hypertension in sheep. Circulation Res. 52: 1.

161. Henderson, L.W. and Koch, K.M., Dinarello, C.A. and Shaldon, S. (1983) Hemodialysis hypotension: the Interleukin hypothesis. Blood Purification 1: 3.

162. Maggiore, Q., Pizzarelli, F., Zoccali, C., Sisca, S., Nicolò, F. and Parlongo, S. (1981) Effect of extracorporeal blood cooling on dialytic arterial hypotension. Proc. Eur. Dial. Transplant. Ass. 18: 597.

163. Sherman, R.A., Faustino, E.F., Bernholc, A.S. and Eisinger, R.P. (1984) Effect of variations in dialysate temperature on blood pressure during hemodialysis. Am. J. Kidney Dis. 4: 66.

164. Coli, U., Landini, S., Lucatello, S., Fracasso, A., Morachiello, P., Righetto, F., Scanferla, F., Onesti, G. and Bazzato, G. (1983) Cold as cardiovascular stabilizing factor in hemodialysis: hemodynamic evaluation. Trans. Am. Soc. Artif. Intern. Organs 29: 71.

165. Mahida, B.H., Dumler, F., Zasuwa, G., Fleig, G., Levin, N.W. (1983) Effect of cooled dialysate on serum catecholamines and blood pressure stability. Trans. Am. Soc. Artif. Intern. Organs 29: 384.

166. Lindholm, T., Thysell, H., Yamamoto, Y., Forsberg, B. and Gullberg, C.A. (1985) Temperature and vascular stability in hemodialysis. Nephron 39: 130.

167. Sherman, R.A., Rubin, M.P., Cody, R.P. and Eisinger, R.P. (1985) Amelioration of hemodialysis-associated hypotension by the use of cool dialysate. Am. J. Kidney Dis. 5: 124.

168. Maggiore, Q., Pizzarelli, F., Sisca, S., Catalano, C. and Delfino, D. (1984) Vascular stability and heat in dialysis patients. Contr. Nephrol. 41: 398.

169. Maggiore, Q., Pizzarelli, F., Sisca, S., Zoccali, C., Parlongo, S., Nicolò, F. and Creazzo, G (1982) Blood temperature and vascular stability during hemodialysis and hemofiltration. Proc. Trans. Am. Soc. Artif. Internal Organs 28: 523.

170. Absolom, D.R., Policova, Z., Neumann, A.W. and Zingg, W. (1983) The effect of temperature on the extent of platelet adhesion to foreigh surfaces. Trans. Am. Soc. Artif. Intern. Organs 29: 425.

171. Schaefer, K., von Herrath, D. and Hüfler, M. (1983) Failure to show a temperature-dependent vascular stability during hemofiltration. Intern. J. Artif. Organs 6: 75–76.

172. Vanholder, R., Piron, M. and Ringoir, S. (1984) Absence of a beneficial haemodynamic effect of bicarbonate versus acetate haemodialysis. Proc. EDTA-ERA 21: 195.

173. Pizzarelli, F., Sisca, S., Zoccali, C., Parlongo, S., Nicolò, F., Greazzo, G., Delfino, D. and Maggiore, Q. (1983) Blood temperature and cardovascular stability in hemofiltration. Int. J. Artif. Organs 6: 37.

174. Enia, G., Catalano, C., Pizzarelli, F., Greazzo, G., Zaccuri, F., Mundo, A., Iellamo, D. and Maggiore, Q. (1984) The effect of dialysate temperature on haemodialysis

leucopenia. Proc. EDTA-ERA 21: 167.
175. Dinarello, C.A. (1984) Interleukin-1. Rev. Infect. Dis. 6: 51.
176. Craddock, P.R., Fehr, J., Dalmasso, A.P., Brigham, K.I. and Jacob, H.S. (1977) Hemodialysis leukopenia: pulmonary vascular leukostasis resulting from complement activation by dialyzer cellophane membranes. J. Clin. Invest. 59: 879.
177. Craddock, P.R., Hammershmidt, D.E., White, J.G., Dalmasso, A.P. and Jacob, H.S. (1977) Complement (C5a)-induced granulocyte aggregation in vitro: a possible mechanism for complement-mediated leukostasis and leukopenia. J. Clin. Invest. 60: 260.
178. Walker, J.F., Lindsey, M., Sibbald, W.J. et al. (1984) 'Cuprophane hypersensitivity'. The cardiopulmonary phenomenon and its modification in an animal model. Trans. Am. Soc. Artif. Internal Organs 30: 168.
179. Arnaout, M.A., Hakim, R.M., Todd, R.F., Dana, N. and Colten, H.R. (1985) Increased expression of an adhesion-promoting surface glycoprotein in the granulocytopenia of hemodialysis. N. Engl. J. Med. 312: 457.
180. Condon, C.J. and Freeman, R.M. (1970) Zinc metabolism in renal failure. Ann. Intern. Med. 73: 531.
181. Chenoweth, D.E., Goodman, M.G. and Wiegle, W.O. (1982) Demonstration of a specific receptor for human C5a anaphylatoxin on murine macrophages. J. Exp. Med. 156: 68.
182. Goodman, M.G., Chenoweth, D.E. and Wiegle, W.O. (1982) Induction of interleukin-1 secretion and enhancement of humoral immunity by binding of human C5a to macrophage surface C5a receptors. J. Exp. Med. 156: 912.
183. Dinarello, C.A. and Wolff, S.M. (1982) Molecular basis of fever in humans. Am. J. Med. 72: 799.
184. Rossi, V., Rivario, F., Ghezzi, P., Mantovani, L. (1985) Interleukin-I induces prostacyclin synthesis in vascular cells. Science: in press.
185. Port, F.K., Weingast, J.A., van de Kerkhove, K., Eiger, S.M. and Kluger, M.J. (1985) Release of pyrogens during clinical hemodialysis. Trans. Amer. Soc. Artif. Intern. Organs 31: in press.
186. Gutierrez, A., Alvestrand, A., Wahren, J. and Bergström, J. (1985) Blood-membrane interaction without dialysis induces increased protein catabolism in normal man. 22nd Congress of the European Dialysis and Transplant Association, Brussels, 1985, abstract book, p. 107.
187. Hakim, R.M. and Lowrie, E.G. (1982) Hemodialysis-associated neutropenia and hypoxemia: the effect of dialyzer membrane materials. Nephron 32: 12.
188. Hakim, R.M., Fearon, D.T. and Lazarus, J.M. (1984) Biocompatibility of dialysis membranes: effects of chronic complement activation. Kidney Int. 26: 194.
189. Lonneman, G., Bingel, M., Koch, K.M., Shaldon, S. and Dinarello, C. (1985) Increased Interleukin-I activity in peritoneal dialysis effluent of CAPD patients with impaired peritoneal clearance. Annual Meeting of the International Society of Hemofiltration, Abstract book, New York.
190. Minetti
191. Röckel, A., Hennemann, H., Sternagel-Haase, A. and Heidland, A. (1979) Uraemic sympathetic neuropathy after haemodialysis and transplantation. Europ. J. Clin. Invest. 9: 23.
192. Lazarus, J.M., Hampers, C.L., Lowrie, E.G. and Merrill, J.P. (1973) Baroreceptor activity in normotensive and hypertensive uremic patients. Circulation 47: 1015.
193. Pickering, T.G., Gribbin, B. and Oliver, D.O. (1972) Baroreflex sensitivity in patients on long-term haemodialysis. Clin. Sci. 43: 645.
194. Lilley, J.J. Golden, J. and Stone, R.A. (1976) Adrenergic regulation of blood pressure in chronic renal failure. J. Clin. Invest. 57: 1190.
195. Koch, K.M., Baldamus, C.A., Ernst, W., Fassbinder, W., Georges, J. and Brecht, H.M. (1980) Autonome Kreislaufregulation in der Urämie. Klin Wochenschr 58: 1037.
196. Nies, A.S., Robertson, D. and Stone, W.J. (1979) Hemodialysis hypotension is not the

result of uremic peripheral autonomic neuropathy. J. Lab. Clin. Med. 94: 395.

197. Cohn, J.N., Combos, F.A. and Tristani, F.F. (1966) Disturbed baroreceptor and peripheral vascular control in chronic uremia. Clin. Res. 14: 374.

198. Kersh, E.S., Kronfield, S.J., Unger, A., Popper, R.W. Cantor, S. and Cohn, K. (1974) Autonomic insufficiency in uremia as a cause of hemodialysis-induced hypotension. N. Engl. J. Med. 290: 650.

199. Rascher, W., Schömig, A., Kreye, V.A. and Ritz, E. (1982) Diminished vascular response to noradrenaline in experimental chronic uremia. Kidney Int. 21: 20.

200. Romoff, M.S., Campese, V.M., Lane, K. and Massry, S.G. (1978) Mechanism of autonomic dysfunction in uremia: evidence for reduced end organ response to norepinephrine. Kidney Int. 14: A731.

201. Horler, E., Hennemann, H. and Heidland, A. (1974) Intraneuronaler Stoffwechsel von Noradrenalin bei experimenteller Urämie und Hypertonie. Verh Dtsch Ges Inn Med. 80: 237.

202. Hennemann, H. and Horler, E. (1976) Sympathicopathy in uremia. In *Renal Insufficiency*, A. Heidland (ed.). Stuttgart: Georg Thieme Verlag, p. 41.

203. Winckler, J., Hennemann, H., Heidland, A. and Wiegand, M.E. (1976) Katecholamingehalt adrenerger Nerven in Speicheldrüsen mit gestörter Elektrolytausscheidung bei Urämie. Klin Wochenschr 51: 479.

204. Brecht, H.M. Ernst, W. and Koch, K.M. (1976) Plasma noradrenaline levels in regular haemodialysis patients. Proc. Eur. Dial. Transpl. Ass. 12: 281.

205. Ksiazek, A. (1979) Dopmaine-beta-hydroxylase activity and catecholamine lev ls in the plasma of patients with renal failure. Nephron 24: 170.

206. McGrath, B.P., Ledingham, J.G.G. and Benedict, C.R. (1978) Catecholamines in peripheral venous plasma in patients on chronic haemodialysis. Clin. Sci. Mol. Med. 55: 89.

207. Baldamus, C.A., Mantz, P., Kachel, H.G., Koch, K.M. and Schoeppe, W. (1984) Baroreflex in patients undergoing hemodialysis and hemofiltration. Contr. Nephrol. 41: 409.

208. Tomiyama, O., Shiigai, T., Ideura, T., Tomita, K., Mito, Y., Shinohara, S. and Tekeuchi, J. (1980) Baroreflex sensitivity in renal failure. Clin. Sci. 58: 21.

209. Ewing, D.J. and Winney, R. (1975) Autonomic function in patients with chronic renal failure on intermittent haemodialysis. Nephron 15: 424.

210. Hung, J., Harris, P.J., Uren, R.E., Tiller, D.J. and Kelly, D.T. (1980) Uremic cardiomyopathy — effect of hemodialysis of left ventricular function in end-stage renal failure N. Engl. J. Med. 302: 547.

211. Prosser, D. and Parsons, V. (1975) The case for a specific uraemic myocardopathy. Nephron 15: 4.

212. Raab, W. (1944) Cardiotoxic substances in the blood and heart muscle in uremia (their nature and action). J. Lab. Clin. Med. 29: 715.

213. Bailey, G.L., Hampers, C.L. and Merrill, J.P. (1967) Reversible cariomyopathy in uremia. Trans. Am. Soc. Artif. Intern. Organs 13: 263.

214. Ianhez, L.E., Lowen, J. and Sabbage, E. (1975) Uremic myocardiopathy. Nephron 15: 17.

215. Drueke, L., Pailleur, A.J., Mailhac, B. et al. (1977) Congestive cardiomyopathy in ureamic patients on long term hemodialysis. Br. Med. J. 1: 350.

216. Gueron, M., Berlyne, G.M., Nord, E. and Ben Ari, J. (1975) The case against the existence of a specific uraemic myocardiopathy. Nephron 15: 2.

217. Nixon, J.V. Mitchell, J.H., McPaul, J.J., Jr. and Henrich, W.L. (1983) Effect of hemodialysis on left ventricular function. J. Clin. Invest. 71: 377.

218. Keshaviah, P. and Shapiro, F.L. (1982) A critical examination of dialysis-induced hypotension. Am. J. Kidney Dis. II. 290.

219. Ylikorkala, O., Huttunen, K., Järvi, J. and Viinikka, L. (1982) Prostacyclin and thromboxane in chronic uremia: the effect of hemodialysis. Clin. Nephrol. 18: 83.

220. Kishimoto, T., Yamamoto, T., Yamamoto, K., Yamagami, S., Nishitani, H., Mitzutani,

Y., Yamakawa, M. and Maekawa, M. (1984) Acetate kinetics during hemodialysis and hemofiltration. Blood Purification 2: 81.
221. Van Stone, Z.C. Bauer, Z. and Cavey, Z. (1982) The effect of dialysate sodium concentration an body fluid compartment volume, plasma runin activity and plasma aldosterome concentration in chronic hemodialysis patients. Umer. Z. Kidney Dis. 2: 58–64.

# INDEX

366